# NSEE
# Nursing School Entrance Exams
# Third Edition

# NSEE

## Nursing School Entrance Exams
### Third Edition

By the Staff of Kaplan Test Prep and Admissions

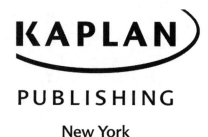

**PUBLISHING**

New York

© 2009 by Kaplan, Inc.

Published by Kaplan Publishing, a division of Kaplan, Inc.
1 Liberty Plaza, 24th Floor
New York, NY 10006

Printed in the United States of America

10 9 8 7 6 5 4 3

ISBN-13: 978-1-4195-5285-4

Kaplan Publishing books are available at special quantity discounts to use for sales promotions, employee premiums, or educational purposes. Please email our Special Sales Department to order or for more information at kaplanpublishing@kaplan.com, or write to Kaplan Publishing, 1 Liberty Plaza, 24th Floor, New York, NY 10006.

# Table of Contents

# How to Use This Book

Congratulations! You've taken the first step to prepare yourself for the nursing school entrance exams. This book contains the information you want and need to do your best and get into the school of your choice. To get you started, this section, Section One, provides you with important information about the test and how best to handle test-day stress.

Chapter One includes test-taking strategies that will boost your confidence on this or any test you take. The tips in this chapter show you how to increase your score.

To minimize your stress on test day, review Chapter Two "Stress Management." Learn the habits that will help you keep cool under any testing conditions.

Before you start your review, find out exactly what your strengths and weaknesses are. The 65-question diagnostic quiz in Chapter Three will help you focus your studies so you don't waste time reviewing topics you have already mastered.

Section Two of this book offers you targeted lessons, strategies, and review questions for each of the topics covered on the nursing school entrance exams. Chapters Four through Eight cover the important subjects of Reading Comprehension, Vocabulary and Spelling, Mathematics, and Science. In short, the lessons and practice in this section will prepare you for success.

Once you have learned about the test, and reviewed the subjects covered, you are ready for more practice. Section Three includes two 250-question practice tests complete with answer keys and detailed answer explanations. By taking these practice tests, you will be able to apply the test-taking strategies you have learned, as well as identify areas in which you have improved and areas that still require further study.

Finally, the Learning Resources found in Section Four will serve as a quick reference for useful information. In addition to a directory of State Boards of Nursing, you will find a study resource.

By using Kaplan's *Nursing School Entrance Exams*, you are taking an important step in getting the score you need to start a successful nursing career. Good luck!

# About the Test

In life, there are some tests that everyone seems to know about. For example, the SAT is typically used for college admissions, the GRE and GMAT are used for graduate and business school admissions, and so on. However, this is not exactly the case with the nursing school entrance exams. In fact, nursing schools across the country use several different tests to determine who is admitted to their programs. So what does this mean?

The answer is simple. Even though there are several different types of exams, they all essentially test the same skills. In short, nursing schools want to know you have basic knowledge and skills in four main subjects: Vocabulary, Reading Comprehension, Mathematics, and Science.

For this reason, Kaplan's *Nursing School Entrance Exams* practice tests have four sections:
- Reading Comprehension
- Vocabulary and Spelling
- Mathematics
- Science (Biology, Chemistry, and Physics)

## ABOUT THE READING COMPREHENSION SECTION

In this section, you will read several passages and answer the questions that follow each of them. All of the questions are multiple-choice, with four answer choices (A–D).

### The Passages

The passages in this section range from very long (up to 850 words), to medium (around 500 words) and short (around 200 words). The passage topics vary, but many of them have a science- or nature-based theme.

### The Questions

There are a total of 45 Reading Comprehension questions in this section. There are four main question types:

- Main Idea
- Detail
- Inference
- Vocabulary-in-Context

To learn more about these question types, refer to Chapter Four, "Reading Comprehension Review."

## ABOUT THE VOCABULARY AND SPELLING SECTION

There are a total of 65 Vocabulary and Spelling questions in this section. All of the questions are multiple-choice, with four answer choices (A–D).

### Vocabulary Questions

These questions test your ability to understand synonyms (words with similar meanings), antonyms (words with opposite meanings), and analogies (relationships between groups of words). There are 15 questions of each type in this section, for a total of 45 Vocabulary questions.

To learn more about the question types, refer to Chapter Five, "Vocabulary and Spelling Review."

### Spelling Questions

These questions test your ability to recognize a misspelled word. The good thing about these questions is that you don't have to know the correct spelling of a word, you only have to recognize an incorrect spelling of a word. There are two types of spelling questions. The first type, of which there are 10 questions, offers you four words, one of which is misspelled. You will have to choose the word that is misspelled. The second type, of which there are 10 questions, offers you three sentences. One of the sentences may or may not have a misspelled word in it. If there is a misspelled word, you select that sentence. If there are no spelling mistakes in any of the three answer choices, you will choose option (D), no mistake.

To learn more about the 20 spelling questions you will find in this section, turn to Chapter Five, "Vocabulary and Spelling Review."

## ABOUT THE MATHEMATICS SECTION

This section of the test covers math topics from basic arithmetic, to algebra and geometry. The 75 questions in this section are all multiple-choice, each with four answer choices (A–D).

### About the Questions

The Math questions are generally of two types:

- Equations
- Word Problems

Equations are straightforward questions that you must solve using basic operations. Word problems are slightly different. You are using the same math skills, however the question appears in the form of a story.

To learn more about solving each type of math question, turn to Chapter Six, "Mathematics Review."

## ABOUT THE SCIENCE SECTION

You may have noticed that this book has two review chapters for science: Life Science and Physical Science. However, on the nursing school entrance exams there is only one section called Science. This section contains 65 questions that cover the topics included in Life Science (biology) as well as the topics included in Physical Science (chemistry and physics). As in previous sections, all Science questions are multiple-choice, with four answer choices (A–D).

## AN IMPORTANT DIFFERENCE

It is important to realize that unlike other sections of the exam in which you can come to a conclusion about the answer quite reasonably, even with limited prior knowledge, the Science section is primarily a test of your knowledge. Although you can make educated guesses on this section, a large part of your success depends upon your knowledge of scientific concepts. When you are ready to review these topics, turn to Chapter Seven and Chapter Eight, "Life Science Review" and "Physical Science Review."

## THE NEXT STEP

Now that you know more about it, you are ready to learn about the ways to succeed on the test. If you want to learn about test-taking and test-day strategies, turn to Chapter One.

## kaptest.com/publishing

The material in this book is up-to-date at the time of publication. However, changes may have been instituted in the test after this book was published.

If there are any important late-breaking developments—or changes or corrections to the Kaplan test preparation materials in this book—we will post that information online at kaptest.com/publishing. Check to see if there is any information posted there regarding this book.

## kaplansurveys.com/books

What did you think of this book? We'd love to hear your comments and suggestions. We invite you to fill out our online survey form at kaplansurveys.com/books. Your feedback is extremely helpful as we continue to develop high-quality resources to meet your needs.

| SECTION ONE |

# The Basics

# Chapter One: **Test-Taking and Test Day Strategies**

The tips in this chapter are designed to help you on your nursing school entrance exam, as well as other tests you may encounter during your career. In addition, you will find a schedule for counting down to test day.

## STRATEGIES FOR ALMOST ANY TEST

When you are faced with so much information to learn in preparation for a test, it can be helpful to know that there are some techniques you can use for any test you are taking. Here are some tips for you to learn and apply on test day. They may seem obvious, but they are easy to forget, so don't let that happen to you.

### You Don't Have to Answer the Questions in Order

On most tests, you are allowed to skip around within each section of the exam. High scorers know this. They move through tests efficiently. They don't dwell on any one question, even a hard one, until they've tried every question at least once.

When you run into questions that look tough, circle them in your test booklet (if you are allowed to write in it) and skip them. Go back and try again after you have answered the easier ones. Remember, in most cases you don't get more points for answering hard questions. If you answer two easy questions correctly in the time it would have taken you to get one hard one right, you just gained points.

There's another benefit in going back to hard ones later. On a second look, questions that initially seemed troublesome can suddenly look quite simple. By answering some easier questions first, you can come back to a harder question with fresh eyes, a new perspective, and more confidence.

### Guessing Advantage

Since most tests don't have a scoring penalty for guessing, you should try to answer every question. If you can determine that one or more answers are definitely wrong, then you should guess from the remaining choices. Even if you aren't sure which one of them is absolutely correct, you've at least increased your chances of success by paring the selection down.

## Answer Sheet Strategies

It sounds simple, but it's extremely important: Don't make mistakes filling out your answer grid. When time is short, it's easy to get confused going back and forth between your test book and grid. If you know the answer, but fill in the wrong bubble on the grid, you won't get points for your answer. To avoid mistakes on the answer grid, try some of the following methods.

### Circle the Questions You Skip

If you are allowed to write in your test booklet, you should put a big circle around any questions you skip. This will help you locate these questions when you are ready to go back to them. Also, if you accidentally skip a box on the grid, you can always check your grid against your book to see where you went wrong.

### Circle Your Answers in Your Test Book When Possible

Again, if you are allowed to write in the test booklet, circling your answers in the test book makes it easier to check your grid. This strategy also makes the next grid strategy possible.

### Grid Five or More Answers at Once

Time is of the essence on most exams. To save time and make sure you are marking your answers in the correct bubbles, transfer your answers after every five questions, or at the end of each reading passage, rather than after every question. That way, you won't keep breaking your concentration to mark the grid. You'll end up with more time to review your answers and you will lower your chances of making a mistake on your answer sheet.

## Keep Track of Time

When you are coming to the end of a test section, you need to be careful about keeping track of how much time you have left to complete everything. You don't want to have your answers in the test booklet and not be able to transfer them to your answer grid because you have run out of time. If it gets down to the wire, and you still have a few questions left, it would be a good idea to start transferring your answers one by one to ensure that every question you answered earns credit.

## Read the Question Carefully Before You Look at the Answers

There is a name for answer choices that look right but aren't: **distracters**. They are easy to choose if you haven't read the question carefully. If you jump right into the answer choices without thinking first about exactly what you're looking for, you're much more likely to fall into one of these traps. Be especially careful of questions that include the word NOT or EXCEPT. If you misread the question and miss these words, you may end up falling into a wrong answer trap.

## PREPARING FOR TEST DAY

We've already covered some of the best strategies for taking any test. Now here's a countdown schedule for test day.

### Three Days Before the Test

Take a full-length practice test. Use the techniques and strategies you've learned in this book. Approach the test strategically, actively, and confidently. We don't recommend taking a full practice test if you have fewer than 48 hours left before exam day. Doing so will probably exhaust you and hurt your score on the actual test.

### Two Days Before the Test

Go over the results of your practice tests. Don't worry too much about your scores or whether you got a specific question right or wrong. The practice tests don't count. But do examine your performance on specific types of questions with an eye on how you might get through each one faster and with more ease on the test to come.

### The Day Before the Test

Our advice is to not do any studying on this day. Instead, organize the things you may need to take to the test:

- A calculator with fresh batteries (Be sure to check with the test administrators to find out if you are allowed to use a calculator on your test.)
- A watch
- A few No. 2 pencils (Pencils with slightly dull points fill the ovals better.)
- Erasers
- Photo ID card
- A snack (There may be a break during the exam and you might be hungry.)

It is also important to know exactly where the test center is located, how you're getting there, and how long it takes to get there. If you can, it's a good idea to visit your test center sometime before the day of the test so you know what to expect—what the rooms are like, how the desks are set up, and so on. Relax the night before the test. Read a good book, take a long, hot shower, or watch something on TV. Go to bed early and get a good night's sleep. Finally, make sure to leave yourself extra time in the morning.

### The Morning of the Test

**After you wake up:**

- Eat breakfast. Make it something substantial, but not anything too heavy or greasy.
- Don't drink a lot of coffee if you're not used to it. Bathroom breaks cut into your time, and too much caffeine may make you jittery.
- Dress in layers so that you can adjust to the temperature of the testing room.
- Read something. Warm up your brain with a newspaper or a magazine. You shouldn't let the test material be the first thing you read that day.
- Be sure to get there early. Allow yourself extra time for traffic, mass transit delays, or detours.

## During the Test

If you find your confidence slipping, remind yourself how well you've prepared. If something goes really wrong, don't panic. If the test booklet is defective—two pages are stuck together or the ink has run—raise your hand, and tell the proctor you need new materials. If you accidentally misgrid your answer page or put your answers in the wrong section, raise your hand and tell the proctor. He or she might be able to arrange for you to regrid your test after it's over—when it won't cost you any time.

## After the Test

**Congratulate yourself.**

Now, you might walk out of the exam thinking you blew it. This is a normal reaction. People tend to remember the questions that stumped them, not the ones they knew. However, we're positive you will perform well and score your best on the exam because you read Kaplan's *Nursing School Entrance Exams*. Be confident that you will be prepared and do well, so you can celebrate when the test is a distant memory.

# Chapter Two: **Stress Management**

Test taking can be stressful, but it doesn't have to be. An important part of taking any exam is having a cool, calm, and collected brain when you are prepping and on the day you take the test. That's what we teach you to do in this chapter, because on test day, few things can hurt your score more than being:

- Sleep deprived or burned out from studying
- In denial over your lack of preparation
- Clueless as to what to expect from the test
- Unaware of what to expect of yourself

This chapter teaches you:

- How to relax
- How to visualize success
- How to build your physical and mental strength

## DEALING WITH TEST STRESS

Your nursing school entrance exam, like all tests, can be scary because it is the *unknown*. You don't know the exact questions that are going to be on it. You don't know how you are going to do. You don't know how your score will stand up at your school of choice. Humans are scared of the unknown. Let this book begin to ease that fear. Let's keep goals attainable. Let's focus on minimizing your unknowns so you can focus on one single thing—doing your best on your nursing school entrance exam.

The main point of this book is to help you exert control over your test experience. You can learn to control your anxiety the same way you can control how to approach a multiple-choice question—by knowing what to expect beforehand and developing strategies to deal with it. We will show you how to relieve stress and mentally prepare for the exam in five specific ways:

1. Identifying sources of stress
2. Visualizing success
3. Exercising away anxiety
4. Eating right
5. Doing isometric exercises

## Sources of Test Stress

Grab a pencil. (Not a pen.) In the space provided, write down your sources of test-related stress. Take 5–10 minutes. The idea is to pin down your sources of anxiety so you can deal with them one by one.

First, read through these common examples. Feel free to use any that apply to you, along with the ones you think up on your own.

- I always freeze up on tests.
- I'm nervous about the math section (or the science section, or the reading section, etc.).
- I need a good/great score to get into my first-choice school.
- I'm afraid of losing my focus and concentration.
- I'm afraid I'm not spending enough time preparing.
- I study like crazy, but nothing seems to stick in my mind.
- I always run out of time and get panicky.

## My Sources of Test Stress

_____

_____

_____

_____

_____

_____

_____

Great. Now read through the list. Take another few minutes. Cross out things or add things. Now rewrite the list in order of most bothersome to least bothersome.

## My Sources of Test Stress, in Order

_____

_____

_____

_____

_____

_____

What was your number one source of stress? Chances are, the top of the list is a fairly accurate description of exactly what you need to tackle. Taking care of the top two or three items on the list should go a long way toward relieving your overall test anxiety. So write down your top three below.

## My Top Three Sources of Test Stress

_____

_____

_____

The rest of this chapter will help you eliminate them.

## Relaxation and Visualization

Now put away your pencil. Sit in a comfortable chair in a quiet setting. If you wear glasses, take them off. Close your eyes and breathe in a deep, satisfying breath of air. Really fill your lungs—to the point where your rib cage is fully expanded and you can't take in any more air. Now exhale the air slowly and completely. Imagine you're blowing out a candle with your last little puff of air. Do this two or three more times, filling your lungs to their maximum capacity and then emptying them totally. Keep your eyes closed, comfortably but not tightly. Let your body sink deeper into the chair as you become even more comfortable.

With your eyes shut and your body in a more relaxed state, you should begin to notice something very interesting. You're no longer dealing with the external worries of the world. Instead, you can concentrate on what happens inside. The more you recognize your own physical reactions to stress and anxiety, the more you can do about them. You may not realize it, but you've begun to regain the ability to stay in control.

Keeping your eyes closed, attempt to visualize TV or movie screens on the back of your eyelids; let relaxing images begin to form on those screens. Allow the images to come easily and naturally; don't force them. The images might be of a special place you've visited before or one you've read about. It can be a fictional location that you create in your imagination, but a real-life memory of a place or situation you know is usually better. Make it as detailed as possible, and notice as much about your surroundings as you can. Stay focused on the images as you sink further into your chair. Breathe easily and naturally. Try to feel the stress and tension drain from your muscles and begin to flow downward, toward your feet and then away from you. Do this for five minutes or so. Start now.

When you are done, slowly open your eyes. Take a moment to check how you're feeling. Notice how comfortable you've become.

Imagine how much easier it would be if you could take the test feeling this relaxed and in this state of ease. You've coupled the images of your special place with sensations of comfort and relaxation. You've also found a way to become relaxed simply by visualizing your own safe, special place.

## Visualize Success

This next part reinforces your *strengths* list and takes visualization one step further. Close your eyes and remember a real-life situation in which you did well on a test. If you can't come up with one, remember a situation in which you did something that you were really proud of—a genuine accomplishment.

Make the memory as detailed as possible. Think about the sights, sounds, smells, and even the tastes associated with this remembered experience. Remember how confident you felt as you accomplished your goal.

Now start thinking about the nursing school entrance exam as an extension of that successful feeling. Keep your thoughts and feelings in line with that previous, successful experience. Don't make comparisons between them. Just imagine taking the test with the same feelings of confidence and relaxed control.

This exercise is a great way to bring the test down to earth. Any feelings of dread you may have associated with the test will be replaced by feelings of accomplishment. Practice your general relaxation technique and this success-oriented relaxation technique together at least three times a week, especially when you feel burned out on test prep. The more you practice relaxation and visualization, the more effective the exercise will be for you.

## Exercise Away Your Anxiety

To be completely prepared for test day, you've got to be in shape—or get in shape—to do your best. Lots of people get out of the habit of regular exercise when they're prepping for an exam. But physical exercise is a very effective way to stimulate both your mind and body, as well as improve your ability to think and concentrate. Along with a good diet and adequate sleep, exercise is an important part of keeping yourself in fighting shape and thinking clearly.

### Hop Like a Frog

Studying uses a lot of energy, but it's all mental. It's important not to forget the importance of using up your physical energy too. When you take a study break, do something active. Take a 5–10 minute exercise break for every 50 or 60 minutes you study. Walk down the block. Do 20 sit-ups. Hop around like a frog. Whatever. The physical exertion helps keep your mind and body in sync. This way, when you finish studying for the night and go to bed, you won't lie there unable to sleep because your brain is exhausted while your body wants to run a marathon.

### Oxygenate Your Brain

Exercise develops your mental stamina and increases the transfer of oxygen to your brain. The brain needs a strong, uninterrupted supply of oxygen to function at its best. Sedentary people have less oxygen in their blood than active people, so their brains receive less oxygen. Your ability to watch TV might not be affected by your brain receiving a little less oxygen, but your ability to think will be.

### Happy Synapses

Exercise also releases your brain's endorphins. Endorphins have no side effects, and they're free! It just takes some exercise to release them. Running, bicycling, swimming, aerobics, and power walking all release endorphins that will occupy the happy spots in your brain's neural synapses.

### Don't Run to Bed

One warning about exercise: It's not a good idea to exercise vigorously right before you go to bed. This could easily cause sleep-onset problems. For the same reason, it's not a good idea to study right up to bedtime. Make time for a buffer period before you go to bed. Take 30 to 60 minutes for yourself and watch some TV, take a long, hot shower, or meditate. Remember our relaxation and visualization tips? This is a good time to do them.

**Squeeze Your Body**

Here's a fast, natural route to relaxation and invigoration. You can do it whenever you get stressed out, including during the test. The idea is that by making your body as tense as possible and relaxing, you are releasing the tension from your body. The entire process takes five minutes from start to finish (maybe a couple of minutes during the test).

- Breathe slowly and easily.
- Close your eyes tightly.
- Squeeze your nose and mouth together so that your whole face is scrunched up. (If it makes you self-conscious to do this in the test room, skip this step.)
- Pull your chin into your chest, and pull your shoulders together.
- Tighten your arms to your body, then clench your fists.
- Pull in your stomach. Squeeze your thighs together, and tighten your calves.
- Stretch your feet, then curl your toes. (Watch out for cramping during this part.)

At this point, every muscle in your body should be tightened. Now, relax your body, one part at a time, in reverse order, starting with your toes. Let the tension drop out of each muscle. This clenching and unclenching exercise will feel silly at first, but it will leave you feeling very relaxed.

## Say No to Drugs, Yes to Eating Right

Using drugs of any kind to prepare for a big test is not a good idea. Mild stimulants, such as coffee, cola, or over-the-counter caffeine pills can help you study longer because they keep you awake, but they can also lead to agitation, restlessness, and insomnia. To reduce stress, eat fruits and vegetables (raw, lightly steamed, or quickly nuked are best); low-fat sources of protein such as fish, skinless poultry, and legumes (lentils, beans, and nuts); and whole grains such as brown rice, whole wheat bread, and pasta (no bleached flour).

Don't eat sweet, high-fat snacks. Simple carbohydrates like sugar make stress worse, and fatty foods lower your immunity. Don't eat salty foods either. They can deplete potassium, which you need for nerve functions.

## Good Stress

We haven't said this yet, but it bears mentioning. A little anxiety is a good thing. You want to be relaxed when you take and prepare for the test, but some stress is healthy. The adrenaline that stress pumps into your bloodstream helps you stay alert and think more clearly. And that's a good thing.

By now you should feel more comfortable about the test. So turn to Chapter Three and complete the Diagnostic Quiz.

# Chapter Three: **Nursing School Entrance Exams Diagnostic Quiz**

Imagine if you were taking an exam that was testing your knowledge of colors and rare flowering plants of South America. Do you think you would spend much time reviewing color swatches and practicing to recognize the differences between green and purple? Or do you think you would spend more time reviewing books on the flowering plants of South America? Chances are, you are probably familiar enough with colors to do well on that part of the test, so you would concentrate on reviewing what you don't know.

That's how this diagnostic test is meant to work. You should take this 65-question test before you review any study materials. This way, your results on this test will give you important information about your strengths and weakness. For example, if you ace all the vocabulary and spelling questions on this test, you can limit the amount of time you spend reviewing Chapter Five. On the other hand, if you struggle with all of the science questions, you should spend more of your time reviewing Chapter Seven and Chapter Eight.

Having an understanding of what you know and what you don't know is an important first step in preparing for a major test. Take this diagnostic test and be sure to review the answer explanations found at the end. Good luck!

# Nursing School Entrance Exams
## Diagnostic Quiz
## Answer Sheet

### Reading Comprehension

1. Ⓐ Ⓑ Ⓒ Ⓓ    4. Ⓐ Ⓑ Ⓒ Ⓓ    7. Ⓐ Ⓑ Ⓒ Ⓓ    10. Ⓐ Ⓑ Ⓒ Ⓓ
2. Ⓐ Ⓑ Ⓒ Ⓓ    5. Ⓐ Ⓑ Ⓒ Ⓓ    8. Ⓐ Ⓑ Ⓒ Ⓓ    11. Ⓐ Ⓑ Ⓒ Ⓓ
3. Ⓐ Ⓑ Ⓒ Ⓓ    6. Ⓐ Ⓑ Ⓒ Ⓓ    9. Ⓐ Ⓑ Ⓒ Ⓓ

### Vocabulary and Spelling

1. Ⓐ Ⓑ Ⓒ Ⓓ    5. Ⓐ Ⓑ Ⓒ Ⓓ    9. Ⓐ Ⓑ Ⓒ Ⓓ     13. Ⓐ Ⓑ Ⓒ Ⓓ
2. Ⓐ Ⓑ Ⓒ Ⓓ    6. Ⓐ Ⓑ Ⓒ Ⓓ    10. Ⓐ Ⓑ Ⓒ Ⓓ    14. Ⓐ Ⓑ Ⓒ Ⓓ
3. Ⓐ Ⓑ Ⓒ Ⓓ    7. Ⓐ Ⓑ Ⓒ Ⓓ    11. Ⓐ Ⓑ Ⓒ Ⓓ    15. Ⓐ Ⓑ Ⓒ Ⓓ
4. Ⓐ Ⓑ Ⓒ Ⓓ    8. Ⓐ Ⓑ Ⓒ Ⓓ    12. Ⓐ Ⓑ Ⓒ Ⓓ    16. Ⓐ Ⓑ Ⓒ Ⓓ

### Mathematics

1. Ⓐ Ⓑ Ⓒ Ⓓ    6. Ⓐ Ⓑ Ⓒ Ⓓ     11. Ⓐ Ⓑ Ⓒ Ⓓ    16. Ⓐ Ⓑ Ⓒ Ⓓ    21. Ⓐ Ⓑ Ⓒ Ⓓ
2. Ⓐ Ⓑ Ⓒ Ⓓ    7. Ⓐ Ⓑ Ⓒ Ⓓ     12. Ⓐ Ⓑ Ⓒ Ⓓ    17. Ⓐ Ⓑ Ⓒ Ⓓ    22. Ⓐ Ⓑ Ⓒ Ⓓ
3. Ⓐ Ⓑ Ⓒ Ⓓ    8. Ⓐ Ⓑ Ⓒ Ⓓ     13. Ⓐ Ⓑ Ⓒ Ⓓ    18. Ⓐ Ⓑ Ⓒ Ⓓ
4. Ⓐ Ⓑ Ⓒ Ⓓ    9. Ⓐ Ⓑ Ⓒ Ⓓ     14. Ⓐ Ⓑ Ⓒ Ⓓ    19. Ⓐ Ⓑ Ⓒ Ⓓ
5. Ⓐ Ⓑ Ⓒ Ⓓ    10. Ⓐ Ⓑ Ⓒ Ⓓ    15. Ⓐ Ⓑ Ⓒ Ⓓ    20. Ⓐ Ⓑ Ⓒ Ⓓ

### Science

1. Ⓐ Ⓑ Ⓒ Ⓓ    5. Ⓐ Ⓑ Ⓒ Ⓓ    9. Ⓐ Ⓑ Ⓒ Ⓓ     13. Ⓐ Ⓑ Ⓒ Ⓓ
2. Ⓐ Ⓑ Ⓒ Ⓓ    6. Ⓐ Ⓑ Ⓒ Ⓓ    10. Ⓐ Ⓑ Ⓒ Ⓓ    14. Ⓐ Ⓑ Ⓒ Ⓓ
3. Ⓐ Ⓑ Ⓒ Ⓓ    7. Ⓐ Ⓑ Ⓒ Ⓓ    11. Ⓐ Ⓑ Ⓒ Ⓓ    15. Ⓐ Ⓑ Ⓒ Ⓓ
4. Ⓐ Ⓑ Ⓒ Ⓓ    8. Ⓐ Ⓑ Ⓒ Ⓓ    12. Ⓐ Ⓑ Ⓒ Ⓓ    16. Ⓐ Ⓑ Ⓒ Ⓓ

GO ON TO THE NEXT PAGE ⇒

KAPLAN

**Questions 1–7 are based on the following passage from a book about wolves, written by a self-taught naturalist who studied them in the wild.**

My precautions against disturbing the wolves were superfluous. It had required me a week to get their measure, but they must have taken mine at our first meeting; and while there was nothing disdainful in their evident assessment of me, they managed to ignore my presence, and indeed my very existence, with a thoroughness which was somehow disconcerting.

Quite by accident I had pitched my tent within ten yards of one of the major paths used by the wolves when they were going to, or coming from, their hunting paths to the westward; and only a few hours after I had taken up my residence, one of the wolves came back from a trip and discovered me and my tent.

He was at the end of a hard night's work and was clearly tired and anxious to go home to bed. He came over a small rise fifty yards from me with his head down, his eyes half-closed, and a preoccupied air about him. Far from being the preternaturally alert and suspicious beast of fiction, this wolf was so self-engrossed that he came straight on to within 15 yards of me, and might have gone right past the tent without seeing it at all, had I not banged an elbow against the teakettle, making a resounding clank. The wolf's head came up and his eyes opened wide, but he did not stop or falter in his pace. One brief, sidelong glance was all he vouchsafed to me as he continued on his way.

By the time this happened, I had learned a great deal about my wolfish neighbors, and one of the facts that had emerged was that they were not nomadic roamers, as is almost universally believed, but were settled beasts and the possessors of a large permanent estate with very definite boundaries. The territory owned by my wolf family comprised more than 100 square miles, bounded on one side by a river but otherwise not delimited by geographical features. Nevertheless there were boundaries, clearly indicated in wolfish fashion.

Once a week, more or less, the clan made the rounds of the family lands and freshened up the boundary markers—a sort of lupine* beating of the bounds. This careful attention to property rights was perhaps made necessary by the presence of two other wolf families whose lands abutted on ours, although I never discovered any evidence of bickering or disagreements between the owners of the various adjoining estates.

I suspect, therefore, that it was more of a ritual activity.

In any event, once I had become aware of this strong feeling of property among the wolves, I decided to use this knowledge to make them at least recognize my existence. One evening, after they had gone off for their regular nightly hunt, I staked out a property claim of my own, embracing perhaps three acres, with the tent at the middle, and including a 100-yard-long section of the wolves' path. This took most of the night and required frequent returns to the tent to consume copious quantities of tea; but before dawn brought the hunters home, the task was done and I retired, somewhat exhausted, to observe the results.

I had not long to wait. At 0814 hours, according to my wolf log, the leading male of the clan appeared over the ridge behind me, padding homeward with his usual air of preoccupation. As usual, he did not deign to look at the tent; but when he reached the point where my property line intersected the trail, he stopped as abruptly as if he had run into an invisible wall. His attitude of fatigue vanished and was replaced by one of bewilderment. Cautiously he extended his nose and sniffed at one of my marked bushes. After a minute of complete indecision he backed away a few yards and sat down. And then, finally, he looked directly at the tent and me. It was a long, considering sort of look.

Having achieved my object—that of forcing at least one of the wolves to take cognizance of my existence—I now began to wonder if, in my ignorance, I had transgressed some unknown wolf law of major importance and would have to pay for my temerity. I found myself regretting the absence of a weapon as the look I was getting became longer, more thoughtful, and still more intent. In an effort to break the impasse I loudly cleared my throat and turned my back on the wolf to indicate as clearly as possible that I found his continued scrutiny impolite, if not actually offensive. He appeared to take the hint. Briskly, and with an air of decision, he turned his attention away from me and began a systematic tour of the area, sniffing each boundary marker once or twice, and carefully placing his mark on the outside of each clump of grass or stone. In 15 minutes he rejoined the path at the point where it left my property and trotted off towards his home, leaving me with a good deal to occupy my thoughts.

*lupine: relating to wolves

GO ON TO THE NEXT PAGE ➤

KAPLAN)

1. According to the author, why were his precautions against disturbing the wolves "superfluous"?

   (A) It was several weeks before he encountered his first wolf.

   (B) Other wild animals posed a greater threat to his safety.

   (C) The wolves noticed him but were not interested in harming him.

   (D) He was not bothered by the wolves until he started interfering with them.

2. The author mentions the wolves' "assessment" of him in order to:

   (A) Account for their strange behavior toward him.

   (B) Convey his initial fear of being attacked.

   (C) Emphasize his ignorance on first encountering them.

   (D) Indicate the need for precautions against disturbing them.

3. In the third paragraph, the author is primarily surprised to find that the wolf:

   (A) Is traveling alone.

   (B) Lacks the energy to respond.

   (C) Is hunting at night.

   (D) Is not more on its guard.

4. The author suggests that boundary marking is a "ritual activity" because:

   (A) The wolves marked their boundaries at regular intervals.

   (B) No disputes over territory ever seemed to occur.

   (C) The boundaries were marked by geographical features.

   (D) The boundaries were marked at the same time each week.

5. The author most likely mentions an "invisible wall" in order to emphasize:

   (A) His delight in attracting the wolf's attention.

   (B) The wolf's annoyance at encountering a challenge.

   (C) The high speed at which the wolf was traveling.

   (D) The sudden manner in which the wolf stopped.

6. The wolf's first reaction on encountering the author's property marking is one of:

   (A) Combativeness

   (B) Confusion

   (C) Anxiety

   (D) Wariness

7. The author turns his back on the wolf primarily in order to:

   (A) Demonstrate his power over the wolf.

   (B) Bring about some change in the situation.

   (C) Compel the wolf to recognize his existence.

   (D) Look for a suitable weapon.

GO ON TO THE NEXT PAGE

**Questions 8–9 are based on the following passage.**

The discovery of helium required the combined efforts of several scientists. Pierre-Jules Cesar Janssen first obtained evidence for the existence of helium during a solar eclipse in 1868 when he detected a new yellow line on his spectroscope while observing the sun. This experiment was repeated by Norman Lockyer who concluded that no known element produced such a line. However, other scientists were dubious, finding it unlikely that an element existed only on the sun. Then, in 1895, William Ramsay discovered helium on Earth after treating clevite, a uranium mineral, with mineral acids. After isolating the resulting gas, Ramsay sent samples to William Crookes and Norman Lockyer who identified it conclusively as the missing element helium.

8.  The passage indicates that Ramsay's chief contribution to the discovery of helium was to:

   (A)  Prove the validity of Janssen's experiment.
   (B)  Find helium in uranium minerals.
   (C)  Identify the element discovered by Crookes as helium.
   (D)  Discover that helium naturally occurs on Earth.

9.  The author of the passage suggests that the results of the work of Janssen and Lockyer were:

   (A)  Repeated incorrectly by other scientists.
   (B)  Thought by others to be the result of flawed methodologies.
   (C)  Met with skepticism by other scientists.
   (D)  Only valid during solar eclipses.

**Questions 10–11 are based on the following passage.**

Diamond is the hardest known material and has long been used in various industrial-shaping processes, such as cutting, grinding, and polishing. Diamond, sapphire, ruby (which is a sapphire with chromium "impurities"), and garnet are increasingly important in various applications. For example, diamond is used in sensors, diaphragms for audio speakers, and coatings for optical materials. Sapphire is used in gallium nitride-based LEDs; ruby is used in check valves; and synthetic garnet is used in lasers intended in applications in medical products.

10.  The main idea of this passage can best be summarized with which of these titles?

   (A)  The Timeless Allure of Precious Stones
   (B)  Nontraditional Uses of Diamonds
   (C)  Industrial Uses for Precious Stones
   (D)  Gem Hardness and Utility

11.  It can be inferred from this passage that:

   (A)  Diamonds are more precious than sapphires.
   (B)  Rubies come from the same type of stone as do sapphires.
   (C)  Garnets are used in various industrial-shaping processes.
   (D)  Precious stones are more costly than ever.

GO ON TO THE NEXT PAGE

**KAPLAN**

## Section 2: Vocabulary and Spelling

1. *Resignation* most nearly means:

   (A) Losing
   (B) Waste
   (C) Acceptance
   (D) Pride

2. *Tangible* most nearly means:

   (A) Real
   (B) Open
   (C) Graphic
   (D) Costly

3. *Feasible* most nearly means:

   (A) Workable
   (B) Breakable
   (C) Imperfect
   (D) Evident

4. *Impure* means the opposite of:

   (A) Harmonious
   (B) Integral
   (C) Unalloyed
   (D) Assiduous

5. *Scale* means the opposite of:

   (A) Enlarge
   (B) Collapse
   (C) Weigh
   (D) Descend

6. *Levity* means the opposite of:

   (A) Inequality
   (B) Gravity
   (C) Laxity
   (D) Credulity

7. Optimistic : Hope ::

   (A) Playwrights : Creativity
   (B) Flying : Fear
   (C) Sculpted : Talent
   (D) Sage : Wisdom

8. Agenda : Meeting ::

   (A) Show : Television
   (B) Map : Plan
   (C) Program : Play
   (D) Organize : Detail

9. Forge : Signature ::

   (A) Originate : Store
   (B) Fake : Meal
   (C) Counterfeit : Money
   (D) Cut : Paper

**Choose the word that is misspelled.**

10. (A) Nuetral
    (B) Perceived
    (C) Efficient
    (D) Analysis

11. (A) Acessible
    (B) Endure
    (C) Magnified
    (D) Comprehension

12. (A) Surreal
    (B) Obsolete
    (C) Negligance
    (D) Infused

GO ON TO THE NEXT PAGE

KAPLAN

In the next four questions, find the sentences that contain a misspelled word. If there are no mistakes, choose (D).

13. (A) The hole is not noticeable.

    (B) We will conduct a formal inquiry.

    (C) Dana is an excelent athlete.

    (D) No mistake.

14. (A) What time will the room be availible?

    (B) Smoking is not allowed in public places.

    (C) We used various fruits in the salad.

    (D) No mistake.

15. (A) Our school cafateria always opens at 8:00 in the morning.

    (B) His proposal for a new park was very interesting.

    (C) The secretary typed very quickly.

    (D) No mistake.

16. (A) Please try not to interupt me when I'm speaking.

    (B) Are you sure this information is accurate?

    (C) This knitting pattern is very complicated.

    (D) No mistake.

## Section 3: Mathematics

1. If $100 + x = 100$, then $x = ?$

   (A) $-100$

   (B) $-10$

   (C) $0$

   (D) $10$

2. The percent decrease from 12 to 9 is equal to the percent decrease from 40 to what number?

   (A) 3

   (B) 10

   (C) 25

   (D) 30

3. On a certain planet, if each year has 9 months and each month has 15 days, how many full years have passed after 700 days on this planet?

   (A) 1

   (B) 2

   (C) 3

   (D) 5

4. $(\frac{1}{5} + \frac{1}{3}) \div \frac{1}{2} = ?$

   (A) $\frac{1}{8}$

   (B) $\frac{1}{4}$

   (C) $\frac{4}{15}$

   (D) $\frac{16}{15}$

GO ON TO THE NEXT PAGE

**KAPLAN**

5. Marty has exactly 5 blue pens, 6 black pens, and 4 red pens in his knapsack. If he pulls out one pen at random from his knapsack, what is the probability that the pen is either red or black?

   (A) 1 out of 5

   (B) 1 out of 3

   (C) 1 out of 2

   (D) 2 out of 3

6. Bill has to type a paper that is $p$ pages long, with each page containing $w$ words. If Bill types an average of $x$ words per minute, how many hours will it take him to finish the paper?

   (A) $60wpx$

   (B) $\dfrac{wx}{60p}$

   (C) $\dfrac{wpx}{60}$

   (D) $\dfrac{wp}{60x}$

7. At a certain school, if the ratio of teachers to students is 1 to 10, which of the following could be the total number of teachers and students?

   (A) 100

   (B) 121

   (C) 144

   (D) 222

8. If $r = 3$ and $s = 1$, then $r^2 - 2s = ?$

   (A) 2

   (B) 4

   (C) 6

   (D) 7

9. A machine caps 5 bottles every 2 seconds. At this rate, how many bottles will be capped in 1 minute?

   (A) 75

   (B) 150

   (C) 225

   (D) 300

10. If $\dfrac{2}{x} + \dfrac{5}{3} = 2$, what is the value of $x$?

   (A) 6

   (B) 2

   (C) $\dfrac{4}{5}$

   (D) $\dfrac{-4}{5}$

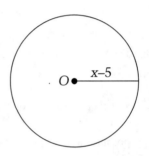

11. In the circle with center $O$ above, for what value of $x$ does the circle have a circumference of $20\pi$?

   (A) 5

   (B) 10

   (C) 15

   (D) 20

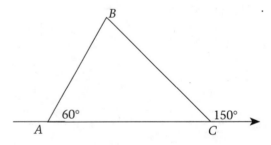

Note: Figure not drawn to scale.

12. In triangle $ABC$ above, if $AB = 4$, then $AC = ?$

   (A) 6

   (B) 7

   (C) 8

   (D) 9

GO ON TO THE NEXT PAGE

13. If a sweater sells for $48 after a 25% markdown, what was its original price?

    (A) $56
    (B) $60
    (C) $64
    (D) $68

14. Which of the following must be equal to 30% of $x$?

    (A) $\dfrac{3x}{1,000}$

    (B) $\dfrac{3x}{100}$

    (C) $\dfrac{3x}{10}$

    (D) $3x$

15. A certain phone call costs 75¢ for the first 3 minutes plus 15¢ for each additional minute. If the call lasted $x$ minutes and $x$ is an integer greater than 3, which of the following expresses the cost of the call, in dollars?

    (A) $0.75(3) + 0.15x$
    (B) $0.75(3) + 0.15(x + 3)$
    (C) $0.75 + 0.15(3 - x)$
    (D) $0.75 + 0.15(x - 3)$

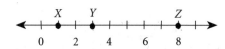

16. On the number line shown above, the length of $YZ$ is how much greater than the length of $XY$?

    (A) 3
    (B) 4
    (C) 5
    (D) 6

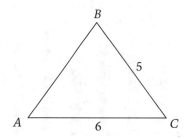

17. If the perimeter of triangle $ABC$ above is 16, what is its area?

    (A) 8
    (B) 9
    (C) 10
    (D) 12

18. $(2 \times 10^4) + (5 \times 10^3) + (6 \times 10^2) + (4 \times 10^1) = ?$

    (A) 20,564
    (B) 25,064
    (C) 25,604
    (D) 25,640

19. If $2n + 3 = 5$, then $4n = ?$

    (A) 1
    (B) 2
    (C) 4
    (D) 8

GO ON TO THE NEXT PAGE

KAPLAN

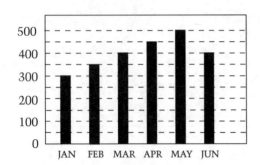

NUMBER OF BOOKS BORROWED
FROM MIDVILLE LIBRARY

20. According to the graph above, the number of books borrowed during the month of January was what fraction of the total number of books borrowed during the first six months of the year?

(A) $\frac{1}{8}$

(B) $\frac{1}{7}$

(C) $\frac{1}{6}$

(D) $\frac{3}{16}$

21. If point $R$ is $(2, 4)$ and point $S$ is $(7, 7)$, what is the length of $\overline{RS}$?

(A) 2

(B) $\sqrt{7}$

(C) $\sqrt{34}$

(D) 9

22. A business is owned by 4 women and 1 man, each of whom owns an equal share. If one of the women sells $\frac{1}{2}$ of her share to the man, and another woman keeps $\frac{1}{4}$ of her share and sells the rest to the man, what fraction of the business will the man own?

(A) $\frac{1}{3}$

(B) $\frac{9}{20}$

(C) $\frac{11}{20}$

(D) $\frac{2}{3}$

## Section 4: Science

1. Animals that consume plants are called:

(A) Saprophytes

(B) Herbivores

(C) Carnivores

(D) Omnivores

2. Which of the following kingdoms is considered the most primitive?

(A) Fungi

(B) Protista

(C) Moneran

(D) Plant

3. A bottle of perfume is opened in the back of a classroom. A short time later the teacher detects the odor. Once the liquid was exposed to the air in the room how did the vapors get from the perfume bottle to the teacher's nose?

(A) Osmosis

(B) Diffusion

(C) Dilution

(D) Dialysis

GO ON TO THE NEXT PAGE ⟹

4. During mitosis, distribution of one copy of each chromosome to each of the resulting cells virtually guarantees

   (A) Reduction of the chromosome number to half of the original chromosome number.

   (B) Formation of daughter cells with identical DNA sequences.

   (C) Cell growth.

   (D) Maximum cell size.

5. Which of the following is the name for the muscular tissue that contracts to permit air to enter the lungs?

   (A) Trachea

   (B) Alveoli

   (C) Esophagus

   (D) Diaphragm

6. Air entering the lungs of a tracheotomy patient through a tracheotomy (a tube inserted directly into the trachea) is colder and drier than normal, which often causes lung crusting and infection. This occurs primarily because the air:

   (A) Enters the respiratory system too rapidly to be filtered.

   (B) Is not properly humidified by the larynx.

   (C) Does not flow through the nasal passageways.

   (D) Does not flow past the mouth and tongue.

7. Which of the following is the location for the exchange of oxygen and carbon dioxide through thin membrane walls?

   (A) Alveoli

   (B) Trachea

   (C) Nasal cavity

   (D) Diaphragm

8. What is the function of a lysosome's membrane?

   (A) It isolates an acidic environment for the lysosome's hydrolytic enzymes from the neutral pH of the cytoplasm.

   (B) It is continuous with the nuclear membrane, thereby linking the lysosome with the endoplasmic reticulum.

   (C) It is used as an alternative site of protein synthesis.

   (D) The cytochrome carriers of the electron transport chain are embedded within it.

9. Oogenesis is the process by which:

   (A) Primary oocytes produce sperm.

   (B) Primary oocytes produce eggs.

   (C) The egg implants in the uterus.

   (D) The egg is released from the ovary.

10. In a neutral atom:

    (A) The number of electrons is greater than the number of protons.

    (B) The number of electrons is less than the number of protons.

    (C) The number of electrons is equal to the number of protons.

    (D) There are no electrons.

11. Which of the following indicates the relative randomness of molecules in the three states of matter?

    (A) Solid > liquid < gas

    (B) Liquid < solid < gas

    (C) Liquid > gas > solid

    (D) Gas > liquid > solid

GO ON TO THE NEXT PAGE

**KAPLAN**

12. Which of the following states has the highest average translational kinetic energy?

    (A) Solid

    (B) Liquid

    (C) Gas

    (D) None of the above

13. An element whose outer shell is only missing a few electrons is called a:

    (A) Metal

    (B) Nonmetal

    (C) Metalloid

    (D) Noble gas

14. Which of the following waves on the electromagnetic spectrum has the highest frequency?

    (A) Microwaves

    (B) X-rays

    (C) Visible light

    (D) Radio waves

15. Which of the following best explains the recoil action of a shooting gun?

    (A) Newton's First Law of Motion

    (B) Newton's Second Law of Motion

    (C) Newton's Third Law of Motion

    (D) Newton's Law of Gravitation

16. Which of the following states the law of charges?

    (A) Like charges repel each other and unlike charges attract each other.

    (B) Unlike charges repel each other and like charges attract each other.

    (C) All charges repel each other.

    (D) All charges attract each other.

END OF TEST. STOP

THE ANSWER KEY APPEARS ON THE FOLLOWING PAGE.

# Diagnostic Quiz: **Answer Key**

| Reading Comprehension | Vocabulary and Spelling | Mathematics | Science |
|---|---|---|---|
| 1. C | 1. C | 1. C | 1. B |
| 2. A | 2. A | 2. D | 2. C |
| 3. D | 3. A | 3. D | 3. B |
| 4. B | 4. C | 4. D | 4. B |
| 5. D | 5. D | 5. D | 5. D |
| 6. B | 6. B | 6. D | 6. C |
| 7. B | 7. D | 7. B | 7. A |
| 8. D | 8. C | 8. D | 8. A |
| 9. C | 9. C | 9. B | 9. B |
| 10. C | 10. A | 10. A | 10. C |
| 11. B | 11. A | 11. C | 11. D |
| | 12. C | 12. C | 12. C |
| | 13. C | 13. C | 13. B |
| | 14. A | 14. C | 14. B |
| | 15. A | 15. D | 15. C |
| | 16. A | 16. A | 16. A |
| | | 17. D | |
| | | 18. D | |
| | | 19. C | |
| | | 20. A | |
| | | 21. C | |
| | | 22. B | |

# Answers and Explanations

## Reading Comprehension

**1.  C**

In the first paragraph, the author explains how the wolves were aware of his presence but ignored him. That's why the author's precautions were superfluous. Answer (C) basically paraphrases that idea: The author's precautions were unnecessary because the wolves weren't interested in him.

**2.  A**

The author's basic point in paragraph one is that he was surprised at the way the wolves behaved toward him: They sized him up quickly right at the beginning and, from then on, ignored him. He found this behavior disconcerting, or *strange*, as (A) puts it.

**3.  D**

In paragraph three, the author describes how the wolf was so preoccupied that he came within 15 yards of his tent without seeing it. It wasn't until the author made noise that the wolf suddenly became aware of its surroundings. Answer (D) paraphrases this idea: that the wolf was not *on its guard*—it was self-absorbed.

**4.  B**

In the middle of paragraph five, the author describes how the wolf family regularly made the rounds of their lands and *freshened up the boundary markers*. He guessed that this was done because there were other wolves living in adjacent areas, although he never saw any sign of trouble between the neighboring wolf families. Then you get the quoted idea: Since he never witnessed any disputes, he figured that it was all basically a ritual activity. Answer (B) catches the idea.

**5.  D**

The phrase *invisible wall* occurs in paragraph seven, and the point is that the wolf, plodding home as preoccupied as usual, was suddenly stopped in its tracks when it encountered the spot where the author had left his own markings. So the idea about the invisible wall is that the wolf

was stopped suddenly (D), as if it had suddenly banged up against it.

**6.  B**

In the very same sentence in paragraph seven, the author says that the wolf, upon finding the author's marks, immediately became bewildered. Answer (B) restates that.

**7.  B**

At the end of paragraph eight, the author states that he turned his back on the wolf *in an effort to break the impasse*. In other words, he did it to bring about a change in the situation (B).

**8.  D**

Ramsay appears toward the middle of the passage after the author mentions that scientists doubted helium exists only on the sun. Since Ramsay's experiment with naturally occurring Earth minerals occurs in the next sentence, the correct answer would be something that cites discovering helium on Earth, and (D) fits this well.

**9.  C**

The passage states that Janssen and Lockyer observed the sun using their spectroscopes and discovered a new yellow line that belonged to an unknown element. Reading the next sentence reveals that Janssen and Lockyer's work was doubted by many other scientists (C).

**10.  C**

The passage here discusses industrial uses for precious stones, so the correct answer choice (C) should pretty much jump out at you.

**11.  B**

The passage notes parenthetically that a ruby is a sapphire with chromium "impurities," so one can logically infer that both gems come from the same kind of stone, choice (B).

## Vocabulary and Spelling

**1. C**

Sometimes, if you are having trouble with a word, such as *resignation* here, try coming up with a different form of the same word—another part of speech—and then working on a synonym for the related word. For instance, if you come up with *resigned*, you might be able to make an easier sentence, such as: He was *resigned* to defeat. And from this you figure out that resignation most nearly means *acceptance*.

**2. A**

Even if you only sort of know the meaning of *tangible*, you might have a sense that something *tangible* can be felt or seen, as oppose to intangible objects, which cannot. From that, you should be able to pick *real* (A) as the closest match.

**3. A**

When the question doesn't provide a context, try to come up with your own. Maybe you've heard something like: "The plan is feasible." Which answer choice best describes a plan? *Feasible* does mean *workable* or viable.

**4. C**

Since the *im-* prefix means *not*, then something *impure* is not pure. The correct answer choice will be a synonym for *pure. Unalloyed* means *not alloyed*, or *pure.* (If you had trouble working out what *unalloyed* means, you could have used word roots: *un-* means *not,* and an *alloy* is a mixture of two or more metals. So, *unalloyed* means *not a mixture,* which is pretty close to *pure* in meaning.)

**5. D**

The answer choices tell you that *scale* is being used as a verb. To scale is to climb up, as in *scale a mountain*. The correct answer choice will mean *climb down. Descend* means to *climb down*. This is the correct answer. If you needed to guess, you could eliminate *collapse* and *weigh*, since they have no clear opposites.

**6. B**

*Levity* means *lightness* and *humor*. The correct answer choice will be a word that means *seriousness* or *lack of humor*. *Gravity* is not only the force that holds us to Earth, but it also means *seriousness*. This is the correct answer.

**7. D**

*Optimistic* means full of hope; *sage* means full of wisdom.

**8. C**

An *agenda* creates a plan for a meeting, and a *program* creates a plan for a play.

**9. C**

One *forges* a *signature* and one *counterfeits money*.

**10. A**

The correct spelling is *neutral*.

**11. A**

The correct spelling is *accessible*.

**12. C**

The correct spelling is *negligence*.

**13. C**

The correct spelling is *excellent*.

**14. A**

The correct spelling is *available*.

**15. A**

The correct spelling is *cafeteria*.

**16. A**

The correct spelling is *interrupt*.

## Mathematics

**1. C**

Subtract 100 from both sides of the equation to find $x = 0$.

**2. D**

Percent change is actual change over original amount. The change from 12 to 9 is 3. The amount being changed from is 12, so $\frac{3}{12}$, or 25% is the percent decrease. 25% of 40 is $40(.25) = 10$, so the percent decrease from 40 to $40 - 10 = 30$ is the same as the percent decrease from 12 to 9. Another way to solve this problem is to set up a proportion: $\frac{12}{9} = \frac{40}{x}$, where $x$ is the number we are looking for. Cross multiply to find $12x = 360$, then divide by 12 to find $x = 30$.

**3. D**

Each month has 15 days, so 700 days is $\frac{700}{15}$ months. Each year has 9 months, so $\frac{700}{15}$ months is $= \frac{700}{15} \div 9 = 5\frac{5}{27}$. This means 5 full years have gone by.

**4. D**

Do what's in parentheses first:

$$\left(\frac{1}{5} + \frac{1}{3}\right) \div \frac{1}{2} = \left(\frac{3}{15} + \frac{5}{15}\right) \div \frac{1}{2}$$
$$= \frac{8}{15} \div \frac{1}{2}$$

Then, to divide fractions, invert the one after the division sign and multiply:

$$\frac{8}{15} \div \frac{1}{2} = \frac{8}{15} \times \frac{2}{1} = \frac{16}{15}$$

**5. D**

Probability is defined as the number of desired events divided by the total number of possible events. There are $5 + 6 + 4 = 15$ pens in the knapsack. If he pulls out 1 pen, there are 15 different pens he might pick, or 15 possible outcomes. The desired outcome is that the pen be either red or black. The group of acceptable pens consists of $4 + 6$, or 10 pens. So the probability that one of these pens will be picked is 10 of 15, or $\frac{10}{15}$, which we can reduce to $\frac{2}{3}$.

**6. D**

Pick numbers for $p$, $w$, and $x$ that work well in the problem. Let $p = 3$ and let $w = 100$. So there are three pages with 100 words per page, or 300 words total. Say he types 5 words a minute, so $x = 5$. Therefore, he types $5 \times 60$, or 300 words an hour. It takes him 1 hour to type the paper. The only answer choice that equals 1 when $p = 3$, $w = 100$, and $x = 5$ is choice (D).

**7. B**

The ratio of teachers to students is 1 to 10, so there might be only 1 teacher and 10 students, or there might be 50 teachers and 500 students, or just about any number of teachers and students that are in the ratio 1 to 10. That means that the teachers and the students can be divided into groups of 11:1 teacher and 10 students in each group. Think of it as a school with a large number of classrooms, all with 1 teacher and 10 students, for a total of 11 people in each room. So, the total number of teachers and students in the school must be a multiple of 11. If you look at the answer choices, you'll notice that 121, choice (B), is the only multiple of 11, so (B) must be correct.

**8. D**

This is a straightforward substitution problem. Plug in the given values and remember your order of operations (PEMDAS). $3^2 - 2(1) = 9 - 2(1) = 9 - 2 = 7$.

**9. B**

If a machine caps 5 bottles every 2 seconds, then it would cap 30 times as many bottles in one minute (since a minute is 60 seconds). $5 \times 30 = 150$ bottles per minute, choice (B).

**10. A**

If $\frac{2}{x} + \frac{5}{3} = 2$, then $\frac{2}{x} = 2 - \frac{5}{3} = \frac{6}{3} - \frac{5}{3} = \frac{1}{3}$. Cross-multiply to find $x = 6$.

### 11. C

The diagram tells you that the radius of the circle is
$x - 5$ and the question tells you that the circumference of
the circle is $20\pi$. Since the circumference of a circle is $2\pi$
times the radius, $20\pi$ must equal $2\pi$ times $(x - 5)$, which
gives you the equation $20\pi = 2\pi(x - 5)$. Solving this
equation gives you $x = 15$, answer choice (C).

### 12. C

Angle $BCA$ is supplementary to the angle marked 150°, so
angle $BCA = 180° - 150° = 30°$. Because the sum of
interior angles of a triangle is 180°, angle $A$ + angle $B$ +
angle $BCA = 180°$; so angle $B = 180° - 60° - 30° = 90°$.
Triangle $ABC$ is a 30-60-90 right triangle, and its sides are in
the ratio $1 : \sqrt{3} : 2$. The side opposite the 30°, $AB$, which we
know has a length of 4, must be half the length of the
hypotenuse, $AC$. Therefore, $AC = 8$, and that's answer
choice (C).

### 13. C

We want to solve for the original price, the whole. The
percent markdown is 25%, so $48 is 75% of the whole.

Percent × Whole = Part

75% × Original Price = $48

Original Price $= \dfrac{\$48}{0.75} = \$64$

### 14. C

Use the formula: Percent × Whole = Part.

30% is $\dfrac{30}{100}$, or $\dfrac{3}{10}$. So $\dfrac{3x}{10}$ = part, and choice (C) is
correct.

### 15. D

The first 3 minutes of the phone call cost 75¢ or $0.75
dollars. If the entire call lasted $x$ minutes, the rest of the call
lasted $x - 3$ minutes. Each minute after the first 3 cost 15¢
or $0.15, so the rest of the call cost $0.15(x - 3)$. Thus, the
cost of the entire call is $0.75 + 0.15(x - 3)$ dollars.

### 16. A

Find the length of each segment, and then subtract the
length of $XY$ from the length of $YZ$. $Y$ is at 3 on the number
line and $Z$ is at 8, so the length of $YZ$ is $8 - 3 = 5$. $X$ is at
1 on the number line and $Y$ is at 3, so the length of $XY$ is
$3 - 1 = 2$. So the length of $YZ$ is $5 - 2 = 3$ greater than the
length of $XY$.

### 17. D

To find the area you need to know the base and height. If
the perimeter is 16, then $AB + BC + AC = 16$, that is,
$AB = 16 - 5 - 6 = 5$. Because $AB = BC$, this is an isosceles
triangle. If you drop a line from vertex $B$ to $AC$, it will divide
the base in half. This divides up the triangle into two smaller
right triangles:

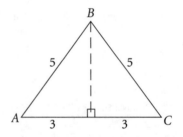

These right triangles each have one leg of 3 and a
hypotenuse of 5; therefore, they are 3-4-5 right triangles.
The missing leg (which is also the height of triangle $ABC$)
must have a length of 4. We now know that the base of
$ABC$ is 6, and the height is 4, so the area is $\dfrac{1}{2} \times 6 \times 4$, or
12, answer choice (D).

### 18. D

$2 \times 10^4 = 20{,}000$. $5 \times 10^3 = 5{,}000$. $6 \times 10^2 = 600$.
$4 \times 10^1 = 40$. So the sum is 25,640.

### 19. C

All you have to do here is solve the equation, but instead of
solving it for $n$, you have to solve it for $4n$. If $2n + 3 = 5$,
then you can subtract 3 from both sides of the equation to
get $2n = 2$. Multiplying both sides of this equation by 2
gives you $4n = 4$, choice (C).

**20. A**

Looking at the graph, you can see that the number of books borrowed in January was 300. To find the total number of books borrowed during the first six months of the year, add the values of each bar:

$300 + 350 + 400 + 450 + 500 + 400 = 2{,}400$ books.

So the number of books borrowed in January is $\frac{1}{8}$ of the total number of books borrowed during the first 6 months of the year.

**21. C**

The distance between two points $(x_1, y_1)$ and $(x_2, y_2)$ can be found by using the distance formula:

$\sqrt{(x_2 - x_1)^2 + (y_2 - y_1)^2}$. Plug in the numbers from the question.

$\sqrt{(7-2)^2 + (7-4)^2} = \sqrt{5^2 + 3^2} = \sqrt{25+9} = \sqrt{34}$

The correct answer is choice (C).

**22. (B)**

Rather than dealing with fractions of the business, let's say that there are 100 total shares. At the beginning of the problem, the 4 women each own 20 shares and the man owns 20 shares. One woman sells $\frac{1}{2}$ of her part of the business, 10 shares, to the man. Another woman sells $1 - \frac{1}{4} = \frac{3}{4}$ of her part of the business which is $20\left(\frac{3}{4}\right) = 15$ shares to the man. Now the man owns $20 + 10 + 15 = 45$ shares out of the total 100 shares in the business.

$\frac{45}{100} = \frac{9}{20}$, so the man owns $\frac{9}{20}$ of the business.

## Science

**1. B**

Animals that consume plants are called herbivores.

**2. C**

The Moneran kingdom is considered the most primitive kingdom.

**3. B**

Diffusion is the tendency of molecules or ions to move from areas of higher concentration to areas of lower concentration until the concentration is uniform throughout the system. Diffusion explains how gases in the air spread out when released from one location where the concentration of their molecules is higher than in the space surrounding their source.

**4. B**

Mitosis is often used interchangeably with cell division. Technically, mitosis is the process of chromosomal replication that results in two daughter nuclei with identical DNA sequences.

**5. D**

The diaphragm is a muscular band of tissue that contracts to permit air to enter the lung.

**6. C**

When a patient breathes through a tracheotomy, the air entering the respiratory system bypasses a very important area—the nasal cavities. In an individual breathing normally, the extensive surfaces of the nasal passageways warm and almost completely humidify the air, and particles are filtered out by nasal air turbulence. Since the air reaching the lungs of a tracheotomy patient has not been warmed or humidified, lung crusting and infection often result.

**7. A**

The alveoli are the location for the exchange of oxygen and carbon dioxide at the lungs.

**8. A**

Lysosome acid has an acidic interior to enhance the activity of lysomal enzymes that degrade biomolecules. The lysomal membrane separates the acidic interior of the lysome from the rest of the cell, which has a neutral pH.

**9. B**

Oogenesis is the process whereby primary oocytes undergo meiosis to produce one egg (or ovum) and two or three polar bodies.

**10. C**

In a neutral atom, the number of electrons is equal to the number of protons.

**11. D**

Because gas molecules have the greatest freedom to move around, gases have the greatest disorder. Liquids are more dense than gases and therefore the molecules experience stronger intermolecular attractions and are less free to move around. The arrangement of molecules in solids is the least random.

**12. C**

The random motion of a gas holds the most translational kinetic energy.

**13. B**

An element whose outer shell is only missing a few electrons is called a nonmetal.

**14. B**

Of the wave states listed, X-rays have the highest frequency in the electromagnetic spectrum (gamma rays have an even higher frequency).

**15. C**

The recoil action of a shooting gun is explained by Newton's Third Law of Motion; that is, for every action there is an equal and opposite reaction.

**16. A**

The law of charges states that like charges repel each other and unlike charges attract each other.

# INTERPRETING THE RESULTS OF THE DIAGNOSTIC QUIZ

Because this is a diagnostic quiz, it's important not to calculate your overall score and move on. How you did on this quiz is not a clear reflection on how you will perform on test day. Remember, its purpose is to help you diagnose your strengths and weaknesses.

## Strengths and Weaknesses

Take a minute or so to list the areas of the Nursing School Entrance Exams Diagnostic Quiz you were good at. They can be general (math) or specific (addition of negative numbers). Put down as many as you can think of.

## Strong Test Subjects

_____

_____

_____

_____

_____

_____

Now, take more time to list areas of the test you need to improve on, are just plain bad at, or have failed at.

## Weak Test Subjects

_____

_____

_____

_____

_____

Taking stock of your strengths and weaknesses lets you know the areas you don't have to worry about and the ones that will demand extra attention and effort. It helps to know where to put the extra effort. You will feel better (and do better) when you face up to what you need to work on instead of neglecting it.

As you work through this book, refer back to your weaknesses list. Check off your weaknesses as you tackle each one of them. (Math? Nerves? Reading Comprehension?) Now we're going to focus on what you're good at. Sharpen your pencil. Go to your strengths list. Copy the general items on that list below. You're going to make them more specific. For example, if you listed math as a broad topic you feel strong in, you would get specific by including areas of this subject about which you are particularly knowledgeable.

If any new strengths come to mind, jot them down. Focus all of your attention and effort on your strengths. Don't underestimate yourself or your abilities. Give yourself full credit. At the same time, don't list strengths you don't really have. You'll only be fooling yourself.

## Strengths: From General to Specific

_____

_____

_____

_____

_____

## General Strength Specifics

_____

_____

_____

_____

_____

## Specifics

_____

_____

_____

_____

_____

After you've stopped, look over your list. Did you write down more things than you thought you knew? Is it possible you know more than you've given yourself credit for? Could that mean you've found a number of areas in which you feel strong?

You just took an active step toward helping yourself. Increased feelings of confidence work wonders on test day. If you are ready to begin your review, turn to Section Two now.

# Review

# Chapter Four: **Reading Comprehension Review**

You may be thinking you don't need to review the lessons in this chapter. You already know how to read, right? After all, you have already read the first three chapters of this book! However, there is a big difference between knowing how to read, and being able to interpret, understand, and remember everything you read. The lessons in this chapter teach you how to be a more efficient reader. In turn, the strategies section of this book shows you how to handle the kinds of reading comprehension questions you are likely to face on your nursing school entrance exam. Don't forget to complete the review questions at the end of this chapter to make sure you have understood everything you have read so far!

## READING LESSON

As you probably know, the way you read during a test is not exactly how you read in everyday life. In general, you usually read to learn or for pleasure. It's a pretty safe bet that you are not reading test passages for fun. If you do enjoy them, great! However, it should be clear that you are not reading these passages for enjoyment. You are reading them to answer questions and earn points. Here are some tips on how to get the most out of the passages you are reading.

### Mark It Up

If you are allowed to write in the test booklet, use this to your advantage. You do not need to take a lot of notes, but do not leave the passage and surrounding space blank. Use it to keep track of the main idea of the whole passage or specific paragraphs. Your notes will help you find the information you need to answer the questions later.

### Focus on the First Third of the Passage

Although you may not find the passages on the test interesting, they are well organized. This means the author is very likely to present important information at the beginning of the passage. Chances are you will be able to answer the main idea questions based on the first third of the passage.

## Use the Paragraph Topics

The first two sentences of each paragraph should tell you what it's about. The rest of the paragraph is likely to be more detail heavy. Just as you should pay more attention to the beginning of the passage, you should also pay more attention to the beginning of each paragraph.

## Don't Worry If You Get Stuck

If there's something in the passage you don't understand, don't waste time reading it over and over again. As long as you have a general idea of where the details are, you don't have to know what they are. Remember, later you can go back and look at paragraphs or notes you have made. This is another example of why marking up passages is so useful. You can circle or underline details that seem important. Furthermore, as long as you have made a note of the paragraph topic, you should be able to go back and find details within it. Details will always be located in the paragraph that deals with the general topic.

### Summarizing, Researching, and Making Inferences

The following skills will also help you with Reading Comprehension sections on test day.

**Summarizing:** For the purpose of the test, summarizing means being able to analyze a single phrase to capture what the entire passage is about.

**Researching:** Research is important in helping you answer detail questions. Researching means knowing where to look for the details. Generally, if you jot down paragraph topics, you should have a good idea where to locate the details.

**Inferring:** Making an inference means coming to a conclusion based on information that is hinted at, but not directly stated.

## How to Read a Passage

You may not know it, but how we read depends upon why we're reading. When you're reading a Reading Comprehension passage on an exam, your goal is to correctly answer each question about that passage. Contrary to what you might expect, to reach that goal, you don't need to read the passage word by word. Instead, your best bet is to carefully skim the passage.

### Serious Skimming

Each Reading Comprehension passage is written with a distinct purpose: The author wants to make a point, describe a situation, or convince you of his or her ideas. As you're reading, ask yourself the following questions:

- What is this passage about?
- What is the point of this passage?
- What is the author trying to say?
- Why did he or she write this?
- What are the two or three most important things in this passage?

By asking these questions, you are doing what is called active reading—and it's the key to staying focused on the page. Active reading does not necessarily mean reading the passage word-for-word. Rather, it means reading lightly but with a focus—in other words, serious skimming. This way, you can quickly find the main ideas and identify the tone of the passage. The questions themselves will help you fill in the details by directing you back to important information and specific details in the passage.

Getting hung up on details is a major Reading Comprehension pitfall. You need to grasp the outline, but you don't need to get all the fine features.

### Components of the Seriously Skim Technique

- Skim the passage to get the writer's drift. Don't read the passage thoroughly. It's a waste of time.
- As you skim, search for important points. Don't wait for important information to jump out at you.
- Don't get caught up in details. The questions will often supply them for you or tell you exactly where to find them.

## Kinds of Reading Comprehension Questions

When you read passages on a test, you're reading for a specific purpose: to be able to correctly answer as many questions as possible. Fortunately, most tests tend to use the same kinds of Reading Comprehension questions over and over again, so whatever the passage is about and however long it may be, you can expect the same four basic question types:

- Main Idea
- Detail
- Inference
- Vocabulary-in-Context

### Main Idea Questions

Main Idea questions test how well you understand the passage as a whole. They ask about:

- The main point or purpose of a passage or individual paragraphs
- The author's overall attitude or tone
- The logic underlying the author's argument
- How ideas relate to each other in the passage

If you're stumped on a Main Idea question, even after reading the passage, do the Detail questions first. They can help you fill in the Main Idea.

### Detail Questions

Detail questions ask about localized bits of information—usually specific facts or details from the passage. These questions may give you a line reference—a clue to where in the passage you'll find your answer. Beware of answer choices that seem to reasonably answer the question but don't make sense in the context of the passage or that are true but refer to a different section of the text.

Detail questions test:

- Whether you understand significant information that's stated in the passage
- Your ability to locate information within a text
- Your ability to differentiate between main ideas and specific details

### Inference Questions

Some Reading Comprehension questions begin with, "it can be inferred that the author…". To infer is to draw a conclusion based on reasoning or evidence. For example, if you wake up in the morning and there's three feet of fresh snow on the ground, you can safely infer that it snowed during the night.

Often, writers will use suggestion or inference rather than stating ideas directly. But they will also leave you plenty of clues so you can figure out just what they are trying to convey. Inference clues include word choice (diction), tone, and specific details. For example, say a passage states that a particular idea was perceived as revolutionary. You might infer from the use of the word *perceived* that the author believes the idea was not truly revolutionary but seen that way.

Thus, Inference questions test your ability to use information in the passage to come to a logical conclusion. The key to inference questions is to stick to the evidence in the text. Most inference questions have pretty strong clues, so avoid any answer choices that seem far-fetched. If you can't find any evidence in the passage, then it probably isn't the right answer.

Make sure you read Inference questions carefully. Multiple answer choices may seem true; however if particular answers can't be inferred from the passage, and don't correspond to the passage as a whole or the specific part of the passage cited in the question, then they can't be the correct answer.

**Vocabulary-in-Context Questions**

Because vocabulary is tested in a separate section of the nursing school entrance exams, you probably won't encounter too many Vocabulary-in-Context questions. Just in case this type of question does appear on your test, we've provided you with some information that will help you.

Vocabulary-in-Context questions test your ability to infer the meaning of a word from the context in which it appears. The words tested are usually fairly common words with more than one meaning. That's the trick.

Many of the answer choices will be definitions of the tested word, but only one will work in context. Sometimes one of the answer choices will jump out at you. It will be the most common meaning of the word in question—but it's rarely right. You can think of this as the obvious choice. Say curious is the word being tested. The obvious choice is inquisitive. But curious also means odd; if that is the context the word appears in, that's the correct answer.

Using context to find the answer will help keep you from falling for this kind of trap. But you can also use these obvious choices to your advantage. If you get stuck on a Vocabulary-in-Context question, you can eliminate the obvious choice and guess from the remaining answers.

# READING COMPREHENSION STRATEGIES

Here are some of the strategies that will help you on test day.

## Kaplan's 5-Step Method for Reading Comprehension Questions

From the lesson you learned that skimming is a vital component of Kaplan's 5-Step Method for Reading Comprehension Questions. Once you have skimmed the passage, apply our system of attacking the questions.

- Read the question stem.
- Locate the material you need.
- Predict the answer.
- Scan the answer choices.
- Select your answer.

### Step 1. Read the Question Stem

You can't answer the question correctly if you haven't read it. It's as simple as that. So make sure to really read it carefully. Make sure you understand exactly what the question is asking. Is it a Main Idea question? Detail? Inference? Vocabulary? Are you looking for an overall main idea or a specific piece of information? Are you trying to determine the author's attitude or the meaning of a particular word?

### Step 2. Locate the Material You Need

If you are given a line reference, read the material surrounding the line mentioned. It will clarify exactly what the question is asking and provide you with the context you need to answer the question correctly.

If you're not given a line reference, scan the text to find the section of the text the question applies to, then quickly reread those few sentences. Keep the main point of the passage in mind.

### Step 3. Predict the Answer

Don't spend time making up a precise answer. You need only a general sense of what you're after so you can recognize the correct answer quickly when you read the choices.

### Step 4. Scan the Answer Choices

Scan the choices, looking for one that fits your idea of the right answer. If you don't find an ideal answer, quickly eliminate wrong choices by checking over the passage again. Rule out choices that are too extreme or go against common sense. Get rid of answers that sound reasonable but don't make sense in the context of the passage or the question. Don't pick far-fetched inferences, and make sure there is evidence for your inference in the passage. Remember, to infer the correct answer, look at what is strongly implied in the passage.

### Step 5. Select Your Answer

You've eliminated the obvious wrong answers. One of the remaining choices should fit your ideal. If you're left with more than one contender, consider the passage's main idea, and make an educated guess.

## Long Passage Strategies

Some of the passages on your nursing school entrance exam are going to be longer. There are a few things to keep in mind when you read the long passages. Consider these as strategies that will help you master the section.

### Question Order

For longer passages, Reading Comprehension questions are usually organized in a specific order. In general, order of questions corresponds with the passage; so it is safe to assume the first few questions ask about the beginning of the passage, the center questions about the middle, and the last few questions about the end.

## Map It

Longer passages cover many aspects of a topic. For example, the first paragraph might introduce the subject, the second paragraph might present one viewpoint, and the third paragraph might argue for a different viewpoint. Within each of these paragraphs, there are several details that help the author convey a message.

Because there is a lot to keep track of, it is always smart to mark up long passages if you can.

- Write simple notes in the margin as you read.
- Underline key points.
- Write down the purpose of each paragraph.
- Concentrate on places where the author expresses an opinion. Most Reading Comprehension questions hinge on opinions and viewpoints, not facts.

These notes are your passage map, which can help you find the part of the passage that contains the information you need. The process of creating your passage map also forces you to read actively. Because you are constantly trying to identify the author's viewpoint, as well as the purpose of each sentence and paragraph, you will be working hard to understand what's happening in the passage. This translates into points on the test.

Now that you have read the lesson and strategies for Reading Comprehension questions, it's time to answer some review questions to make sure you have understood what you've read.

## REVIEW QUESTIONS

The following questions are not meant to mimic actual test questions. Instead, these questions will help you review the concepts and terms covered in this chapter.

1. True or False? The reason you are reading should affect how you read.

2. Fill in the blank. The main idea of a passage is usually found _____.

3. Match the words with their definitions.

    ____ Summarizing

    ____ Researching

    ____ Inferring

    A. Knowing where to look for details.

    B. Coming to a conclusion based on information that is hinted at.

    C. Analyzing a single phrase to capture the meaning.

4. Write at least four questions you should be asking yourself when reading.

    _____

    _____

    _____

    _____

    _____

5. All of the following are types of Reading Comprehension questions EXCEPT:

    (A) Detail

    (B) Inference

    (C) Underlining

    (D) Main Idea

6. True or False? Detail questions test your ability to differentiate between main ideas and specific details.

7. Fill in the blank. _____ questions test your ability to draw a conclusion based on reasoning.

8. When you are mapping a passage, you should do all of the following EXCEPT:

    (A) Write simple notes in the margin as you read.

    (B) Write down the purpose of each paragraph.

    (C) Underline key points.

    (D) Concentrate on places where the author goes into specific detail about an element of the passage.

9. True or False? The order of questions generally follows the order of the passage.

10. Write Kaplan's 5-Step Method for Reading Comprehension Questions in order.

    1. _____

    2. _____

    3. _____

    4. _____

    5. _____

# REVIEW ANSWERS

1.  True. You wouldn't read your favorite novel in the same manner you would read a Reading Comprehension passage. Remember, you are reading to earn points, not for enjoyment or to learn anything.

2.  The main idea is usually found in the first third of a passage.

    The correct definitions are:
    -   Summarizing means analyzing a single phrase to capture what the entire passage is about.
    -   Researching means knowing where to look for details.
    -   Inferring means coming to a conclusion based on information that is hinted at.

4.  Your answers may vary, but here are some possible answers:
    -   What is this passage about?
    -   What is the point of this?
    -   What is the author trying to say?
    -   Why did the author write this?
    -   What are the two or three most important things in this passage?

5.  Underlining is not a question type.

6.  True. Detail questions test your ability to differentiate between main ideas and specific details.

7.  Inference questions test your ability draw a conclusion based on reasoning.

8.  The correct answer is (D), because you should not concentrate on places where the author goes into specific detail. Instead, you should concentrate on places where the author expresses an opinion.

9.  True. The order of the questions generally follows the order of the passage.

10. The correct order is:
    1.  Read the question stem.
    2.  Locate the material you need.
    3.  Predict the answer.
    4.  Scan the answer choices.
    5.  Select your answer.

# Chapter Five: **Vocabulary and Spelling Review**

Even though it might not seem that vocabulary and spelling would be important parts of the nursing school entrance exams, they are crucial to score your best. There isn't really a way to teach spelling and vocabulary (after all, a lot of it has to do with memorization), but this chapter covers the essentials for succeeding on test day.

## VOCABULARY LESSON

### Your Vocabulary

To get a sense of your vocabulary strength, take a few minutes to go through the following list of words and see how many you know. Write your definition to the right of each word. To see how many words you defined correctly, check the definitions listed immediately following.

*Resolute* _____

*Terse* _____

*Vanquish* _____

*Cautious* _____

*Lethargic* _____

*Sullen* _____

*Distraught* _____

*Legible* _____

*Fawn* (v.) _____

*Jeer* (n.) _____

*Adrift* _____

*Query* _____

*Impure* _____

*Disinterested* _____

*Pathetic* _____

**Here are the definitions:**

| | |
|---|---|
| *Resolute:* | Determined |
| *Terse:* | Short, abrupt |
| *Vanquish:* | To defeat or conquer in battle |
| *Cautious:* | Careful in actions and behaviors |
| *Lethargic:* | Sluggish, inactive, apathetic |
| *Sullen:* | Depressed, gloomy |
| *Distraught:* | Extremely troubled; agitated with anxiety |
| *Legible:* | Possible to read or decipher |
| *Fawn (v.):* | To act in a servile manner |
| *Jeer (n.):* | Taunt, ridicule |
| *Adrift:* | Wandering aimlessly; afloat without direction |
| *Query:* | A question; to call into question |
| *Impure:* | Lacking in purity; containing something unclean |
| *Disinterested:* | Impartial; unbiased |
| *Pathetic:* | Sad, pitiful, tending to arouse sympathy |

If you got six definitions or fewer right, you should start working on building your vocabulary as soon as possible. The techniques and tools in this chapter will teach you ways to improve your vocabulary and help you to make the most out of words you already know. If you got between seven and eleven definitions right, your vocabulary is about average. We recommend using the techniques and tools discussed below to further improve your skills. If you got more than eleven definitions right, your vocabulary is above average. You can always polish it further, though.

## A Vocabulary-Building Plan

A great vocabulary can't be built overnight, but you can begin building a good vocabulary with a little bit of time and effort. Here's our best advice on how to do that.

### Look It Up

Challenge yourself to find at least five words a day that are unfamiliar to you. You could find these words listening to a news broadcast, or reading a magazine or novel. In fact, books that you choose to read for enjoyment normally contain three to five words per page that are unfamiliar to you. Write down these words, look them up in the dictionary, and record their definitions in a notebook.

But don't only write the word's definition. Below your definition, use the word in a sentence. This will help you to remember the word and anticipate possible context questions.

### Study Word Roots and Prefixes

Many tricky vocabulary words are made up of prefixes and suffixes that can help you figure out at least part of the definition—which, thankfully, is often enough to help you get the right answer. For instance, if you know that the prefix *bio-* means "life," you might be able to decode the definition of *biodegradable*, which means *able to be broken down by living things*. Fortunately, many word roots may already be familiar if you've studied a foreign language, particularly a Romance language such as French, Spanish, or Italian.

### Think Like a Thesaurus

On any test it's better to know a little bit about a lot of words than to know a lot about a few words. So, try to think like a thesaurus rather than a dictionary. For instance, instead of studying the dictionary definition of lackluster, you can study *lackluster* in a thesaurus along with words like the following: *drab, dull, flat, lifeless, lethargic, listless, sluggard, somnolent.* Instead of just learning one word, learn them together and you'll get 12 words for the price of one definition.

## Personalize the Way You Study Vocabulary

It's important to figure out a study method that works for you and stick to it. But realize that most students don't learn best by reading passively from lists. The following techinques are surefire ways to improve your study habits.

### Use Flashcards

Write down new words or word groups and run through them whenever you have some spare time. Write the word or word group on one side of an index card and a short definition on the other side.

### Make a Vocabulary Notebook

List words in the left-hand column and their meanings in the right-hand column. Cover up or fold over the page to test yourself. See how many words you can define from memory.

### Create Memory Devices

That is, try to come up with hooks to lodge new words into your head. Create visual images, silly sentences, rhymes, whatever, to build associations between words and their definitions.

## Trust Your Hunches

Vocabulary knowledge is not an all-or-nothing proposition. Don't write off a word you see just because you can't recite its definition. There are many levels of vocabulary knowledge.

- Some words you know so well you can rattle off their dictionary definitions.
- Some words you "sort of " know. You can't define them precisely and you probably wouldn't use them yourself, but you understand them when you see them in context.
- Some words you barely recognize. You know you've heard them before, but you're not sure where.
- Some words you've never, ever seen before.

If the word before you falls in the second or third category, go with your hunch. The following techniques may help you to get a better fix on the word.

## Try To Recall Where You've Heard the Word Before

If you can recall a phrase in which the word appears, that may help you choose the correct answer. Take a look at the following example. Remember that you don't need to know the dictionary definition to solve a question like this one. A sense of where you've heard a word before may be sufficient.

1. *Clandestine* most nearly means:

    (A) Amicable
    (B) Spirited
    (C) Auspicious
    (D) Secret

You may not have known the definition of *clandestine*, but you may have heard the word used in phrases like *"clandestine activity "* on the news or in spy films. In that case, you may have gotten a sense of the meaning, which is "covert" or "secret." Choice (D) is the correct answer.

## Think Positive and Negative

Sometimes just knowing the "charge" of a word—that is, whether a word has a positive or negative sense—will be enough to earn you points on a test. Take the word *auspicious*. Let's assume you don't know its dictionary definition. Ask yourself: Does *auspicious* sound positive or negative? How about *callow*? Negative words often just sound negative. Positive words, on the other hand, tend to sound more friendly. If you said that *auspicious* is positive, you're right. It means "favorable or hopeful." And if you thought that *callow* is negative, you're also right. It means "immature or unsophisticated."

You can also use prefixes to help determine a word's charge. *Mal-, de-, dis-, dys-, un-, in-, im-,* and *mis-* often indicate a negative, while *pro-, ben-, magn-,* and *eu-* are often positives. Some words are neutral and don't have a charge. But if you can get a sense of the word's charge, you can probably answer some questions on that basis alone.

In the example below, begin by getting a sense of the "charge" of the word in italics.

> *Rankle* most nearly means:
>
> (A) Exhort
> (B) Impress
> (C) Relieve
> (D) Irk

Word sense is a very subjective thing, but in this case, most people—even if they can't come up with an exact definition of *rankle*—can just tell by the sound of the word that it has some sort of negative connotation. In this case, just having that sense should be enough for you to pick the correct answer.

Choices (B) and (C) are clearly too positive for either to be the right answer. And choice (A) is neither positive nor negative, which also can't be right if you're sure the word is negative. *Rankle*, like *irk*, means to annoy or irritate. So you shouldn't become *rankled* if you don't know the exact definition of a word. Try to come up with the word's charge instead. It may be enough to find the correct answer.

Now that you know a little more about building a vocabulary, it's time to learn more about the kinds of vocabulary questions you will face on test day.

## Question Type 1: Synonyms

A synonym is a word that is similar in meaning to another word. *Fast* is a synonym for *quick*. *Garrulous* is a synonym for *talkative*. On the nursing school entrance exams, a synonym question will read: "*Fast* most nearly means…." It will be followed by four answer choices.

> Genuine most nearly means:
>
> (A) Authentic
> (B) Valuable
> (C) Ancient
> (D) Damaged

## Question Type 2: Antonyms

Antonyms are words that have the opposite meaning of one another. *Slow* is the antonym of *fast*; *taciturn* is the antonym of *garrulous*. An antonym question will read: "*Generous* means the opposite of…."

## Question Type 3: Analogies

Analogy questions ask you to compare two words and then extend the relationship to another set of words. Simply put, an analogy is a comparison. When you say, "She's as slow as molasses," or "He eats like a horse," you're making an analogy. In the first example, you're comparing the person in question with molasses, and in the second example, you're comparing the person with a horse. Analogies look like this:

Talkative : Loquacious :: Thrifty : Miserly

The ":" and "::" are translated as:

Talkative **IS TO** loquacious **AS** thrifty **IS TO** miserly.

The symbols are used to show the relationship of the words to each other. Remember, on your nursing school entrance exam, analogies may use the symbol or may be written out in words. Here's a sample analogy question.

> Edifice : Building ::
> (A)  Shack : Bungalow
> (B)  Tome : Book
> (C)  Magazine : Newspaper
> (D)  Couch : Bench

One set of words—*edifice* and *building*—is given. The second set is missing. Your job is to find the second set of words among the answer choices with the same corollary relationship that exists in the first set. In this case, the answer is (B). An *edifice* is a grander word for a *building* and a *tome* is a grander word for a *book*.

Analogies may seem pretty weird at first glance. However, once you become familiar with the format, you'll find that they are pretty straightforward and very predictable. With practice, you can learn to get analogy questions right even when you don't know all of the vocabulary words involved. Here are some other helpful things to know about analogies.

## The Classic Bridges

Relationships between items in analogy questions need to be strong and definite, so there are some bridges that appear again and again. We call these classic bridges. Get to know these bridges; you'll be able to identify them quickly and save yourself a lot of time getting to the correct answer choice on analogy questions. As you read through each one, use the space provided to come up with an example of your own.

### Bridge 1: Character

One word characterizes the other.

*Quarrelsome* : *Argue*… Someone quarrelsome is characterized by a tendency to argue.

*Vivacious* : *Energy*… Someone vivacious is characterized by a lot of energy.

Your example: _____

### Bridge 2: Lack

One word describes what someone or something lacks (or does not have).

*Coward* : *Bravery*… A coward lacks bravery.

*Braggart* : *Modesty*… A braggart lacks modesty.

Your example: _____

### Bridge 3: Function

One word names an object; the other word defines its function or what it is used for.

*Scissors* : *Cut*… Scissors are used to cut.

*Pen* : *Write*… A pen is used to write

Your example: _____

### Bridge 4: Degree

One word is a greater or lesser degree of the other word.

*Loud* : *Deafening*… Something is extremely loud is deafening.

*Apartment* : *Mansion*… An apartment provides housing on a lesser degree than a mansion. (Including the specific "lesser degree" might help you hone in on the right answer choice.)

Your example: _____

### Bridge 5: Example

One word is an example of, or type of, the other word.

*Measles* : *Disease*… Measles is a type of disease.

*Baseball* : *Sport*… Baseball is a type of sport.

Your example: _____

**Bridge 6: Group**

One word is the group form of the other word.

*Forest : Trees…* A forest is made up of many trees.

*Bouquet : Flowers…* A bouquet is made up of many flowers.

Your example: _____

# SPELLING LESSON

Spelling is a difficult skill to teach. We'll start by reviewing two types of questions you may face on test day. Then, you'll see a list of the most commonly misspelled words, as well as a list of words that are often confused for one another or used interchangeably. Use these lists as well as the spelling rules found in this lesson to improve your spelling skills.

## Two Types of Spelling Questions

There are essentially two types of spelling questions on your nursing school entrance exam. The first type is a multiple-choice question that gives you a list of four words. Only one of the words is spelled incorrectly; to answer the question correctly, you will have to choose the word that is misspelled.

Here's an example:

(A) Regret
(B) Unpleasent
(C) Solemn
(D) Cautious

In this case, the correct answer is (B). The correct spelling is unpleasant.

The other type is also a multiple-choice question. However, instead of giving you a list of just four words, you are provided four sentences, and one of the sentences contains a misspelled or misused word. This question type can be tricky. Take a look at the following example to find out why.

(A) I was genuinely surprised to hear the good news.
(B) The girl was upset when she was asked to meet with principle of the school.
(C) My favorite cuisine is Mexican food.
(D) Growing up, my brother was extremely timid and shy.

The correct answer is (B). You may say to yourself that every word is spelled correctly, which is partially true. In this case, the word *principle* is spelled correctly. However, it is the wrong word for the sentence. The head of a school is a *principal*, so (B) contains the misspelled word. The following lists of frequently misspelled words and words commonly confused for one another are a good place to begin your review.

## Frequently Misspelled Words

**Absence:** One *a*, two *e*'s.

**Accommodate, accommodation:** Two *c*'s, two *m*'s

**Accompany:** Two *c*'s.

**All right:** Two words. *Alright* is *NOT* all right.

**A lot:** Always two words, never one; do not confuse with *allot*.

**Argument:** No *e* after the *u*.

**Calendar:** *A*, *e*, then another *a*.

**Campaign:** Remember the *aig* combination.

**Cannot:** Usually spelled as a single word, except where the meaning is "able not to."

- CORRECT: One cannot ignore the importance of conformity.
- CORRECT: Anyone can not pay taxes, but the consequences may be serious.

**Comparative, comparatively:** Yes, *comparison* has an *i* after the *r*. These words don't.

**Conscience:** Spell it with *science*.

**Correspondent, correspondence:** No dance.

**Definite:** Spell it with *finite*, not *finate*.

**Develop, development:** No *e* after the *p*.

**Embarrass:** Two *r*'s, two *s*'s.

**Every day (adv.):** Two words with *every* modifying *day*. Note that there is also an adjective.

**Everyday (adj.):** Meaning *commonplace*, *usual*.

- ADVERB: We see this error *every day*.
- ADJECTIVE: Getting stuck behind an elephant in traffic is no longer an *everyday* occurrence in Katmandu.

**Exaggerate:** One *x*, two *g*'s.

**Foreign:** Think of the *reign* of a *foreign* king.

**Grammar:** No *e*.

**Grateful:** Spell it with *grate*.

**Harass:** One *r*, two *s*'s.

**Independent, independence:** No dance.

**Indispensable:** It's something you are not *able* to dispense with.

**Judgment:** No *e* on the end of *judge*.

**Leisure:** Like *pleasure* but with an *i* instead of *a*.

**License:** In alphabetical order: *c* then *s*, not *lisence*.

**Maintenance:** *Main*, then *ten*, then *ance* (reverse alphabetical order for your vowels preceding *n*).

**Maneuver:** Memorize the unusual *eu* combo.

**No one:** Two words. Don't be mislead by *nobody, nothing, everyone, someone,* and *anyone*.

**Noticeable:** Notice that this one keeps the *e* when adding the suffix.

**Occur, occurred, occurrence:** Double the *r* when you add a suffix beginning with a vowel.

**Parallel, unparalleled:** Two *l*'s, then one.

**Parenthesis (pl. parentheses):** Likewise, many other words of Greek origin are spelled with *-is* in the singular and *-es* in the plural; among the more common are *analysis, diagnosis, prognosis, synthesis, thesis*.

**Perseverance:** Only two *r*'s—*sever*, not *server*. Remember that the *a* in the suffix keeps it from being all *e*'s.

**Professor, professional:** One *f*.

**Pronunciation:** Never mind *pronounce* and *pronouncement: pronunciation* has no *o* in the second syllable.

**Questionnaire:** Two *n*'s, one *r*.

**Regardless:** Not *irregardless*, an unacceptable yoking of *irrespective* and *regardless*.

**Responsible, responsibility:** While the French and Spanish cognates end in *-able*, it's *-ible* in English.

**Separate:** Look for *a rat* in separate.

**Unanimous:** *Un-* and then *-an-*.

**Vacuum:** One *c*, two *u*'s.

## Words Commonly Confused for One Another

*Accept* or *except? Alter* or *altar? Discrete* or *discreet?* Even if you know the difference between these words, when you're under pressure and short on time, it's easy to get confused. So, here's a quick review of some of the most common troublemakers.

**Accept (v.):** To take or receive. The CEO accepted the treasurer's resignation.

**Except (prep.):** Leave out. The Town Council approved all elements of the proposal except the tax increase.

**Adverse (adj.):** Unfavorable. This plan would have an adverse impact on the environment.

**Averse (adj.):** Opposed or reluctant. I am averse to doing business with companies that don't treat their employees fairly.

**Advice (n.):** Recommendation as to what should be done. I would like your advice about how to handle this situation.

**Advise (v.):** To recommend what should be done. I will be happy to advise you.

**Affect (v.):** To have an impact or influence on. The expansion of Pyramid Shopping Mall will certainly affect traffic on the access roads.

**Effect (n.):** Result, impact. The proposal will have a deleterious effect on everyone's quality of life. **(v.):** To cause, implement. The engineers were able to effect a change in the train's performance at high speeds.

**Altar (n.):** An elevated structure, typically intended for the performance of religious rituals. The court refused to allow the construction of an altar on public property.

**Alter (v.):** To change. It should be a simple matter to alter one's will.

**Among (prep.):** Used to compare three or more items or entities. We can choose from among dozens of styles.

**Between (prep.):** Used to compare two items or entities. We can choose between these two styles.

**Assent (n.):** Agreement; **(v.):** to agree. Peter has given his assent to the plan.

**Assure (v.):** To convince or guarantee. He has assured me that this is a safe investment.

**Ensure (v.):** To make certain. Please ensure that this is a safe investment.

**Insure (v.):** To guard against loss. There is no way to insure this investment.

**Bazaar (n.):** A market. I found these fantastic trinkets at the bazaar.

**Bizarre (adj.):** Very strange, weird. No one knew how to respond to such a bizarre question.

**Cite (v.):** To quote, to refer. The article cited our annual report.

**Sight (n.):** Something seen or visible; the faculty of seeing. What an amazing sight!

**Site (n.):** Location; **(v.):** to place or locate. This is the perfect site for a new office.

**Complement (n.):** Something that completes; **(v.):** to go with or complete. This item really complements our product line.

**Compliment (v.):** To flatter; **(n.):** a flattering remark. That was a sincere compliment.

**Continual (adj.):** Repeated regularly and frequently. Alan's continual telephone calls finally wore Rosa down and she agreed to a meeting.

**Continuous (adj.):** Extended or prolonged without interruption. The continuous banging from the construction site gave me a severe headache.

**Decent (adj.):** Proper, acceptable. You can trust Lena to do what is decent.

**Descent (n.):** Downward movement. The rapid descent of the balloon frightened its riders.

**Discrete (adj.):** Separate, not connected. These are two discrete issues.

**Discreet (adj.):** Prudent, modest, having discretion; not allowing others to notice. I must be very discreet about looking for a new job while I am still employed here.

**Disinterested (adj.):** Impartial, objective. We need a disinterested person to act as an arbitrator in this dispute.

**Uninterested (adj.):** Not interested. Charles is uninterested, but he'll come along anyway.

**Eminent (adj.):** Outstanding, distinguished. The eminent Dr. Blackwell will teach a special seminar in medical ethics this fall.

**Imminent (adj.):** About to happen, impending. Warned of imminent layoffs, Loretta began looking for another job.

**Incidence (uncountable noun: occurrence):** Frequency. The incidence of multiple births is on the rise.

**Incident (pl.: incidents) (countable noun: events, cases):** An occurrence of an event or situation. She preferred to forget the whole incident.

**Personal (adj.):** Private or pertaining to the individual. Please mark the envelope "personal and confidential."

**Personnel (n.):** Employees. This year we had a 5% increase in personnel.

**Precede (v.):** To come before. The list of resources should precede the financial worksheet.

**Proceed (v.):** To go forward. Although Jules will be absent, we will proceed with the meeting as planned.

**Principal (n.):** Head of a school or organization, primary participant, main sum of money; **(adj.):** main, foremost, most important. Joshua is one of the principals of the company.

**Principle (n.):** A basic truth or law. I have always run my business based on the principle that honesty is the best policy.

**Reign (v.):** To exercise power; **(n.):** period in which a ruler exercised power or a condition prevailed. Under the reign of King Richard, order was restored.

**Rein (n.):** A means of restraint or guidance; **(v.)** to restrain, control. You need to rein in your intern, Carol—she's taking on much too much responsibility and doesn't seem to know what she's doing.

**Than (conj.):** Used to compare. I will be more successful this time because I am more experienced than before.

**Then (adv.):** I was very naïve back then.

**Weather (n.):** Climatic conditions, state of the atmosphere. The bad weather is going to keep people away from our grand opening.

**Whether (conj.):** Used to refer to a choice between alternatives. I am not sure whether I will attend the grand opening or not.

# VOCABULARY STRATEGIES

Here are some strategies that will help you on test day.

## Kaplan's 3-Step Method for Synonyms

- Define the stem word.
- Find the answer choice that best fits your definition.
- If no choice fits, think of other definitions for the stem word and go through the choices again.

Let's use the Kaplan 3-Step Method for the sample synonym question found earlier in the chapter.

> *Genuine* most nearly means:
>
> (A) Authentic
> (B) Valuable
> (C) Ancient
> (D) Damaged

### Step 1. Define the Stem Word

What does *genuine* mean? Something genuine is something real, such as a real Picasso painting, rather than a forgery. Your definition might be something like this: *Something genuine can be proven to be what it claims to be.*

### Step 2. Find the Answer Choice That Best Fits Your Definition

Go through the answer choices one by one to see which one fits best. Your options are: *authentic, valuable, ancient,* and *damaged.* Something genuine could be worth a lot or not much at all, old or new, or in good shape or bad. The only word that really means the same thing as *genuine* is (A) *authentic.*

### Step 3. If No Choice Fits, Think of Other Definitions for the Stem Word and Go Through the Choices Again

In the example above, one choice fits. Now, take a look at the following example:

> Grave most nearly means:
>
> (A) Regrettable
> (B) Unpleasant
> (C) Serious
> (D) Careful

When you applied Step 1 to this example, maybe you defined grave as a burial location. You looked at the choices, and didn't see any words like *tomb* or *coffin*. What to do? Use the idea presented in Step 3; go back to the stem word, and think about other definitions. Have you ever heard the word *grave* used any other way? If someone were in a "grave situation" what would that mean? *Grave* can also mean *serious* or *solemn*, so (C) *serious* fits perfectly. If none of the answer choices seems to work with your definition, there may be a second definition you haven't considered yet.

## Avoiding a Pitfall

Kaplan's 3-Step Method for Synonyms should be the basis for tackling every question, but there are a few other things you need to know to perform your best on synonym questions. Fortunately, there is only one pitfall to watch out for.

### Choosing Tempting Wrong Answers

Test makers choose wrong answer choices very carefully. Sometimes that means throwing in answer traps that will tempt you, but aren't right. Be a savvy test taker; don't fall for these distracters!

What kinds of wrong answers are we talking about here? In synonym questions, there are two types of answer traps to watch out for: answers that are almost right, and answers that sound like the stem word. Let's illustrate both types to make the concept concrete.

*Delegate* most nearly means:

(A) Delight
(B) Assign
(C) Decide
(D) Manage

*Favor* most nearly means:

(A) Award
(B) Prefer
(C) Respect
(D) Improve

In the first example, choices (A), and (C) might be tempting, because they all start with the prefix *de-*, just like the stem word, *delegate*. It's important that you examine all the answer choices, because otherwise you might choose (A) and never get to the correct answer, which is (B). In the second example, you might look at the word *favor* and think, oh, that's something positive. It's something you do for someone else. It sounds a lot like choice (A), *award*. Maybe you pick (A) and move on. If you do that, you would be falling for a trap! The correct answer is (B) *prefer*, since *favor* is being used as a verb, and *to favor* someone or something is to like it better than something else—in other words, to prefer it. If you don't read through all of the choices, you might be tricked into choosing a wrong answer.

At this point, you have a great set of tools for answering most synonym questions. You know how to approach them and you know some traps to avoid. But what happens if you don't know the word in the question? Here are some techniques to help you figure out the meaning of a tough vocabulary word and answer a difficult synonym question.

### What to Do if You Don't Know the Word

- Look for familiar roots and prefixes.
- Use your knowledge of foreign languages.
- Remember the word used in a particular context.
- Figure out the word's charge.

Let's examine each technique more closely:

### Look for Familiar Roots and Prefixes

Having a good grasp of how words are put together will help you tremendously on synonym questions, particularly when you don't know a vocabulary word. If you can break a word into pieces you do understand, you'll be able to answer questions you might have thought too difficult to tackle. Look at the words below. Circle any prefixes or roots you know.

Benevolence

Insomnia

Inscribe

Conspire

Verify

*Bene-* means good; *somn-* has to do with sleep; *scribe* has to do with writing; *con-* means doing something together; and *ver-* has to do with truth. So, if you were looking for a synonym for *benevolence*, you'd definitely want to choose a positive, or "good" word.

### Use Your Knowledge of Foreign Languages

Remember, any knowledge of a foreign language, particularly if it's one of the Romance languages (French, Spanish, Italian), can help you decode lots of vocabulary words. Look at the example words below. Do you recognize any foreign language words in them?

Facilitate

Dormant

Explicate

In Italian, *facile* means easy; in Spanish, *dormir* means to sleep; and in French, *expliquer* means to explain. A synonym for each of these words would have something to do with what they mean in their respective language.

### Remember the Word Used in a Particular Context

Sometimes a word might look strange to you when it is sitting on the page by itself, but if you think about it, you realize you've heard it before in a phrase. If you can put the word into context, even if that context is cliché, you're on your way to deciphering its meaning.

*Illegible* most nearly means:

(A) Illegal

(B) Twisted

(C) Unreadable

(D) Eligible

Have you heard this word in context? Maybe someone you know has had his or her handwriting described as illegible. What is illegible handwriting? The correct answer is (C). Remember to try to think of a definition first, before you look at the answer choices. Some of the answer choices in this example are tricks. Which wrong answers are tempting, meant to remind you of the question word?

Here's another example:

*Laurels* most nearly means:

(A) Vine

(B) Honor

(C) Lavender

(D) Cushion

Is "don't rest on your laurels" a phrase you've ever heard or used? What do you think it might mean? The phrase "don't rest on your laurels" originated in ancient Greece, where heroes were given wreaths of laurel branches to signify their accomplishments. Telling people not to rest on their laurels is the same thing as telling them not to get too smug; rather than living off the success of one accomplishment, they should strive for improvement.

### Figure Out the Word's Charge

Even if you know nothing about the word, have never seen it before, don't recognize any prefixes or roots, and can't think of any word in any language that it sounds like, you can still take an educated guess by trying to define the word's charge. Remember the discussion found earlier in the chapter about deciding if a word has a positive or negative charge? Well, on all synonym questions, the correct answer will have the same charge as the stem word, so use your instincts about word charge to help you when you're stuck on a tough word.

Not all words are positive or negative; some are neutral. But, if you can define the charge, you can probably eliminate some answer choices on that basis alone. Word charge is a great technique to use when answering antonym questions, too.

## Kaplan's 3-Step Method for Antonyms

- Define the word. Then, think of a word that means the opposite.
- Find the answer choice that best fits your definition.
- If no choice fits, think of other definitions for the stem word and go through the choices again.

Let's practice with an example:

*Dear* means the opposite of:

(A) Beloved

(B) Close

(C) Cheap

(D) Family

### Step 1. Define the Word. Then, Think of a Word That Means the Opposite

*Dear* is a pretty familiar word. You know it from the beginning of a letter as in "Dear Aunt Sue." So, you might define *dear* as *a term for someone you love*. The opposite might be *a term for someone you hate or dislike*. Use roots, context, or word charge to help you if you don't know the definition of the question word.

### Step 2. Find the Answer Choice That Best Fits Your Definition

When we look at the answer choices—*beloved*, *close*, *cheap*, *family*—none of them fits our definition of the opposite of *dear*, which is *someone disliked* or *hated*. Since dear is an "easy" word, we have to figure that perhaps our definition is a little off. We have to refocus it.

### Step 3. If No Choice Fits, Think of Other Definitions for the Stem Word and Go Through the Choices Again

When we use the term "Dear Aunt Sue," or "Dear Sir," what are we saying about that person? We say that we care about them and think that they are valuable—they are worth a lot to us. When people pay a lot of money for something, it is often expressed as, "they paid dearly." In other words, the purchase was worth a lot, and had a lot of value. Okay, so let's use valuable as our new definition of *dear*. Our antonym would then be the opposite of *valuable—worthless*, perhaps. Which of the answer choices comes closest to worthless? Choice (C), *cheap* is closest to *worthless*. That's the correct answer.

The rules that applied for attempting to find a synonym for a word applies to antonyms as well—the difference is that once you have defined the word, you are going to look for its opposite. When you don't find an obvious answer choice for a word you know, you can suspect that there is an alternate meaning for that word. Use your knowledge of the word's primary meaning and see if you can expand on it to arrive at the correct answer.

You can also use your knowledge of word roots, familiarity with the word in context, and the word's charge to help you select the answer to antonym questions. When looking at a word's charge on antonym questions, don't forget you're looking for words with the opposite charge. If the question word has a positive charge, your answer choice should have a negative one, and vice versa.

## Kaplan's 3-Step Method for Analogies

- Build a bridge.
- Predict your answer choice, and select an answer.
- Adjust your bridge if necessary.

You might remember from earlier in the chapter that a bridge is a sentence you create to express the relationship between the words in an analogy. Building a bridge helps you zone in on the correct answer and prevents you from falling for traps that will lead you to the wrong answer. Let's use Kaplan's 3-Step Method for a sample analogy question found earlier in the chapter.

> Edifice : Building ::
> (A) Shack : Bungalow
> (B) Tome : Book
> (C) Magazine : Newspaper
> (D) Couch : Bench

### Step 1. Build a Bridge

In every analogy question, there's a strong, definite connection between the two stem words. Your first task is to figure out this relationship. A bridge is a short sentence that relates the two words in the question, and every pair of words will have a strong bridge that links them.

### Step 2. Predict Your Answer Choice and Select an Answer

You know that an edifice is another word for a building. Now you need to determine which answer choice relates two items in the same way. Use your bridge to do that. The bridge was: An edifice is another word for a building. Apply the same bridge to the incomplete pair:

A _____ is another word for _____.

So, when we predict the answer choice, we come up with two words that mean the same thing. A tome is a type of book.

Take a moment to look at the incorrect answer choices:

> Shack : Bungalow
> Magazine : Newspaper
> Couch : Bench

The choices are all related in some way, but not in the way the bridge is defined. Building a strong bridge is essential to predicting an answer, selecting a correct answer choice, and avoiding traps. What if your bridge doesn't work? Sometimes you may find that even though you came up with a bridge, none of the answer choices fit. In this case, your bridge is either too broad or too narrow. You'll need to refocus it. That's where Step 3 comes in.

**Step 3. Adjust Your Bridge if Necessary**

Using the previous example, let's see how you can adjust a weak bridge.

Edifice : Building ::
(A) Shack : Bungalow
(B) Tome : Book
(C) Magazine : Newspaper
(D) Couch : Bench

Let's say you created this bridge: "An edifice and a building *can both be* lived in." Then you went to the answer choices and plugged in the bridge:

(A) A shack and a bungalow *can both be* lived in.
(B) A tome and a book *can both be* read.
(C) A magazine and a newspaper *can both be read.*
(D) A couch and a bench *can both be* sat on.

You could say that nearly every choice fits. In this case, the bridge was too general, so you'll need to adjust your bridge. What would a good adjustment be? Try to create a relationship between the words that is as specific as possible; the more specific your bridge is, the fewer choices will match it. A good bridge for this pair might be: "An edifice is another word for a building." Now try plugging that bridge into the answer choices.

(A) A shack is another word for a bungalow. **No.**
(B) A tome is another word for a book. **Yes.**
(C) A magazine is another word for a newspaper. **No.**
(D) A couch is another word for a bench. **No**

It should now be easier to see the correct answer: edifice : building :: tome : book, which is choice (B).

## SPELLING STRATEGIES

Unfortunately, there aren't any steps for answering spelling questions. However, there are a few rules you can memorize along with the lists found earlier in the lesson. Sounding things out may help, or it may not, especially if you are not certain of the word's pronunciation. However, remember: *i* before *e*, except after *c,* and except when it sounds like *a* as in *neighbor* and *weigh*.

Example: *Society, transient, feign*

When a word of more than one syllable ends in a single vowel and a single consonant, the word's emphasis is on the final syllable; to add a suffix that begins with a vowel, the consonant preceding should be doubled.

Example:   *Occur, occurring*

   *Prefer, preferred*

If the final syllable has no accent, do not double the consonant.

Example:     *Benefit + -ing = Benefiting*

If a word ends with a silent *e*, drop the *e* before adding a suffix that begins with a vowel.

Example:     *Hope, hoping*

                  *Like, liking*

Do not drop the *e* when the suffix begins with a consonant.

Example:     *Manage, management*

                  *Like, likeness*

                  *Use, useless*

When *y* is the last letter in a word and the *y* is preceded by a consonant, change the *y* to *i* before adding any suffix other than those beginning with *i*.

Example:     *Pretty, prettier*

                  *Hurry, hurried*

                  *Deny, denied*

Spelling is one area where knowing your own strengths and weaknesses is important. If you tend to have trouble spelling, you may decide to go against your instinct when selecting an answer choice. In other words, if a word looks right to you, but you know you are a terrible speller, you may guess that the word is actually spelled incorrectly. Vice versa, if a word sounds wrong to you, but you admit you're not sure of its pronunciation, you may decide that word is actually correct. Finally, if you are not certain whether or not a word is spelled correctly, take your best guess and move on.

Now that you have read the lessons and strategies, test how much you learned by answering the following review questions.

## REVIEW QUESTIONS

The following questions are not meant to mimic actual test questions. Instead, these questions will help you review the concepts and terms covered in this chapter.

1. True or False? Determining a word's charge is to make answer work an effective strategy for spelling questions.

2. Synonym questions test your knowledge of words with:

   (A) Similar meanings
   (B) Opposite meanings
   (C) Similar spellings
   (D) Alternative spellings

3. Write at least four of the classic bridges.

   _____

   _____

   _____

   _____

   _____

4. True or false? In spelling, if the final syllable has no accent, you do not double the consonant when adding the suffix -*ing*.

5. Fill in the blank. The rule is: *i* before *e*, except after *c*, _____.

6. True or False? To figure out a word's charge to answer antonym questions, you should always look for an answer choice that has the same charge as the question.

7. *Ghastly* most nearly means:

   (A) Fun
   (B) Lazy
   (C) Torrid
   (D) Awful

8. *Acute* means the opposite of:

   (A) Conspicuous
   (B) Relevant
   (C) Aloof
   (D) Dull

9. Abdicate : Throne ::

   (A) Rule : Nation
   (B) Revolt : Government
   (C) Defeat : Candidate
   (D) Resign : Office

10. Choose the word that is misspelled:

   (A) Regulation
   (B) Catergory
   (C) Conflagration
   (D) Incident

## REVIEW ANSWERS

1. False. You should determine a word's charge (deciding whether a word is positive, negative, or neutral) in order to find a synonym or antonym of a word.

2. (A)  Synonyms test your knowledge of words with similar meanings.

3. Your answers may include any four of the following:
   Bridge 1: Character
   Bridge 2: Lack
   Bridge 3: Function
   Bridge 4: Degree
   Bridge 5: Example
   Bridge 6: Group

4. True. For example, *benefit* becomes *benefiting*.

5. The rule is: *i* before *e*, except after *c*, except when it sounds like *a* as in *neighbor* and *weigh*.

6. False. Because you are looking for the opposite of the word in the question, you should look for a word with an opposite word charge among the answer choices.

7. (D)  *Ghastly* most nearly means *awful*.

8. (D)  *Dull* is the opposite of *acute*.

9. (D)  To abdicate a throne is to give up any claim to it. When a king abdicates, he willingly passes his hereditary right to rule his country to the next in line for the throne. Answer (D) is the only choice to match this bridge. When a politician gives up *office*, he or she voluntarily *resigns*.

10. (B)  The correct spelling is *category*.

# Chapter Six: **Mathematics Review**

Mathematics is likely to be the longest section on your nursing school entrance exam. It also happens to be the subject most test takers feel is their weakest. This chapter offers a review of mathematics, from the most fundamental operations of addition and subtraction through the types of basic algebra and geometry you are likely to encounter on test day. You will also find strategies for answering math questions, as well as questions to reinforce principles you have reviewed.

## MATHEMATICS LESSON

### Arithmetic

The math skills tested on your nursing school entrance exam include basic computation, using integers, fractions, decimals, and percentages. You need to have a firm grasp of arithmetic concepts such as number properties, factors, divisibility, units of measure, ratio and proportion, percentages, and averages. These skills may be tested in basic operations or in word problems. Even if you feel that you know them, spend time on this section. The more you practice, the more comfortable you will feel working with numbers on your test.

First, take a look at a few definitions.

| Number Type: | Definition: | Examples: |
|---|---|---|
| **Real Numbers** | *Any number that can name a position on a number line, regardless of whether that position is negative or positive.* | |
| **Rational Numbers** | *Any number that can be written as a ratio of two integers, including integers, terminating decimals, and repeating decimals.* | $5 = \frac{5}{1}$, $2 = \frac{2}{1}$, $0 = \frac{0}{1}$, $-6 = \frac{-6}{1}$<br><br>$2\frac{50}{100}$, or $\frac{250}{100}$<br><br>$\frac{1}{3}$ (.33333) |
| **Integers** | *Any of the positive counting numbers (which are also known as natural numbers), the negative numbers, and zero.* | Positive integers: 1, 2, 3…<br>Negative integers: −1,− 2, −3…<br>Neither negative nor positive: zero |
| **Fractions** | *A **fraction** is a number that is written in the form $\frac{A}{B}$ where A is the numerator and B is the denominator. An **improper fraction** is a number that is greater than 1 (or less than −1) that is written in the form of a fraction. An improper fractions can be converted to a **mixed number,** which consists of an integer (positive or negative) and a fraction.* | $\frac{-5}{6}$, $\frac{3}{17}$, $\frac{1}{2}$, $\frac{899}{901}$<br><br>$\frac{-65}{64}$, $\frac{9}{8}$, $\frac{57}{10}$<br><br>$-1\frac{1}{64}$, $1\frac{1}{8}$, $5\frac{7}{10}$ |
| **Positive/Negative** | *Numbers greater than zero are positive numbers; numbers less than zero are negative; zero is neither positive nor negative.* | Positive: 1, 5, 900<br>Negative: −64, −40, −11, $\frac{-6}{13}$ |
| **Even/Odd** | *An even number is an integer that is a multiple of 2. NOTE: Zero is an even number. An odd number is an integer that is not a multiple of 2.* | Even numbers: −6, −2, zero, 4, 12, 190<br>Odd numbers: −15, −1, 3, 9, 453 |
| **Prime Numbers** | *An integer greater than 1 that has no factors other than 1 and itself; 2 is the only even prime number.* | 2, 3, 5, 7, 11, 13, 59, 83 |
| **Consecutive Numbers** | *Numbers that follow one after another, in order, without any skipping.* | Consecutive integers: 3, 4, 5, 6<br>Consecutive even integers: 2, 4, 6, 8, 10<br>Consecutive multiples of 9: 9, 18, 27, 36 |
| **Factors** | *A positive integer that divides evenly into a given number with no remainder.* | The complete list of factors of 12:<br>1, 2, 3, 4, 6, 12 |
| **Multiples** | *A number that a given number will divide into with no remainder.* | Some multiples of 12:<br>zero, 12, 24, 60 |

## Odds and Evens

| | |
|---|---|
| Even ± Even = Even | $2 + 2 = 4$ |
| Even ± Odd = Odd | $2 + 3 = 5$ |
| Odd ± Odd = Even | $3 + 3 = 6$ |
| Even × Even = Even | $2 \times 2 = 4$ |
| Even × Odd = Even | $2 \times 3 = 6$ |
| Odd × Odd = Odd | $3 \times 3 = 9$ |

## Positives and Negatives

There are few things to remember about positives and negatives.

Adding a negative number is basically subtraction.

$6 + (-4)$ is really $6 - 4$ or $2$.

$4 + (-6)$ is really $4 - 6$ or $-2$.

Subtracting a negative number is basically addition.

$6 - (-4)$ is really $6 + 4$ or $10$.

$-6 - (-4)$ is really $-6 + 4$ or $-2$.

Multiplying and dividing positives and negatives is like all other multiplication and division, with one catch. To figure out whether your product is positive or negative, simply count the number of negatives you had to start. If you had an odd number of negatives, the product is negative. If you had an even number of negatives, the product is positive.

$$6 \times (-4) = -24 \text{ (1 negative} \rightarrow \text{negative product)}$$

$$(-6) \times (-4) = 24 \text{ (2 negatives} \rightarrow \text{positive product)}$$

$$(-1) \times (-6) \times (-4) = -24 \text{ (3 negatives} \rightarrow \text{negative product)}$$

Similarly,

$$-24 \div 3 = -8 \text{ (1 negative} \rightarrow \text{negative quotient)}$$

$$-24 \div (-3) = 8 \text{ (2 negatives} \rightarrow \text{positive quotient)}$$

## Absolute Value

Absolute value describes how far a number on the number line is from zero. It doesn't matter in which direction the number lies—to the right on the positive side, or to the left on the negative side.

For example, the absolute value of both 3 and −3 is 3.

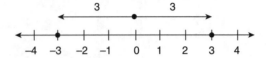

To find the absolute value of a number, simply strip the number within the vertical lines of its sign.

$$|4| = 4$$
$$|-4| = 4$$

When absolute value expressions contain different arithmetic operations, perform the operation first, and then strip the sign from the result.

$$|-6 + 4| = |-2| = 2$$
$$|(-6) \times 4| = |-24| = 24$$

## Factors and Multiples

To find the prime factorization of a number, keep breaking it down until you are left with only prime numbers.

To find the prime factorization of 168:

$$168 = 4 \times 42$$
$$= 4 \times 6 \times 7$$
$$= 2 \times 2 \times 2 \times 3 \times 7$$

To find the greatest common factor (GCF) of two integers, break down both integers into their prime factorizations and multiply all prime factors they have in common. The greatest common factor is the largest factor that goes into each integer.

For example, if you're looking for the greatest common factor of 40 and 140, first identify the prime factors of each integer.

$$40 = 4 \times 10$$
$$= 2 \times 2 \times 2 \times 5$$
$$140 = 10 \times 14$$
$$= 2 \times 5 \times 2 \times 7$$
$$= 2 \times 2 \times 5 \times 7$$

Next, see what prime factors the two numbers have in common and then multiply these common factors.

Both integers share two 2s and one 5, so the GCF is $2 \times 2 \times 5$ or 20.

If you need to find a common multiple of two integers, you can always multiply them. However, you can use prime factors to find the least common multiple (LCM). To do this, multiply all of the prime factors of each integer as many times as they appear. Don't worry if this sounds confusing, it becomes pretty clear once it's demonstrated. Take a look at the example to see how it works.

To find a common multiple of 20 and 16:

$20 \times 16 = 320$

320 is a common multiple of 20 and 16, but it is not the *least* common multiple.

To find the least common multiple of 20 and 16 first find the prime factors of each integer:

$20 = 2 \times 2 \times 5$

$16 = 2 \times 2 \times 2 \times 2$

Now, multiply each prime integer the greatest number of times it appears in each integer:

$2 \times 2 \times 2 \times 2 \times 5 = 80$

## The Order of Operations

You need to remember the order in which arithmetic operations must be performed. PEMDAS (or Please Excuse My Dear Aunt Sally) may help you remember the order.

Please = Parentheses

Excuse = Exponents

My Dear = Multiplication and Division (from left to right)

Aunt Sally = Addition and Subtraction (from left to right)

$$3^3 - 8(3 - 1) + 12 \div 4$$
$$= 3^3 - 8(2) + 12 \div 4$$
$$= 27 - 8(2) + 12 \div 4$$
$$= 27 - 16 + 3$$
$$= 11 + 3$$
$$= 14$$

## Divisibility Rules

If you've forgotten—or never learned—divisibility rules, spend a little time with this chart. Even if you remember the rules, take a moment to refresh your memory. There are no easy divisibility rules for 7 and 8.

| Divisible by | The Rule | Example: 558 |
|---|---|---|
| 2 | The last digit is even. | A multiple of 2 because 8 is even. |
| 3 | The sum of the digits is a multiple of 3. | A multiple of 3 because $5 + 5 + 8 = 18$, which is a multiple of 3. |
| 4 | The last 2 digits comprise a 2-digit multiple of 4. | NOT a multiple of 4 because 58 is not a multiple of 4. |
| 5 | The last digit is 5 or zero. | NOT a multiple of 5 because it doesn't end in 5 or zero. |
| 6 | The last digit is even AND the sum of the digits is a multiple of 3. | A multiple of 6 because it's a multiple of both 2 and 3. |
| 9 | The sum of the digits is a multiple of 9. | A multiple of 9 because $5 + 5 + 8 = 18$, which is a multiple of 9. |
| 10 | The last digit is zero. | NOT a multiple of 10 because it doesn't end in zero. |

## Properties of Numbers

Here are some essential laws or properties of numbers.

### Commutative Property for Addition

When adding two or more terms, the sum is the same regardless of which number is added to which.

$$3 + 2 = 2 + 3$$
$$a + b = b + a$$

### Associative Property for Addition

When adding three terms, the sum is the same, regardless of which two terms are added first.

$$2 + (5 + 3) = (2 + 5) + 3$$
$$a + (b + c) = (a + b) + c$$

### Commutative Property for Multiplication

When multiplying two or more terms, the result is the same regardless of which number is multiplied by which.

$$2 \times 4 = 4 \times 2$$
$$ab = ba$$

### Associative Property for Multiplication

When multiplying three terms, the product is the same regardless of which two terms are multiplied first.

$$2 \times (4 \times 3) = (2 \times 4) \times 3$$
$$a \times (b \times c) = (a \times b) \times c$$

### Distributive Property of Multiplication Over Addition

When multiplying groups, the product of the first number, and the sum of the second and third number, is equal to the sum of the product of the first and second number, as well as the product of the first and third number.

$$a(b + c) = ab + ac$$
$$3 \times (7 + 18) = 3 \times 7 + 3 \times 18$$

## Fractions and Decimals

Generally, it's a good idea to reduce fractions when solving math questions. To do this, simply cancel all factors that the numerator and denominator have in common.

$$\frac{28}{36} = \frac{4 \times 7}{4 \times 9} = \frac{7}{9}$$

To add fractions, get a common denominator and then add the numerators.

$$\frac{1}{4} + \frac{1}{3} = \frac{3}{12} + \frac{4}{12} = \frac{3 + 4}{12} = \frac{7}{12}$$

To subtract fractions, get a common denominator and then subtract the numerators.

$$\frac{1}{4} - \frac{1}{3} = \frac{3}{12} - \frac{4}{12} = \frac{3 - 4}{12} = \frac{-1}{12}$$

To multiply fractions, multiply the numerators and multiply the denominators.

$$\frac{1}{4} \times \frac{1}{3} = \frac{1 \times 1}{4 \times 3} = \frac{1}{12}$$

To divide fractions, invert the second fraction and multiply. In other words, multiply the first fraction by the reciprocal of the second fraction.

$$\frac{1}{4} \div \frac{1}{3} = \frac{1}{4} \times \frac{3}{1} = \frac{1 \times 3}{4 \times 1} = \frac{3}{4}$$

## Comparing Fractions

To compare fractions, multiply the numerator of the first fraction by the denominator of the second fraction to get a product. Then, multiply the numerator of the second fraction by the denominator of the first fraction to get a second product. If the first product is greater, the first fraction is greater. If the second product is greater, the second fraction is greater.

Here's an example:

$$\text{Compare } \frac{2}{5} \text{ and } \frac{5}{8}$$

1. Multiply the numerator of the first fraction by the denominator of the second.

   $2 \times 8 = 16$

2. Multiply the numerator of the second fraction by the denominator of the first.

   $5 \times 5 = 25$

3. The second product is greater, therefore, $\frac{5}{8}$ (the second fraction), is greater than $\frac{2}{5}$.

To convert a fraction to a decimal, divide the numerator by the denominator.

To convert $\frac{8}{25}$ to a decimal, divide 8 by 25.

$$\frac{8}{25} = 0.32$$

To convert a decimal to a fraction, first set the decimal over 1. Then, move the decimal point over as many places as it takes until it is immediately to the right of the digit farthest to the right. Count the number of places that you moved the decimal. Then, add that many zeros to the 1 in the denominator.

$$0.3 = \frac{0.3}{1} = \frac{3.0}{10} \text{ or } \frac{3}{10}$$

$$0.32 = \frac{0.32}{1} = \frac{32.0}{100} \text{ or } \frac{8}{25}$$

## Common Percent Equivalencies

Being familiar with the relationships among percents, decimals, and fractions can save you time on test day. Don't worry about memorizing the following chart. Simply use it to review relationships you already know (e.g., $50\% = 0.50 = \frac{1}{2}$) and to familiarize yourself with some that you might not already know. To convert a fraction or decimal to a percent, multiply by 100%. To convert a percent to a fraction or decimal, divide by 100%.

| Fraction | Decimal | Percent |
|:---:|:---:|:---:|
| $\frac{1}{20}$ | 0.05 | 5% |
| $\frac{1}{10}$ | 0.10 | 10% |
| $\frac{1}{8}$ | 0.125 | 12.5% |
| $\frac{1}{6}$ | $0.16\overline{6}$ | $16\frac{2}{3}\%$ |
| $\frac{1}{5}$ | 0.20 | 20% |
| $\frac{1}{4}$ | 0.25 | 25% |
| $\frac{1}{3}$ | $0.33\overline{3}$ | $33\frac{1}{3}\%$ |
| $\frac{3}{8}$ | 0.375 | 37.5% |
| $\frac{2}{5}$ | 0.40 | 40% |
| $\frac{1}{2}$ | 0.50 | 50% |
| $\frac{3}{5}$ | 0.60 | 60% |
| $\frac{2}{3}$ | $0.66\overline{6}$ | $66\frac{2}{3}\%$ |
| $\frac{3}{4}$ | 0.75 | 75% |
| $\frac{4}{5}$ | 0.80 | 80% |
| $\frac{5}{6}$ | $0.83\overline{3}$ | $83\frac{1}{3}\%$ |
| $\frac{7}{8}$ | 0.875 | 87.5% |

## Rounding

You might be asked to estimate or round a number on the test. Rounding might also help you determine an answer choice. There are a few simple rules to rounding. Look at the digit to the right of the number in question. If it is a 4 or less, leave the number in question as it is and replace all the digits to the right with zeros.

For example, round off 765,432 to the nearest 100. The 4 is the hundreds digit, but you have to look at the digit to the right of the hundreds digit, which is the tens digit, or 3. Since the tens digit is 3, the hundreds digit remains the same and the tens and ones digits both become zero. Therefore, 765,432 rounded to the nearest 100 is 765,400.

If the digit to the right of the number in question is 5 or greater, increase the number by 1 and replace all the digits to the right with zeros.

For example, 837 rounded to the nearest 10 is 840. If 2,754 is rounded to the nearest 100, it is 2,800.

## Place Units

Rounding requires that you know the place unit value of the digits in a number.

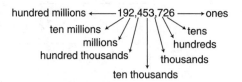

## Symbols of Inequality

An inequality is a mathematical sentence in which two expressions are joined by symbols such as $\neq$ (not equal to), $>$ (greater than), $<$ (less than), $\geq$ (greater than or equal to), $\leq$ (less than or equal to). Examples of inequalities are:

| | |
|---|---|
| $5 + 3 \neq 7$ | 5 plus 3 is not equal to 7 |
| $6 > 2$ | 6 is greater than 2 |
| $8 < 8.5$ | 8 is less than 8 and a half |
| $x \leq 9 + 6$ | $x$ is less than or equal to 9 plus 6 |
| $c \geq 10$ | $c$ is greater than or equal to 10. ($c$ is an algebraic variable. That means, it varies, and could be any number greater than or equal to 10.) |

## Exponents and Roots

An exponent indicates the number of times that a number (or variable) is to be used as a factor. On your nursing school entrance exam you'll usually deal with numbers or variables that are squares (a variable multiplied by itself) and cubes (a variable multiplied by itself 3 times).

You should remember the squares of 1 through 10.

| Square = A number raised to the exponent 2 (also known as the second power) | | Cube = A number raised to the exponent 3 (also known as the third power) | |
|---|---|---|---|
| $2^2$ | $2 \times 2 = 4$ | $2^3$ | $2 \times 2 \times 2 = 8$ |
| $3^2$ | $3 \times 3 = 9$ | $3^3$ | $3 \times 3 \times 3 = 27$ |
| $4^2$ | $4 \times 4 = 16$ | $4^3$ | $4 \times 4 \times 4 = 64$ |
| $5^2$ | $5 \times 5 = 25$ | $5^3$ | $5 \times 5 \times 5 = 125$ |
| $6^2$ | $6 \times 6 = 36$ | | |
| $7^2$ | $7 \times 7 = 49$ | | |
| $8^2$ | $8 \times 8 = 64$ | | |
| $9^2$ | $9 \times 9 = 81$ | | |
| $10^2$ | $10 \times 10 = 100$ | | |

To add or subtract terms consisting of a coefficient (the number in front of the variable) multiplied by a power (a power is a base raised to an exponent), both the base and the exponent must be the same. As long as the bases and the exponents are the same, you can add the coefficients.

$x^2 + x^2 = 2x^2$ can be added. The base ($x$) and the exponent (2) are the same.

$3x^4 - 2x^4 = x^4$ can be subtracted. The base ($x$) and the exponent (4) are the same.

$x^2 + x^3$ cannot be combined. The exponents are different (2) and (3).

$x^2 + y^2$ cannot be combined. The bases are different ($x$) and ($y$).

To multiply terms consisting of coefficients multiplied by powers having the same base, multiply the coefficients and add the exponents.

$$2x^5 \times (8x^7) = (2 \times 8)(x^{5 + 7}) = 16x^{12}$$

To divide terms consisting of coefficients multiplied by powers having the same base, divide the coefficients and subtract the exponents.

$$6x^7 \div 2x^5 = (6 \div 2)(x^{7-5}) = 3x^2$$

To raise a power to an exponent, multiply the exponents.

$$(x^2)^4 = x^{2 \times 4} = x^8$$

A square root of a non-negative number is a number that, when multiplied by itself, produces the given quantity. The radical sign $\sqrt{\phantom{x}}$ is used to represent the positive square root of a number, so $\sqrt{25} = 5$, since $5 \times 5 = 25$.

To add or subtract radicals, make sure the numbers under the radical sign are the same. If they are, you can add or subtract the coefficients outside the radical signs.

$$2\sqrt{2} + 3\sqrt{2} = 5\sqrt{2}$$

$\sqrt{2} + \sqrt{3}$ cannot be combined.

To simplify radicals, factor out the perfect squares under the radical, take the square root of the perfect square, and put the result in front of the radical sign.

$$\sqrt{32} = \sqrt{16 \times 2} = 4\sqrt{2}$$

To multiply or divide radicals, multiply (or divide) the coefficients outside the radical. Multiply (or divide) the numbers inside the radicals.

$$\sqrt{x} \times \sqrt{y} = \sqrt{xy}$$

$$3\sqrt{2} \times 4\sqrt{5} = 12\sqrt{10}$$

$$\frac{\sqrt{x}}{\sqrt{y}} = \sqrt{\frac{x}{y}}$$

$$12\sqrt{10} \div 3\sqrt{2} = 4\sqrt{5}$$

To take the square root of a fraction, break the fraction into two separate roots and take the square root of the numerator and the denominator.

$$\sqrt{\frac{16}{25}} = \frac{\sqrt{16}}{\sqrt{25}} = \frac{4}{5}$$

## The Power of 10

When a power of 10 (that is, the base is 10) has an exponent that is a positive integer, the exponent tells you how many zeros to add after the 1. For example, 10 to the 12th power ($10^{12}$) has 12 zeros.

When the exponent of a power of 10 is positive, the exponent indicates how many zeros the number would contain if it were written out. For example, $10^4 = 10,000$ (4 zeros) since the product of 4 factors of 10 is equal to 10,000.

When multiplying a number by a power of 10, move the decimal point to the right the same number of places as the number of zeros in that power of 10.

$$0.0123 \times 10^4 = 123$$

When dividing by a power of 10 with a positive exponent, move the decimal point to the left.

$$43.21 \div 10^3 = 0.04321$$

Multiplying by a power with a negative exponent is the same as dividing by a power with a positive exponent. Therefore, when you multiply by a number with a positive exponent, move the decimal to the right. When you multiply by a number with a negative exponent, move the decimal to the left.

For example:

$$10^3 = 1.000 = 1,000$$

## Percents

Remember these formulas: Part = Percent × Whole or Percent = $\dfrac{\text{Part}}{\text{Whole}}$

### From Fraction to Percent

To find part, percent, or whole, plug the values you have into the equation and solve.

$$44\% \text{ of } 25 = 0.44 \times 25 = 11$$

42 is what percent of 70?

$$42 \div 70 = 0.6$$

$$0.6 \times 100\% = 60\%$$

To increase or decrease a number by a given percent, take that percent of the original number and add it to or subtract it from the original number.

To increase 25 by 60%, first find 60% of 25.

$$25 \times 0.6 = 15$$

Then, add the result to the original number.

25 + 15 = 40

To decrease 25 by the same percent, subtract the 15.

25 − 15 = 10

## Average, Median, and Mode

$$\text{Average} = \frac{\text{Sum of the Terms}}{\text{Number of the Terms}}$$

The formula to calculate the average of 15, 18, 15, 32, and 20 is:

$$\frac{15 + 18 + 15 + 32 + 20}{5} = \frac{100}{5} = 20.$$

When there are an odd number of terms, the median of a group of terms is the value of the middle term, with the terms arranged in increasing order.

Suppose that you want to find the median of the terms 15, 18, 15, 32, and 20. First, put the terms in order from small to large: 15, 15, 18, 20, 32. Then, identify the middle term. The middle term is 18.

When there is an even number of terms, the median is the average of the two middle terms with the terms arranged in increasing order.

Suppose that you want to find the mode of the terms 15, 18, 15, 32, and 20. The mode is the value of the term that occurs most; 15 occurs twice, so it is the mode.

## Ratios, Proportions, and Rates

Ratios can be expressed in different forms.

One form is $\frac{a}{b}$.

If you have 15 dogs and 5 cats, the ratio of dogs to cats is $\frac{15}{5}$. (The ratio of cats to dogs is $\frac{5}{15}$.) Like any other fraction, this ratio can be reduced; $\frac{15}{5}$ can be reduced to $\frac{3}{1}$. In other words, for every three dogs, there's one cat.

Another form of expressing ratios is $a:b$.

The ratio of dogs to cats is 15:5 or 3:1. The ratio of cats to dogs is 5:15 or 1:3.

Pay attention to what ratio is specified in the problem. Remember that the ratio of dogs to cats is different from the ratio of cats to dogs.

To solve a proportion, cross-multiply and solve for the variable.

$$\frac{x}{6} = \frac{2}{3}$$

$$3x = 12$$

$$x = 4$$

A rate is a ratio that compares quantities measured in different units. The most common example is miles per hour. Use the following formula for such problems:

$$\text{Distance} = \text{Rate} \times \text{Time or } D = R \times T$$

Remember, although not all rates are speeds, this formula can be adapted to any rate.

## Units of Measurement

You will most likely see at least a few questions that include units of measurement on the test. You are expected to remember these basic units of measurement. Spend some time reviewing the list below.

### Distance

1 foot = 12 inches

1 yard = 3 feet = 36 inches

**Metric:** 1 kilometer = 1,000 meters. 1 meter = 10 decimeters = 100 centimeters = 1,000 millimeters (Remember the root *deci* is 10; the root *centi* is 100, the root *milli* is 1,000)

### Weight

1 pound = 16 ounces

**Metric:** A gram is a unit of mass. A kilogram is 1,000 grams.

### Volume

1 cup = 8 ounces

2 cups = 1 pint

1 quart = 2 pints

4 cups = 1 quart

1 gallon = 4 quarts

**Metric:** A liter is a unit of volume. A kiloliter is 1,000 liters.

You must be careful when approaching a problem that includes units of measurement. Be sure that the units are given in the same format. You may have to convert pounds to ounces or feet to yards (or vice versa) to arrive at the correct answer choice.

## A Word About Word Problems

You can expect to see a lot of word problems on the test. Some of them however, will just be asking you to perform arithmetic equations. Your job is to find the math within the story.

Here's an example:

> A grocery store charges $0.99 for a liter of milk, $1.49 for a half pound of tomatoes, $0.49 for a jar of tomato sauce, and $1.25 for a box of pasta. If Reggie buys 2 liters of milk, 1 pound of tomatoes, a jar of tomato sauce, and 2 boxes of pasta, what is his bill?
>
> (A) $7.90
> (B) $7.95
> (C) $6.36
> (D) $8.36

If you sort through the story, you realize that the question is asking you to add the amounts of each item that Reggie bought. Read the question carefully to make sure you have the correct number of each item he bought, then add the amounts.

$0.99 \times 2 = 1.98$ (The price of two liters of milk.)

$1.49 \times 2 = 2.98$ (The price given was per half pound; Reggie bought 1 full pound.)

$0.49$ (The price of one jar of sauce.)

$1.25 \times 2 = 2.50$ (The price of two boxes of pasta.)

Now, add these numbers together to get the total.

```
  1.98
  2.98
  0.49
  2.50
_____
$7.95 (B)
```

Often, word problems can seem tricky because it may be hard to figure out precisely what you are being asked to do. It can be difficult to translate English into math. The following table lists some common words and phrases that turn up in word problems, along with their mathematical translation.

| When you see: | Think: |
|---|---|
| Sum, plus, more than, added to, combined total | + |
| Minus, less than, difference between, decreased by | − |
| Is, was, equals, is equivalent to, is the same as, adds up to | = |
| Times, product, multiplied by, of, twice, double, triple | × |
| Divided by, over, quotient, per, out of, into | ÷ |

## ALGEBRA

Algebra has been called math with letters. Just like arithmetic, the basic operations of algebra are addition, subtraction, multiplication, division, and roots. Instead of numbers though, algebra uses letters to represent unknown or variable numbers. Why would you work with a variable? Let's look at an example.

> You buy 2 bananas from the supermarket for 50 cents total.
> How much does one banana cost?

That's a simple equation, but how would you write it down on paper if you were trying to explain it to a friend?

Perhaps you would write: $2 \times ? = 50$ cents.

Algebra gives you a systematic way to record the question mark.

$2 \times b = 50$ cents or $2b = 50$ cents, where $b =$ the cost of 1 banana in cents.

Algebra is a type of mathematical shorthand. The most commonly used letters in algebra are $a$, $b$, $c$ and $x$, $y$, $z$.

The number 2 in the term $2b$ is called a **coefficient**. It is a constant that does not change.

To find out how much you paid for each banana, you could use your equation to solve for the unknown cost.

$$2b = 50$$

$$\frac{2b}{2} = \frac{50}{2}$$

$$b = 25$$

## Algebraic Expressions

An expression is a collection of quantities made up of constants and variables linked by operations such as + and −.

Let's go back to our fruit example. Let's say you have 2 bananas and you give one to your friend. You could express this in algebraic terms as:

$2b - b$

$2b - b$ is an example of an algebraic expression, where $b = 1$ banana.

In fact, this example is a binomial expression. A **binomial** is an expression that is the sum of two terms. A term is the product of a constant and one or more variables. A **monomial** expression has only one term; a **trinomial** expression is the sum of three terms; a **polynomial** expression is the sum of two or more terms.

$2b = $ monomial

$2b - b = $ binomial

$2(b + x) = $ binomial

$2 + b^2 + y = $ trinomial or polynomial

On the test an algebraic expression is likely to look something like this:

$(11 + 3x) - (5 - 2x) = ?$

In addition to algebra, this problem tests your knowledge of positives and negatives, and the order of operations (PEMDAS).

The main thing you need to remember about **expressions** is that you can only combine like terms.

Let's talk about fruit once more. Let's say in addition to the 2 bananas you purchased you also bought 3 apples and 1 pear. You spent $4.00 total. If $b$ is the cost of a banana, $a$ is the cost of an apple, and $p$ is the cost of a pear, the purchase can be expressed as $2b + 3a + p = 4.00$.

However, let's say that once again you forgot how much each banana cost. You could NOT divide $4.00 by 6 to get the cost of each item. They're different items.

While you cannot solve expressions with unlike terms, you *can* simplify them. For example, to combine monomials or polynomials, simply add or subtract the coefficients of terms that have the exact same variable. When completing the addition or subtraction, do not change the variables.

$$6a + 5a = 11a$$
$$8b - 2b = 6b$$
$$3a + 2b - 8a = 3a - 8a + 2b = -5a + 2b \text{ or } 2b - 5a$$

Coefficient = The number that comes before the variable. In 6*x*, 6 is the coefficient.

Variable = The variable is the letter that stands for an unknown. In 6*x*, *x* is the variable.

Term = The product of a constant and one or more variables.

Monomial = One term: 6*x* is a monomial.

Polynomial = Two or more terms: 6*x* – *y* is a polynomial.

Trinomial = Three terms: 6*x* – *y* + *z* is a trinomial.

To review:

$6a + 5a^2$ cannot be combined. Why not? The variables are not exactly alike; that is, they are not raised to the same exponent. (One is *a*, the other is $a^2$.)

$3a + 2b$ cannot be combined. Why not? The variables are not the same. (One is *a*, the other is *b*.)

Multiplying and dividing monomials is a little different. Unlike addition and subtraction, you can multiply and divide terms that are different. When you multiply monomials, multiply the coefficients of each term. (In other words, multiply the numbers that come before the variables.) Add the exponents of like variables. Multiply different variables together.

$$(6a)(4b) = (6 \times 4)(a \times b)$$
$$= 24ab$$

$$(6a)(4ab) = (6 \times 4)(a \times a \times b)$$
$$= (6 \times 4)(a^{1+1} \times b)$$
$$= 24a^2b$$

Use the FOIL method to multiply and divide binomials. FOIL stands for **F**irst **O**uter **I**nner **L**ast.

$$(y + 1)(y + 2) = (y \times y) + (y \times 2) + (1 \times y) + (1 \times 2)$$
$$= y^2 + 2y + y + 2$$
$$= y^2 + 3y + 2$$

## Equations

The key to solving equations is to do the same thing to both sides of the equation until you have your variable isolated on one side of the equation and all of the numbers on the other side.

$$8a + 4 = 24 - 2a$$

First, subtract 4 from each side so that the left side of the equation has only variables.

$$8a + 4 - 4 = 24 - 2a - 4$$
$$8a = 20 - 2a$$

Then, add $2a$ to each side so that the right side of the equation has only numbers.

$$8a + 2a = 20 - 2a + 2a$$
$$10a = 20$$

Finally, divide both sides by 10 to isolate the variable.

$$\frac{10a}{10} = \frac{20}{10}$$
$$a = 2$$

### Treat Both Sides Equally

Always perform the same operation to both sides to solve for a variable in an equation.

Sometimes you're given an equation with two variables and asked to solve for one variable in terms of the other. This means that you must isolate the variable for which you are solving on one side of the equation and put everything else on the other side. In other words, when you're done, you'll have $x$ (or whatever the variable you're looking for is) on one side of the equation and an expression on the other side.

Solve $7x + 2y = 3x + 10y - 16$ for $x$ in terms of $y$.

Since you want to isolate $x$ on one side of the equation, begin by subtracting $2y$ from both sides.

$$7x + 2y - 2y = 3x + 10y - 16 - 2y$$
$$7x = 3x + 8y - 16$$

Then, subtract $3x$ from both sides to get all the $x$'s on one side of the equation.

$$7x - 3x = 3x + 8y - 16 - 3x$$
$$4x = 8y - 16$$

Finally, divide both sides by 4 to isolate $x$.

$$\frac{4x}{4} = \frac{8y - 16}{4}$$
$$x = 2y - 4$$

## Substitution

If a problem gives you the value for a variable, just plug the value into the equation and solve. Make sure that you follow the rules of PEMDAS and are careful with your calculations.

If $x = 15$ and $y = 10$, what is the value of $4x(x - y)$?

Plug 15 in for $x$ and 10 in for $y$.

$4(15)(15 - 10) = ?$

Then, find the value.

$(60)(5) = 300$

## Inequalities

Solve **inequalities** like you would any other equation. Isolate the variable for which you are solving on one side of the equation and everything else on the other side of the equation.

$4a + 6 > 2a + 10$

$4a - 2a > 10 - 6$

$2a > 4$

$a > 2$

The only difference here is that instead of finding a specific value for $a$, you get a range of values for $a$. That is, $a$ can be any number greater than 2. The rest of the math is the same.

There is, however, one *crucial* difference between solving equations and inequalities. **When you multiply or divide an inequality by a negative number, you must change the direction of the sign.**

$-5a > 10$

$\dfrac{-5a}{-5} > \dfrac{10}{-5}$

$a < -2$

If this seems confusing, think about the logic. You're told that $-5$ times something is greater than 10. This is where your knowledge of positives and negatives comes into play. You know that negative $\times$ positive = negative and negative $\times$ negative = positive. Since $-5$ is negative and 10 is positive, $-5$ has to be multiplied by something negative to get a positive product. Therefore, $a$ has to be *less* than $-2$, not *greater* than it. If $a > -2$, then any value for $a$ that is greater than $-2$ should make $-5a$ greater than 10. Say $a$ is 20; $-5a$ would be $-100$ which is certainly NOT greater than 10.

## Algebra Word Problems

Understanding algebra word problems is probably one of the most useful math skills you can have. The great thing about word problems is that they're not only important on test day, they're also useful in everyday life. Whether you're figuring out how much a piece of clothing will cost you with sales tax, or calculating your earnings, algebraic word problems help you figure out unknown amounts.

## Word Problems with Formulas

Some of the more challenging word problems may involve translations with mathematical formulas. For example, you might see questions dealing with averages, rates, or areas of geometric figures. (More about geometry later.) For example:

> If a truck driver travels at an average speed of 50 miles per hour for 6.5 hours, how far will the driver travel?

To answer this question, you need the distance formula:

$$\text{Distance} = \text{Rate} \times \text{Time or } D = R \times T$$

Once you know the formula, you can plug in the numbers:

$D = 50 \times 6.5$

$D = 325$ miles

Here's another example:

> Thomas took an exam with 60 questions on it. If he finished all the questions in two hours, how many minutes on average did he spend answering each question?

To answer this question, you need the average formula:

$$\text{Average} = \frac{\text{Sum of Terms}}{\text{Number of Terms}}$$

Then plug in the numbers:

$$x = \frac{(2 \text{ hours} \times 60 \text{ minutes})}{60 \text{ questions}} = \frac{120}{60} = 2 \text{ minutes per question}$$

You may have noticed there's a trick in this question as well. Do you see it? The time it took for Thomas to finish the exam is given in *hours*, but the question is asking how many *minutes* each question took. Be sure to read each the question carefully so you don't fall for tricks like this.

## Working With A Question

Sometimes you do not need to use a formula to solve a word problem. You need to know how to work with the question. Remember to translate the words into math.

| When you see: | Think: |
|---|---|
| Sum, plus, more than, added to, combined total | + |
| Minus, less than, difference between, decreased by | − |
| Is, was, equals, is equivalent to, is the same as, adds up to | = |
| Times, product, multiplied by, of, twice, double, triple | × |
| Divided by, over, quotient, per, out of, into | ÷ |
| What, how much, how many, a number | $x, n, a, b$, etc. |

## GEOMETRY

You will definitely see some basic geometry on your nursing school entrance exam. You can count on seeing questions that test your knowledge of lines and angles, triangles, and circles. You'll also see a little coordinate geometry. You might also see geometry in word problems that don't include diagrams.

If you're concerned about your geometry skills, take some time to review this section, spending more time with the subjects that are less familiar to you.

## Lines and Angles

There are 180° in a straight line.

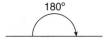

180°

## Line Segments

Some of the most basic geometry problems deal with line segments. A **line segment** is a piece of a line, and it has an exact measurable length. A question might give you a segment divided into several pieces, provide the measurements of some of these pieces, and ask you for the measurement of the remaining piece.

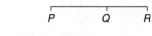

If $PR = 12$ and $QR = 4$, $PQ =$

$PQ = PR - QR$

$PQ = 12 - 4$

$PQ = 8$

The point exactly in the middle of a line segment, halfway between the endpoints, is called the midpoint of the line segment. To bisect means to cut in half, so the **midpoint** of a line segment bisects that line segment.

$M$ is the midpoint of $AB$, so $AM = MB$.

## Angles

A **right angle** measures 90° and is usually indicated in a diagram by a little box. The figure above is a right angle. Lines that intersect to form right angles are said to be **perpendicular.**

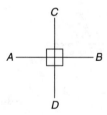

In the figure above, line $AB$ and line $CD$ are perpendicular.

Angles that form a straight line add up to 180°. In the figure above, $a + b = 180$.

The angle marked $b$ is less than 90°; it is an **acute angle**. The angle marked $a$ is greater than 90°. Angles greater than 90° are called **obtuse**.

Right angle = 90°

Acute angle < 90°

Obtuse angle > 90°

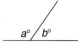

When two lines intersect, adjacent angles are **supplementary**, meaning they add up to 180°. In the figure above $a + b = 180$.

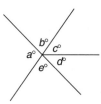

Angles around a point add up to 360°. In the figure above $a + b + c + d + e = 360$.

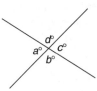

When lines intersect, angles across the vertex (the middle point) from each other are called vertical angles and are equal to each other. Above, $a = c$ and $b = d$.

## Parallel Lines

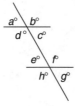

When parallel lines are crossed by a transversal:

- Corresponding angles are equal (for example $a = e$, $d = h$)
- Alternate interior angles are equal ($d = f$)
- Same side interior angles are supplementary ($c + f = 180$)
- All four acute angles are equal, as are all four obtuse angles ($a, c, e, g$ are equal, $b, d, f, h$ are equal)

## Triangles

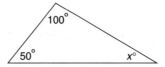

The three interior angles of any triangle add up to 180°. In the figure above $x + 50 + 100 = 180$, so $x = 30$. By finding the sum of the two angles, $x$ can be calculated. The sum of $100 + 50 = 150$, so $x = 180 - 150$.

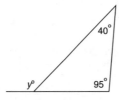
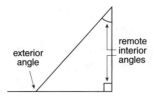

An exterior angle of a triangle is equal to the sum of the remote interior angles. In this figure, the exterior angle labeled $y°$ is equal to the sum of the remote interior angles so $y = 40 + 95 = 135$.

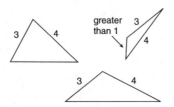

The length of one side of a triangle must be **greater than the positive difference and less than the sum** of the lengths of the other two sides. For example, if it is given that the length of one side is 3 and the length of another side is 4, then the length of the third side must be greater than $4 - 3 = 1$ and less than $4 + 3 = 7$.

### Triangles—Area and Perimeter

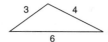

The **perimeter** of a triangle is the sum of the lengths of its sides. The perimeter of the triangle in the figure above is $3 + 4 + 6 = 13$.

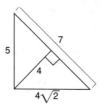

Area of triangle $= \frac{1}{2}$(base)(height) or $A = \frac{1}{2}bh$.

The height is the perpendicular distance between the side that is chosen as the base and the opposite vertex. In this triangle, 4 is the height when 7 is chosen as the base.

Area $= \frac{1}{2}bh = \frac{1}{2}(7)4 = 14$

**Similar Triangles:** Similar triangles have the same shape: **corresponding angles are equal** and **corresponding sides are proportional**. The triangles below are similar because they have the same angles. The 3 corresponds (or relates to) the 4 and the 6 corresponds to the unknown $s$. Because the triangles are similar, therefore, you can set up a proportion to solve for $s$.

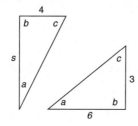

$\frac{3}{4} = \frac{6}{s}$

$3s = 24$

$s = 8$

**Special Triangles**

**Isosceles Triangles:** An isosceles triangle is a triangle that has **two equal sides**. Not only are two sides equal, but the angles opposite the equal sides, called base angles, are also equal to one another.

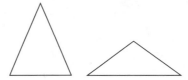

So, if you were asked to determine angle $a$ in the isosceles triangle below, you could set up an equation. Since the sum of the degrees in a triangle is 180, and you are given one angle of 40°, then: $2a = 180 - 40$, $2a = 140$, $\frac{2a}{2} = \frac{140}{2}$, $a = 70°$.

**Equilateral Triangles:** Equilateral triangles are triangles in which all **three sides are equal**. Since the sides are equal, all the angles are also equal. If all three angles are equal, and the sum of the angles in a triangle is 180°, how many degrees is each angle in an equilateral triangle?

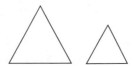

$$\frac{180}{3} = 60$$

The answer is 60°.

**Right Triangles:** A right triangle is a triangle with a right angle. (Remember, a right angle equals 90°.) Every right triangle has exactly two acute angles. The sides opposite the acute angles are called the legs. The side opposite the right angle is called the hypotenuse. Since it is opposite the largest angle, the hypotenuse is the longest side of a right triangle.

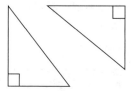

## The Pythagorean Theorem

The Pythagorean theorem states the following:

$$\text{leg1}^2 + \text{leg2}^2 = (\text{hypotenuse})^2$$

The theorem can also be written out as:

$$a^2 + b^2 = c^2$$

The following right angle has legs with lengths of 2 and 3:

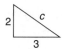

If one leg is 2 and the other leg is 3, then:

$$2^2 + 3^2 = c^2$$
$$4 + 9 = c^2$$
$$13 = c^2$$
$$c = \sqrt{13}$$

Your knowledge of squares and square roots will really come in handy when using the Pythagorean therorem.

## Quadrilaterals

A quadrilateral has 4 sides. The perimeter of a quadrilateral (or any polygon) is the sum of the lengths of its sides.

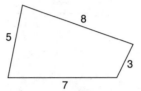

The perimeter of the quadrilateral in the figure above is: $5 + 8 + 3 + 7 = 23$.

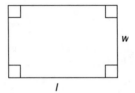

A **rectangle** is a parallelogram containing four right angles. Opposite sides are equal. The formula to find the area of a rectangle is: Area = (length)(width), which is sometimes abbreviated as $A = lw$. In the diagram above, $l$ = length and $w$ = width, so area = $lw$ and perimeter = $2(l + w)$.

A **square** is a rectangle with four equal sides. The formula to calculate the area of a square is: Area = (side)$^2$. Notice this can also be written as $A = lw$. However, since $l = w$ in a square, you can use the notation $s^2$ (see notation below).

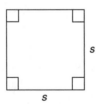

In the diagram above, $s$ = length of a side, so area = $s^2$ and perimeter = $4s$.

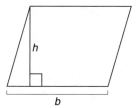

A parallelogram is a quadrilateral with two sets of parallel sides. Opposite sides are equal, as are opposite angles. The formula for the area of a parallelogram is:

$$\text{Area} = (\text{base})(\text{height}) \text{ or } A = bh$$

In the diagram above, $h$ = height and $b$ = base, so you can use the formula: $A = bh$.

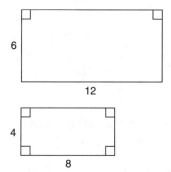

If two rectangles (or squares, since squares are special rectangles) are similar, then the corresponding angles are equal (90°) and corresponding sides are in proportion. In the figures above, the two rectangles are similar because all the angles are right angles, and each side of the larger rectangle is $1\frac{1}{2}$ times the corresponding side of the smaller rectangle.

## Circles

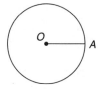

A **circle** is a figure in which each point is an equal distance from its center. In the diagram, $O$ is the center of the circle.

The **radius** ($r$) of a circle is the direct distance from its center to any point on the circle. All radii of one circle have equal lengths. In the figure above, $OA$ is the radius of circle $O$.

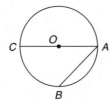

A **chord** is a line segment that connects any two points on a circle. Segments *AB* and *AC* are both chords. The largest chord that may be drawn in a circle is the diameter of that circle.

The **diameter** (*d*) of a circle is a chord that passes through the circle's center. All diameters are the same length and are equal to twice the radius. In the figure above, *AC* is a diameter of circle *O*.

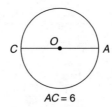

$$AC = 6$$

The **circumference** of a circle is the distance around it. It is equal to $\pi d$, or $2\pi r$. In this example Circumference $= \pi d = 6\pi$

The **area** of a circle equals $\pi$ times the square of the radius, or $\pi r^2$. In this example, since *AC* is the diameter, $r = \dfrac{6}{2} = 3$ and area $= \pi r^2 = \pi(3^2) = 9\pi$.

## Coordinate Geometry

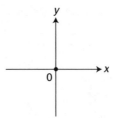

Coordinate geometry has to do with plotting points on a graph. The diagram above represents the coordinate axes—the perpendicular number lines in the coordinate plane. The horizontal line is called the *x*-axis. The vertical line is called the *y*-axis. In a coordinate plane, the point *O* at which the two axes intersect is called the origin, or (0, 0).

The pair of numbers, written inside parentheses, specifies the location of a point in the coordinate plane. These are called coordinates. The first number is the *x*-coordinate, and the second number is the *y*-coordinate. The origin is the zero point of both axes, with coordinates (0, 0).

Starting at the origin:

- To the right: *x* is positive.
- To the left: *x* is negative.
- Up: *y* is positive.
- Down: *y* is negative.
- The two axes divide the coordinate plane into 4 quadrants. When you know what quadrant a point lies in, you know the signs of its coordinates. A point in the upper left quadrant, for example, has a negative *x*-coordinate and a positive *y*-coordinate.

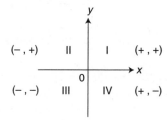

If you were asked the coordinates of a given point, you would start at the origin, count the number of units given to the right or left on the *x*-axis, and then do the same up or down on the *y*-axis.

If you had to plot given points you would start at the origin, count the number of units given on the *x*-axis, and then on the *y*-axis. To plot (2, −3) for example, you would count 2 units to the right along the *x*-axis, then three units down along the *y*-axis.

## TABLES, CHARTS, AND GRAPHS

You are likely to see some type of table, chart, or graph on the test. You will have to gather information from these graphics and use them to solve accompanying questions.

Keep in mind that no matter which type of graphic representation you see, labels or keys must be given to identify the material. By carefully reading the labels, we can understand what information is contained and in what manner it is organized. Remember, a table, chart, or graph is a visual way of organizing information.

## Line Graphs

A line graph presents information by plotting points on an *xy* coordinate system, then connecting them with a line. Because you can plot more than one line, a line graph is widely used to communicate relationships. Also, since the lines clearly indicate rising or decreasing trends, a line graph is a great way to show growth or decline trends.

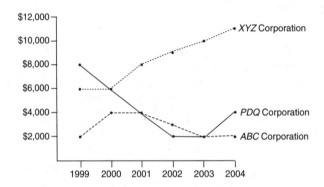

Notice that the previous graph is not titled. Charts, tables, and graphs on the test may not have titles. However, we can use the information found on the *x*- and *y*-axes to decode or make sense of the graph. The *x*-axis is labeled 1999–2004. Therefore, each marking represents one year from 1999 to 2004. The *y*-axis is marked in units of increasing dollar value. Each unit going up the *y*-axis increases $2,000. The lines themselves are labeled *ABC* Corporation, *PDQ* Corporation, and *XYZ* Corporation. Therefore, we can see the dollar amount of each company at a particular point in time during the period of 1999–2004. A line connects these points to show an upward, or downward trend.

## Bar Graphs

A bar graph is also called a histogram or histograph. In it, numerical values are shown in bars of varying length. This type of graph is also a good, clear way to show comparisons.

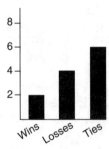

The bar graph below labels the various bars on the horizontal axis "wins," "losses," or "ties." The vertical axis shows units of 2. This bar graph represents the numerical value of a team's wins, losses, and ties. See how far each vertical bar extends on the vertical axis. The bar representing wins of Team 1 is at the 2 unit; the team has 2 wins. The bar representing Team 1 losses is at 4 units; the team has 4 losses. The bars representing ties are at 6 units; both teams have 6 ties.

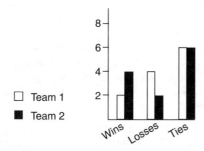

A bar graph has the added benefit of illustrating multiple comparisons in a way that is still visually clear. The previous bar graph includes a second set of bars. These bars, the shaded bars, represent the performance of another team. By placing the two sets of bars side by side, we can easily see that Team 2 won more games than Team 1, it lost fewer, and it tied the same number of games.

A bar graph can be vertical or horizontal. Decode it the same way you would a line graph, by reading the labels on the *x*- and *y*-axes which tell what the bars represent and the value of the units given.

## Tables

Tables compare information in rows and columns. Because information appears side by side, tables are a good way to present detailed information to compare.

|          | Mon | Tues | Wed | Thurs | Fri |
|----------|-----|------|-----|-------|-----|
| New York | 70° | 72°  | 65° | 71°   | 80° |
| Boston   | 65° | 70°  | 60° | 63°   | 72° |
| L.A.     | 81° | 82°  | 85° | 80°   | 80° |
| Miami    | 80° | 85°  | 86° | 81°   | 84° |

Labels in the far left column and on the top row will identify the information in the table. The left column in the table above, for example, contains the names of cities. The top row is labeled with days of the week. Let's say you were looking for the temperature in New York on Thursday. You would find the row labeled New York and the column labeled Thursday. The box that aligns with these two axes gives you the temperature in New York on Thursday, 71°.

Tables may also use pictures rather than numbers. Either way, when you are looking for information in a table, find the row corresponding to the information you are looking for. Then, read across and find the vertical column that corresponds to the second detail you are looking for. The box at which these details meet will give you your data.

## Pie Charts

A pie chart is a circle cut into parts. You can think of it as showing the pieces of a pie or how the pie is divided. Thus, a pie chart is a good chart to use when showing the distribution of a whole, or into which parts a whole is divided. On a pie chart, the portions or pieces of the pie will be labeled. The labels will explain what the different sections represent and the percentage of the whole each section comprises.

NOTE: The whole pie always equals 100%. That does not mean that the numbers shown in a pie chart will equal 100. However, you should think of a pie chart as 100% with each section representing a part (percentage) of the whole.

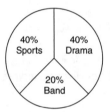

The pie chart above shows the various after-school activities of students in a class. The whole pie represents the whole class. As the labels indicate, 40% of the students participate in sports, 40% participate in the drama club, and 20% participate in the band.

While pie charts are a great way to show how a whole is divided, they can be difficult to use if the pie is divided into sections that are too small.

The following pie chart shows an example of when NOT to use a pie chart. It is meant to show the after-school activities of an entire class, but breaking the sections down into such small pieces makes the chart difficult to use.

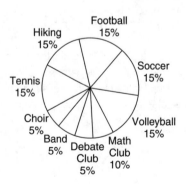

## MATHEMATICS STRATEGIES

Multiple-choice questions are the kind of questions you are most likely to see on your nursing school entrance exam. They are simply questions followed by answer choices. All the questions in this book are followed by four answer choices, although the number of choices on the test may vary depending on the exam your school requires. Fortunately, on this question type the correct answer is right in front of you—you just have to pick it out. Just like on any other exam, the key to working quickly and efficiently through the math section is to think about the question before you start looking for the answer. Kaplan has developed a special process for tackling math questions.

### Kaplan's 4-Step Method for Math Questions

- Read the question.
- Decide to skip or do the problem.
- Look for the fastest approach.
- Make an educated guess.

### Step 1: Read the Question

This is obvious. If you try to solve the question without knowing all the facts, you'll most likely come up with the wrong answer.

### Step 2: Decide to Skip or Do the Problem

If a question leaves you seriously scratching your head, circle it and move on. Spend your time on the questions you can do, and then at the end of the section, if you have more time, go back to the difficult problems. Remember, easy questions are usually worth as much as difficult ones.

### Step 3: Look for the Fastest Approach

All the information you will need to answer the question is right there in front of you. You never need outside knowledge to answer a question. Your job is to figure out the best way to use that information. There's more than one way to use given information. Look for shortcuts. Sometimes the most obvious way of finding a solution is also the longest way. Take the following question for example:

> At a diner, Joe orders 3 doughnuts and a cup of coffee and is charged $2.25. Stella orders 2 doughnuts and a cup of coffee and is charged $1.70. What is the price of 2 doughnuts?
>
> (A) $0.55
> (B) $0.60
> (C) $1.10
> (D) $1.30

The cost of doughnuts and coffee could be translated into two distinct equations using the variables $d$ and $c$. You could start by finding $c$ in terms of $d$, then you could plug the values into the other equation.

If you stop for a minute, and look for a shortcut, you'll see there's a faster way: The difference in price between 3 doughnuts and a cup of coffee and 2 doughnuts and a cup of coffee is the price of one doughnut. So the cost of one doughnut can be figured out by subtracting the two costs:

$$\$2.25 - \$1.70 = \$0.55.$$

Notice that's choice (A)? Don't get caught in the trap! The price of one doughnut is $0.55, but if you read the question carefully you'll see that it's asking for the price of two doughnuts, which is $1.10. Choice (C) is the correct answer.

### Step 4: Make an Educated Guess

In the previous example, you were able to find the correct answer through several simple steps. However, if you've tried solving a problem and are stuck, cut your losses. Eliminate any wrong answer choices you can, make an educated guess, and move on.

## Kaplan's Other Strategies

There are also other special Kaplan strategies you might use, such as picking numbers and backsolving.

### Picking Numbers

This strategy is based on the idea that instead of always trying to wrap your head around abstract variables, you can pick numbers for them. This way you end up making calculations with real numbers and you can really see the answer. The strategy of picking numbers works especially well with even/odd questions. For example:

> If $a$ is an odd integer and $b$ is an even integer, which of the following must be odd?
>
> (A) $2a + b$
> (B) $a + 2b$
> (C) $ab$
> (D) $a^2b$

By picking numbers to represent $a$ and $b$, you may come to the solution more easily. When you are adding, subtracting, or multiplying even and odd numbers, you can generally assume that what happens with one pair of numbers happens with similar pairs of numbers. Let's say, for the time being, that $a = 3$ and $b = 2$. Plug those values into the answer choices, and there's a good chance that only one choice will be odd:

$$(A) \ 2a + b = 2(3) + 2 = 8$$
$$(B) \ a + 2b = 3 + 2(2) = 7$$
$$(C) \ ab = (3)(2) = 6$$
$$(D) \ a^2b = (3^2)(2) = 18$$

Choice (B) is the only odd answer when the numbers 2 and 3 are used to represent the variables; thus, it is fair to assume that it must be the only odd-answer choice, no matter what odd number you plug in for $a$ and even number you plug in for $b$. The answer is (B).

Picking numbers is a helpful strategy in several other situations, such as when:

- The answer choices for problems involving percentages are all percents.
- The answer choices for word problems are algebraic expressions.

Here are a few rules to remember when picking numbers:

- Pick easy numbers rather than ones that might be used or suggested in the problem. Keep the numbers small and manageable. You should avoid zero and 1; these often give several answers that are possibly correct.
- Remember that you have to try all the answer choices. If more than one works, pick another set of numbers.
- Don't pick the same number for more than one variable.
- Always pick 100 for questions involving percents.

## Backsolving

With some math questions, it's easier to work backward from the answer choices than to try and trudge through the question. Basically, with backsolving, you are plugging the answer choices back into the question until you find a solution. This method works best when the question is a complex word problem and the answer choices are numbers, or when your only other choice is to set up multiple algebraic equations.

Backsolving is not ideal:

- If the answer choices include variables.
- If the answer choices are radicals or fractions (plugging them in takes too much time).

Here's an example of how backsolving works:

A music club draws 27 patrons. If there are 7 more males than females in the club, how many patrons are male?

(A)  8

(B)  10

(C)  14

(D)  17

Try each of the answers as a substitute for the number of males in the club. Plugging in choice (C) gives you 14 males in the club. Since there are 7 more males than females, there are 7 females in the club, but $14 + 7 < 27$, so 14 doesn't work. You know the solution has to be higher, so you can eliminate (A), (B), and (C). Already you've found the right answer. Now, if you plug in (D) you see that it gives you 17 males and 10 females. $17 + 10 = 27$. That's the right answer.

Now that you have reviewed the best math strategies, it's time to test how much you have learned by answering the following review questions.

## REVIEW QUESTIONS

The following questions are not meant to mimic actual test questions. Instead, these questions will help you review the concepts and terms covered in this chapter.

1.  Match the number type with its definition.

    ____ Real numbers

    ____ Rational numbers

    ____ Consecutive numbers

    (A) Any number that can be written as a ratio of two integers, including whole numbers, integers, terminating decimals, and repeating decimals.

    (B) Numbers that follow one after another, in order, without any skipping.

    (C) Any number that can name a position on a number line regardless of whether that position is positive or negative.

2.  Fill in the blank. When you multiply an even number by an odd number the product is _____.

3.  True or false? The product of three negative numbers is positive. _____

4.  Define the term Greatest Common Factor.

    _____

5.  Write the steps of the Order of Operations.

    _____

    _____

    _____

    _____

    _____

6.  True or False? To convert a fraction to a decimal, you divide the numerator into the denominator.

    _____

7.  Write the formula for calculating an average.

    _____

8.  Fill in the blank. In algebra, the _____ is the letter that stands for an unknown.

9.  Write the formula for calculating distance.

    _____

10. Match the term with its definition.

    ____ Supplementary

    ____ Complementary

    ____ Obtuse

    (A) When the measure of an angle is greater than 90° but less than 180°.

    (B) When the measures of two angles add up to 180°.

    (C) When the measures of two angles add up to 90°.

11. Fill in the blank. The three interior angles of any triangle add up to _____.

12. Write the formula for calculating the area of a triangle.

    _____

13. Match the term with its formula for calculating perimeter.

    ____ Square

    ____ Rectangle

    (A) 2 (length + width)

    (B) 4 (side)

14. Write the formula for calculating the area of a circle.

    _____

15. Fill in the blank. The point at which the $x$- and $y$-axes intersect is called the _____.

## REVIEW ANSWERS

1.  (C) Real numbers are any number that can name a position on a number line regardless of whether that position is positive or negative.

    (A) Rational numbers are any number that can be written as a ratio of two integers, including whole numbers, integers, terminating decimals, and repeating decimals.

    (B) Consecutive numbers are numbers that follow one after another, in order, without any skipping.

2.  When you multiply an even number by an odd number the product is even.

3.  False. The product of three negative numbers is negative.

4.  The Greatest Common Factor is the largest factor that goes into two or more numbers.

5.  Parentheses

    Exponents

    Multiplication and Division (from left to right)

    Addition and Subtraction (from left to right)

6.  True. To convert a fraction to a decimal, you divide the numerator into the denominator.

7.  $\text{Average} = \dfrac{\text{Sum of the Terms}}{\text{Number of Terms}}$

8.  In algebra, the variable is the letter that stands for an unknown.

9.  Distance = Rate × Time

10. (B) Supplementary: When the measures of two angles add up to 180°.

    (C) Complementary: When the measures of two angles add up to 90°.

    (A) Obtuse: When the measure of an angle is greater than 90° but less than 180°.

11. The three interior angles of any triangle add up to 180°.

12. Area of a triangle $= \dfrac{1}{2}$ (base × height)

13. (B) Square: 4 (side)

    (A) Rectangle: 2 (length + width)

14. Area of a circle $= \pi r^2$

15. The point at which the x- and y-axes intersect is called the origin.

# Chapter Seven: **Life Science Review**

In preparing for your nursing school entrance exam, it is important to have a grasp of the fundamentals of Life Science. This chapter covers the topic of biology, from the structure of cells through the functions and structure of the human body, and beyond.

## BUILDING BLOCKS FOR THE TEST

Use this chapter as a road map or your core set of building blocks. Just as it's easier to start with addition and work your way up to algebra, it is easier to learn biology starting with cells and then moving up to evolution and diversity. Since our review lessons are already organized this way, you should avoid skipping around in a chapter. Instead, you should review each lesson from beginning to end.

### General Test-Taking Strategies

To prepare yourself for the Life Science portion of the test, you might want to go back to Chapter One and review some tips that are likely to help on any type of question. These include answering easier questions first, making an educated guess, and using the process of elimination to find the right answer.

Basically, for the Life Science questions, your very best option is to study hard and prepare yourself for test day. Don't forget to use the Learning Resources in the back of the book to help you. Once you have read through this chapter and reviewed the basic principles of Life Science, you'll be ready to start reviewing. Use the review questions at the end of this chapter to see how much of the material you have become comfortable with and what topics you might need to study further.

## BIOLOGY LESSON

One way to solve a puzzle is to put together the pieces in larger and larger assemblies until the entire puzzle is complete. Biologists try to gain understanding about living systems in a similar way, by studying life at many levels and then putting all of the pieces together in one complete picture.

Looking at biology from this perspective, molecules are studied for further knowledge of the workings of cells, which explain how tissues, organs, and organisms function. From those facts, we can explain how and why populations and ecosystems operate as they do, as well as evolutionary changes that have created the great diversity of life on Earth today.

In the beginning of this lesson we will discuss molecules and the workings of cells. This will form the foundation for later parts of this lesson, which concern organisms, genetics, ecology, and evolution. By the final section of this lesson, it will be possible to view life not as a set of isolated facts, but as a rich, interconnected network.

## CELLULAR BIOLOGY

### Biological Chemistry

At the elemental level, all life is composed primarily of carbon, hydrogen, oxygen, nitrogen, phosphorous, and sulfur, with traces of other elements such as iron, iodine, magnesium, and calcium—these are all essential components for living organisms. Salts like sodium chloride are also essential components of life. Chemicals that do not contain carbon—such as sodium chloride, nitrogen, and phosphorus—are called **inorganic compounds**.

Chemicals that contain carbon are called **organic compounds**, and include the major types of biological molecules (that is, molecules that support life) found in all organisms, including proteins, lipids, carbohydrates, and nucleic acids. Before we explore these molecules, let's look at a vastly important and seldom-appreciated molecule fundamental for all life: water.

### Water

Life is not possible without water. The presence of liquid water allowed life to evolve and to persist on Earth. The way water molecules are structured gives water unique properties that allow it to play its particular role. Each water molecule is composed of one atom of oxygen and two hydrogen atoms that are attached at an angle. Water's ability to absorb heat means that water remains in a liquid form over a range of temperatures common on our planet. Another important feature of water is that the solid form of water, ice, is less dense than its liquid form. This is due to a special type of bonding that takes place in water called hydrogen bonding.

### Other Biological Molecules

There are a few other biological molecules you should be familiar with. These are carbohydrates, lipids, proteins, enzymes, and nucleic acids. A description of each follows.

## Carbohydrates

**Carbohydrates**, are a main class of biological molecules. Another name for carbohydrates is **saccharides**. Carbohydrates are composed of carbon, hydrogen, and oxygen; they include sugars and starches. The functions of carbohydrates include important roles in energy metabolism and storage, and structural support for cells and organisms. One carbohydrate, **cellulose**, is the material that forms the cell wall of plants, and is the single most abundant biological molecule on Earth. Carbohydrates are a short-term energy source due primarily to their structure.

## Lipids (Fats and Oils)

**Lipids** tend to repel water. Like carbohydrates, lipids are composed of carbon, hydrogen, and oxygen; but lipids are very distinct from carbohydrates in their structure and function. Lipids have much lower oxygen content than carbohydrates and are less oxidized, storing more energy than carbohydrates. Lipids are a long-term energy source. The significance of this is important to understand. When you ingest carbohydrates and then lipids, your body first uses carbohydrates for energy. If you take in more carbohydrates than necessary, the body will store them as fatty acids, which are eventually re-synthesized as triglycerides and can lead to increased cholesterol levels.

## Proteins

Carbohydrates and lipids provide both energy and structure for cells. There is much more to life, however, than these functions. One of the characteristics of life is that it is very active, with cells continually carrying out a broad range of functions in order to grow, reproduce, and survive. **Proteins** provide cells with the ability to carry out these functions; below you will find a list of several of these functions.

| Type of Protein | Functions | Examples |
| --- | --- | --- |
| Hormonal | Chemical messengers | Insulin, glucagon |
| Transport | Transports other substances | Hemoglobin, carrier proteins |
| Structural | Physical support | Collagen |
| Contractile | Movement | Actin, myosin |
| Antibodies | Immune defense | Immunoglobulins, interferons |
| Enzymes | Biological catalysts | Amylase, lipase, ATPase |

## Enzymes

**Enzymes** act as catalysts for all biochemical reactions, making them useful for living organisms. Enzymes increase reaction rates by lowering activation energy. What is activation energy? It is the minimum amount of energy needed to start a reaction. Every chemical reaction begins with reactants, and proceeds to products. The reactants have a certain amount of energy contained in their bonds, and the products contain a unique amount of energy as well.

### Nucleic Acids

**Nucleic acids** are another class of the essential biological molecules found in all living organisms. They act as informational molecules, and include deoxyribonucleic acid (DNA) and ribonucleic acid (RNA). All organisms (except for some viruses, which most people do not classify as truly living) use DNA as their **genome** (an organism's chromosomal set). The structure and function of nucleic acids will be addressed in a separate section about genome expression.

## How Cells Get Energy to Make ATP

One of the essential features of life is the ability to capture and harness energy from the environment and use this energy to build, move, grow, replicate, and even think. What energy is used and where does it come from?

Organisms eat carbohydrates and fats that contain chemical energy, digesting these molecules to trap their chemical energy in a molecule called adenosine triphosphate (ATP). Cells use ATP to do most activities that require energy input to occur. Processes requiring energy input will not occur on their own, catalyzed or not. In fact, without energy input, most of the molecules fundamental to life tend to move in the other direction, toward oxidation and a loss of structure. By capturing food energy and converting it into ATP, life uses energy to drive forward all of the reactions it needs to perform.

Where does the ATP come from? Cells in humans and other organisms use a common set of biochemical reactions to make ATP, including pathways such as **glycolysis**, the **Krebs cycle**, and **electron transport**. It all starts with glucose. In humans, glucose is present in the blood as a fuel for all cells. Cells take in glucose, leading to the glycolytic pathway that is the first step in the path to ATP.

### Glycolysis

A **metabolic pathway** is a linked series of biochemical reactions that have a common purpose. Glycolysis is a very ancient pathway in the evolution of life, present in all of the kingdoms of life, from bacteria to humans. The reason for its importance is that glycolysis is the first biochemical pathway in the capture of energy from glucose, which makes ATP. The **glycolytic pathway** consists of ten steps, each catalyzed by an enzyme uniquely evolved to catalyze that reaction. We will not go into all of the individual reactions or the individual enzymes, but being familiar with the idea of metabolic pathways and the function of glycolysis is a good idea. Glycolysis takes glucose, a sugar molecule with six carbon atoms, and breaks it into two pyruvate molecules, each with three carbons, that capture energy in different ways. Energy is captured to make NADH, an energy carrier the cell uses to make ATP through electron transport.

### Fermentation

In glycolysis, NAD+ is required, and it is converted to NADH. Obviously, NAD+ must be regenerated or glycolysis would run out of it and stop, halting ATP production as well (and probably the life of the cell or organism involved). NAD+ is regenerated in one of two ways. In the first, NADH goes on to the electron transport chain and is used to produce more ATP, as described in the sections that follow; during this process it is converted back to NAD+. The second way to regenerate NAD+ occurs in the absence of oxygen or in anaerobic organisms that do not use oxidative metabolism. This alternate pathway is called **fermentation**.

Fermentation allows glycolysis to continue even in the absence of oxygen. In fermentation, NADH is regenerated back to NAD+ in the absence of oxygen to allow glycolysis to continue to produce ATP, producing either ethanol or lactic acid as by-products.

### Aerobic Respiration

Although glycolysis produces two ATP and two NADH for every molecule of glucose, this is not where the eukaryotic cell extracts most of its energy from glucose. Glycolysis is only the beginning; **aerobic respiration** is the rest of the story. During aerobic respiration, glucose is fully combusted by the cell as an energy source, going through the Krebs cycle and electron transport to trap energy ultimately used to make ATP.

To accomplish this more efficient form of energy production, pyruvate from glycolysis is oxidized all the way to carbon dioxide in a pathway called the Krebs cycle. The **Krebs cycle** and the other steps of oxidative metabolism occur in mitochondria. It is not important to know all the details about the Krebs cycle, but you should understand that the Krebs cycle is a series of reactions linked in a circle that extracts energy from the products of glycolysis to make the high-energy electron carriers. Finally, **electron transport** is the mechanism used to convert the energy held by these carriers into a more useful form that ultimately results in ATP production.

### Photosynthesis

**Photosynthesis** is the foundation of all ecosystems because it is the source of the energy for ecosystems and planet Earth as a whole. Plants are **autotrophs**, or self-feeders, that use photosynthesis to generate their own chemical energy from the energy of the sun. There are also many prokaryotic photosynthetic organisms, such as algae, that contribute significantly to biological production. The chemical energy that plants get from the sun is used to produce the glucose that can be burned in mitochondria to make ATP, which is then used to drive all of the energy-requiring processes in a plant, including the production of proteins, lipids, carbohydrates, and nucleic acids. Animals eat plants to extract this energy for their own metabolic needs. In this way, photosynthesis supports almost all living systems. In plants, photosynthesis occurs in the **chloroplast**, an organelle that is specific to plants. In algae, a prokaryote, there are no chloroplasts, and photosynthesis occurs throughout the cytoplasm. Chloroplasts are found mainly in the cells of the **mesophyl**, green tissue in the interior of leaves. A leaf contains pores in its surface called **stomata** that allow carbon dioxide in and oxygen out, facilitating photosynthesis in the leaf. Chloroplasts have an inner and outer membrane; within the inner membrane there is a fluid called the **stroma**. Photosynthesis involves the reduction of carbon dioxide ($CO_2$) to a carbohydrate. It can be characterized as the reverse of respiration, in that the reduction of $CO_2$ produces glucose instead of the oxidation of glucose making $CO_2$. Oxygen, one of the by-products of photosynthesis, is of keen interest to all of us air-breathers since we need it to survive.

# THE GENOME AND GENE EXPRESSION

Plants, animals, and bacteria may differ in their form, biochemistry, and lifestyle, but they all share a common molecular structure that underlies the inheritance and expression of traits. All living organisms inherit traits from their parents and these traits are encoded by the molecule called DNA. By comparing the features of parents with their children, humans throughout history have known intuitively that animals transfer traits from one generation to another. Many years ago, Gregor Mendel (discussed further in Classical Genetics) pioneered studies of the genetic behavior of traits passed between generations of pea plants. The discovery of the identity of the molecules that store and transfer genetic information is relatively recent, however. **Genes** encode these physical traits. Many scientists once believed that proteins were the main source of genetic material. That theory was based on the fact that nucleic acids such as DNA have such simple components. As such, it was difficult for many scientists to believe DNA could carry such complex information. Through many elegant experiments, however, it was proven that DNA is the foundation of genetic material. Furthermore, with the elucidation of DNA by Watson and Crick in 1953, it became clear how and why DNA has its role as the source of genetic material.

The basic outline of information flow in living organisms is sometimes called the **Central Dogma**. The Central Dogma includes several concepts, which are the foundation of modern molecular biology.

## Principles of Central Dogma

1. DNA contains an organism's genetic material—the genes that are responsible for the physical traits (phenotype) observed in all living organisms.
2. DNA is replicated from existing DNA to produce new genomes.
3. RNA is produced when a gene segment of DNA is read by RNA. Through the process of **transcription**, RNA acquires the same gene sequence.
4. The gene sequence carried by RNA is read and appropriated into a sequence of amino acids, which form protein. This process of protein synthesis is called **translation**.

## DNA Basics

Although DNA is a complex concept, there are key concepts surrounding it you should understand. DNA is a polymer built from simple building blocks called **nucleotides**, of which there are four types: **adenine** (A), **guanine** (G), **thymine** (T), and **cytosine** (C).

### The Genetic Code

Part of the Central Dogma is that DNA contains genes that are transcribed to create messenger RNA, which is in turn translated to make proteins. How do the four base pairs in DNA encode the 20 amino acids found in a protein polypeptide chain? The order of the four base pairs in DNA is the basis of this encoded information, and is called the **genetic code**.

### Mutation

In a **mutation**, nucleotides are added, deleted, or substituted to change the sequence of a gene. In some cases, inappropriate amino acids are created, and a mutated protein is produced. Genetic diseases are caused by gene mutations. There will be more information about mutation later in the lesson.

### RNA

The Central Dogma states RNA is produced while DNA is read during transcription. Like DNA, RNA is a polymer of nucleotides. Both DNA and RNA are nucleic acids; the structure of RNA is very similar to single-stranded DNA. However, there are some important differences between DNA and RNA. These differences include the use of ribose in the RNA backbone rather than deoxyribose; the presence of the base uracil in RNA rather than thymine; and the fact that RNA is usually single stranded, while DNA is usually double stranded.

There are three types of RNA with distinct functions: **messenger** RNA (mRNA), **ribosomal** RNA (rRNA), and **transfer** RNA (tRNA). In short, mRNA encodes gene messages that are to be decoded during protein synthesis to form proteins; rRNA is a part of the structure of ribosomes and is involved in translation (protein synthesis); and tRNA plays a role in protein synthesis.

## CELL STRUCTURE AND ORGANIZATION

### Cell Theory

Modern biology has shown that the cell is so inherent in the way we view life that it is easy to overlook its importance. Cells were unknown until the seventeenth century, after the development of the microscope allowed scientists to see cells for the first time. In 1838, Matthias Schleiden and Theodor Schwann proposed that all life was composed of cells, while Rudolph Virchow proposed in 1855 that cells arise only from other cells. The **cell theory** based on these ideas unifies all biology at the cellular level and may be summarized as follows:

- All living things are composed of cells.
- All biological chemical reactions occur in cells or in association with cells.
- Cells arise only from pre-existing cells.
- Cells carry genetic information in the form of DNA. Genetic material is passed from parent cell to daughter cell.

## Prokaryotic Versus Eukaryotic Cells

### Prokaryotic Cells

**Prokaryotes** include bacteria and cyanobacteria (blue-green algae), which are unicellular organisms with a simple cell structure. These organisms have an outer lipid bilayer cell membrane, but do not contain any membrane-bound organelles, unlike their cousins the eukaryotes. Prokaryotes have no true nucleus and their genetic material consists of a single, circular molecule of DNA concentrated in an area of the cell called the nucleoid region. Bacteria also have a cell wall, cell membrane, cytoplasm, ribosomes, and, sometimes, flagella that are used for locomotion.

Prokaryotes conduct respiration in the cell membrane. This is due to the fact that there are no other membranes present for ATP (energy) synthesis to take place.

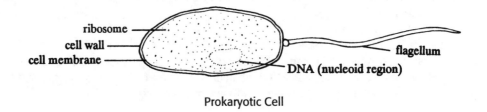

ribosome
cell wall
cell membrane
flagellum
DNA (nucleoid region)

Prokaryotic Cell

### Eukaryotic Cells

All multicellular organisms (for example: you, a tree, a mushroom) and all protists (amoebas or paramecia) are composed of **eukaryotic cells**. A eukaryotic cell is enclosed within a lipid bilayer cell membrane, as are prokaryotic cells. Unlike prokaryotes, however, eukaryotic cells contain organelles, which are membrane-bound structures within a cell with specific functions isolated in separate compartments. The organelle membrane and interior are separated from the rest of the cell, allowing organelles to perform distinct functions isolated from other activities, which is not possible in prokaryotes.

The presence of membrane-enclosed organelles prevents incompatible processes from mixing together, allows stepwise processes to be more strictly regulated, and makes processes more efficient by making them happen in a single, constrained place. **Cytoplasm** is the liquid inside a cell that surrounds organelles.

Although both animal and plant cells are eukaryotic, they differ in a number of ways. For example, plant cells have a cell wall and chloroplasts, while animal cells do not. Centrioles, located in the centrosome, are found in animal cells but not in plant cells.

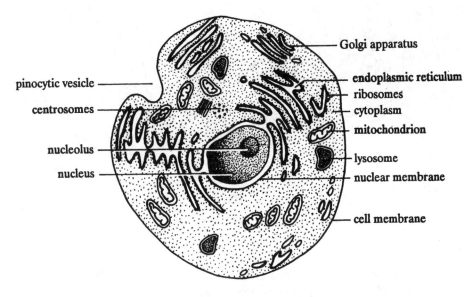

Eukaryotic Cell

| Summary of Cell Properties | | | | |
|---|---|---|---|---|
| *Structure* | *Nucleus?* | *Genetic Material?* | *Cell Wall?* | *Cell Membrane?* |
| Eukaryote | Yes | DNA | Yes/No | Yes |
| Prokaryote | No | DNA | Yes | Yes |
| *Structure* | *Membrane Organelles?* | *Ribosomes?* | | |
| Eukaryote | Yes | Yes | | |
| Prokaryote | No | Yes* | | |

*Ribosomes in prokaryotes are smaller and have a different subunit composition than those in eukaryotes.

## Plasma Membrane

The **plasma membrane** is not an organelle but is an important component of cellular structure. The plasma membrane (also called the **cell membrane**) encloses the cell and exhibits **selective permeability**; it regulates the passage of materials into and out of the cell. To carry out the biochemical activities necessary to sustain life, some molecules must be retained inside the cell and other materials must be kept out of the cell. This is what the selective permeability of the membrane provides.

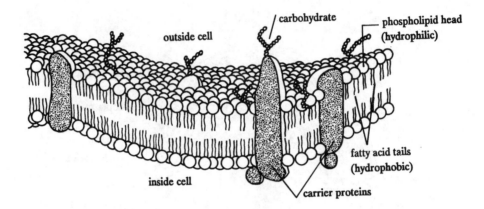

The Plasma Membrane

## Organelles

Eukaryotic cells have specialized membrane-bound structures called **organelles** that carry out particular functions for the cell. Organelles include the nucleus, endoplasmic reticulum, Golgi apparatus, lysosomes, microbodies, vacuoles, mitochondria, and chloroplasts. The lipid bilayer membranes that surround organelles also regulate and partition the flow of material into and out of these compartments, just as the plasma membrane does for the cell and its exterior environment.

### Nucleus

One of the largest organelles of the cell is the **nucleus**. The nucleus is the site in which the genes present in DNA are read to produce messenger RNA (the process of transcription). RNA is then spliced, and the DNA genome is replicated when the cell divides. Other activities like glycolysis and protein synthesis are excluded from the nucleus. The nucleus is surrounded by a two-layer **nuclear membrane** (or nuclear envelope) that maintains a nuclear environment distinct from that of the cytoplasm. Nuclear pores in this membrane allow a selective two-way exchange of materials between the nucleus and cytoplasm, importing some proteins into the nucleus that are involved in transcription, mRNA splicing, and DNA replication, while keeping out other factors like those involved in glycolysis and translation. The dense structure within the nucleus in which ribosomal RNA (rRNA) synthesis occurs is known as the **nucleolus**.

The nucleus also contains DNA genomes that have become complex with proteins called **histones,** which are involved in packaging DNA and regulating access to genes. The term **chromatin** is used to describe DNA that has been packaged with histones. Chromatin becomes condensed through several processes, leading to the development of **chromosomes**, which are the highest level of structure in the genome. Each chromosome contains a fully packaged and immensely long molecule of DNA containing many different genes. The activity of chromosomes during cell division and the role it plays in heredity will be discussed in Classical Genetics.

## Ribosomes

**Ribosomes** are not membrane-bound organelles; rather they are relatively large, complex structures that are the sites of protein production and are synthesized by the nucleolus. They consist of two subunits, one large and one small; each subunit is composed of rRNA and many proteins. Free ribosomes are found in the cytoplasm, while bound ribosomes line the outer membrane of the endoplasmic reticulum. Prokaryotes have ribosomes that are similar in function to eukaryotic ribosomes, although they are smaller.

## Endoplasmic Reticulum

The **endoplasmic reticulum** (ER) is a network of membrane-enclosed spaces connected with the nuclear membrane at various points. The network extends in sheets and tubes through cytoplasm. If this network has ribosomes lining its outer surface, it is termed **rough endoplasmic reticulum** (RER); without ribosomes, it is known as **smooth endoplasmic reticulum** (SER). The ER is involved in the transport of proteins in cells, especially proteins destined to be secreted from the cell. SER is involved in lipid synthesis and the detoxification of drugs and poisons, while RER is involved in protein synthesis.

Proteins that are found in the cytoplasm are made by free ribosomes. Proteins that are secreted, found in the cell membrane, the ER, or the Golgi apparatus, are made by ribosomes on the RER. Proteins synthesized by bound ribosomes cross into the **cisternae** (the interior) of the RER. Small regions of ER membrane bud off to form small round membrane-bound vesicles that contain newly synthesized proteins. These cytoplasmic vesicles are then transported to the Golgi apparatus.

## Golgi Apparatus

The **Golgi** is a stack of membrane-enclosed sacs. It receives vesicles and their contents from the ER and modifies proteins (through glycosylation, the process of modifying proteins with carbohydrate chains, for example). Next, it repackages them into vesicles and ships the vesicles to their next stop, such as lysosomes or the plasma membrane. In cells that are very active in the secretion of proteins, the Golgi is particularly active in the distribution of newly synthesized material to the cell surface. Secretory vesicles, produced by the Golgi, release their contents to the cell's exterior by the process of exocytosis.

## Lysosomes

**Lysosomes** contain hydrolytic enzymes involved in intracellular digestion—the process in which proteins and structures that are worn out or not in use become degraded. Lysosomes fuse with endocytic vacuoles, breaking down material ingested by the cells. They also aid in renewing a cell's components by breaking them down and releasing their molecular building blocks into the cytosol for reuse.

## Microbodies

**Microbodies** can be characterized as specialized containers for metabolic reactions. The two most common types of microbodies are **peroxisomes** and **glyoxysomes**. Peroxisomes break fats down into small molecules that can be used for fuel; they are also used in the liver to detoxify compounds, such as alcohol, that may be harmful to the body. Glyoxysomes, on the other hand, are usually found in the fat tissue of germinating seedlings. Until seedlings are mature enough to use photosynthesis to produce their own supply of sugars, they use glyoxysomes to convert fats into sugars.

## Vacuoles

**Vacuoles** are membrane-enclosed sacs within the cell. Contractile vacuoles in freshwater protists pump excess water out of the cell. Plant cells have a large, central vacuole called the tonoplast, which is part of their endomembrane system. In plants, the tonoplast functions as a place to store organic compounds, such as proteins, and inorganic ions, such as potassium and chloride.

## Mitochondria

**Mitochondria** are sites of aerobic respiration within the cell and are important suppliers of energy. Each mitochondrion has an outer and inner phospholipid bilayer membrane. The outer membrane has many pores and acts as a sieve, allowing molecules through on the basis of their size. The area between the inner and outer membranes is known as the intermembrane space. The inner membrane has many convolutions called **cristae**, as well as a high protein content that includes the proteins of the electron transport chain. The area bound by the inner membrane is known as the **mitochondrial matrix**, and is the site of many reactions that occur during cell respiration—including ATP production.

Mitochondria are somewhat unusual in that they are semiautonomous. They contain their own circular DNA and ribosomes, which enable them to produce some of their own proteins, and they self-replicate through binary fission. They are believed to have developed from early prokaryotic cells that evolved from a symbiotic relationship with the ancestors of eukaryotes and still retain vestiges of this earlier independent life.

## Chloroplasts

**Chloroplasts** are found only in algal and plant cells. With the help of one of their primary components, chlorophyll, they function as the site where photosynthesis transpires. They contain their own DNA and ribosomes, exhibit the same semiautonomy as mitochondria, and are also believed to have evolved via symbiosis. For more information about chloroplasts, see the section titled **Photosynthesis**.

## Cytoskeleton

Cells are not blobs of gelatin enclosed by a membrane bag. Cells have shape, and in some cases they move actively and change their shape. Cells gain mechanical support, maintain their shape, and carry out cell motility functions with the help of their **cytoskeleton**. This structure is composed of **microtubules**, **microfilaments**, **intermediate fibers**, as well as chains and rods of proteins that all have distinct functions and activities.

**Microtubules** are hollow rods made of polymerized tubulin proteins. Microtubules radiate throughout cells, providing support and a framework for organelle movement within the cell.

**Cilia** and **flagella** are specialized arrangements of microtubules that extend from certain cells and are involved in cell motility.

Cell movement and support are maintained in part through the action of solid rods composed of actin subunits; these are termed **microfilaments**. Muscle contraction, for example, is based on the interaction of actin with myosin in muscle cells. Microfilaments move materials across the plasma membrane; they are active, for instance, in the contraction phase of cell division and in amoeboid movement.

**Intermediate fibers** are a collection of fibers involved in the maintenance of cytoskeletal integrity. Their diameters fall between those of microtubules and microfilaments.

## Membrane Transport Across the Plasma

It is crucial for a cell to control what enters and exits it. In order to preserve this control, cells use the mechanisms described below.

### Osmosis

**Osmosis** is the simple diffusion of water from a region of lower solute concentration to a region of higher solute concentration. Water flows to equalize the solute concentrations. If a membrane is impermeable to a particular solute, then water will flow across the membrane until the differences in the solute concentration have been equilibrated. Differences in the concentration of substances to which the membrane is impermeable affect the direction of osmosis. Water diffuses freely across the plasma membrane. When the cytoplasm of the cell has a lower solute concentration than the extracellular medium, the medium is said to be **hypertonic** to the cell; water will flow out, causing the cell to shrink. On the other hand, when the cytoplasm of a cell has a higher solute concentration than the extracellular medium, the medium is **hypotonic** to the cell, and water will flow in, causing the cell to swell. Finally, when solute concentrations are equal inside and outside, the cell and the medium are said to be **isotonic**. There is no net flow of water in either direction.

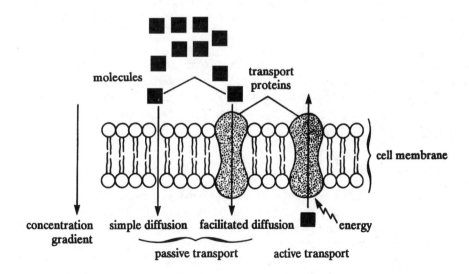

Movement Across Membranes

### Permeability—Diffusion Through the Membrane

Traffic through the membrane is extensive, but the membrane is selectively permeable; substances do not cross its barrier indiscriminately. A cell is able to retain many small molecules and exclude others. The sum total of movement across the membrane is determined by the **passive diffusion** of material directly through the membrane and selective transport processes through the membrane that require proteins. Most molecules cannot passively diffuse through the plasma membrane. The hydrophobic core of the membrane impedes diffusion of charged and polar molecules. Hydrophobic molecules such as hydrocarbons can readily diffuse through the membrane, however. The ability of cells to get the oxygen needed to fuel electron transport depends on two factors: the ability of oxygen to diffuse through membranes **into** the cell and the passive diffusion **out of** the cell membrane and into the blood stream. Although it is polar, water is also able to readily diffuse through the membrane. If two molecules are equally soluble, then the smaller molecule will diffuse through the plasma membrane faster. Small, polar, uncharged molecules can pass through easily, but the lipid bilayer is not permeable to large, uncharged polar molecules such as glucose.

### Diffusion and Transport

**Diffusion** is the net movement of dissolved particles across concentration gradients, from a region of higher concentration to a region of lower concentration. **Passive diffusion** does not require proteins since it occurs directly through the membrane. Since molecules are moving down a concentration gradient, no external energy is required.

The net movement of dissolved particles across concentration gradients—with the help of carrier proteins in the membrane—is known as **facilitated diffusion**. This process does not require energy. Ion channels are one example of membrane proteins involved in facilitated diffusion. During this process, channels act as a passage for ions to flow through the membrane and into another concentration gradient. Ions will not flow through the membrane on their own. Some channels are always open for ions to flow through, while other ion channels open only in response to specific stimuli, such as a change in the voltage across the membrane or the presence of a molecule like a neurotransmitter.

Transport proteins aid in the process of **active transport,** which is the net movement of dissolved particles against their concentration gradient. This process requires energy and is necessary to maintain membrane potentials in specialized cells such as neurons. The most common forms of energy to drive active transport are ATP or a concentration gradient of another molecule. Active transport is used for uptake of nutrients against a gradient.

### Transport Proteins

Molecules that do not diffuse through the membrane can often get in or out of the cell with the aid of proteins in the membrane. Hydrophilic substances avoid contact with the lipid bilayer and still traverse the membrane by passing through transport proteins. There are three types of transport proteins: uniport, symport, and antiport. Uniport proteins carry a single solute across the membrane. Symport proteins translocate two different solutes simultaneously in the same direction; transport occurs only if both solutes bind to the proteins. Antiport proteins exchange two solutes by transporting one into the cell and the other out of the cell.

# ORGANISMAL BIOLOGY

Living organisms must maintain constant interior conditions in a changing environment. The interior environment that cells must maintain includes water volume and salt concentration, as well as appropriate levels of oxygen, carbon dioxide, toxic metabolic waste products, and essential nutrients. Organisms must respond to their environment to avoid harm and seek out beneficial conditions; they must also reproduce. Single-cell organisms like prokaryotes or protists have relatively simple ways to meet these needs, while multicellular organisms have evolved more complex body plans that provide a variety of solutions to the common problems all organisms face. As multicellular organisms have over time evolved into larger and more complex forms, their cells have become removed from the external environment and specialized toward one specific function. These specialized cells form **tissues**, cells with a common function and often a similar form. Cells from different tissues come together to form **organs**, large anatomical structures made from several tissues working together toward a common goal. Organs, in turn, are part of various systems that are the basis for digestion, respiration, circulation, immune reactions, excretion, and reproduction, among others.

## Reproduction

One of the essential functions for all living things is the ability to reproduce, to produce offspring that will allow a species to continue. An individual organism can survive without reproducing, but if an entire species does not reproduce, it will not survive past a single generation. The reproduction of eukaryotes can occur either asexually or sexually. Prokaryotes have a different mechanism called **binary fission** for reproduction.

## Cell Division

One of the inherent features in reproduction is cell division. Prokaryotic cells divide and reproduce through the relatively simple process of binary fission. Eukaryotic cells divide by one of two mechanisms: mitosis or meiosis. **Mitosis** is a process in which cells divide to produce two daughter cells with the same genomic complement as the parent cell; in the case of humans there are two copies of the genome in each cell. Mitotic cell division can be a means of asexual reproduction; it is also the mechanism for the growth, development, and replacement of tissues. **Meiosis** is a specialized form of cell division involved in sexual reproduction that produces male and female gametes (sperm and ova, respectively). Meiotic cell division creates cells with a single copy of the genome in preparation for sexual reproduction. During reproduction, gametes join to create a new organism with two copies of the genome, one from each parent.

## Prokaryotic Cell Division and Reproduction

Prokaryotes are single-celled organisms and their mechanism for cell division, binary fission, is also their means of reproduction. As with all forms of cell division, one of the key steps is DNA replication. Prokaryotes have no organelles and only one chromosome in a single, long circular DNA strand. The single prokaryotic chromosome is attached to the cell membrane and replicated as the cell grows. With two copies of the genome attached to the membrane after DNA replication, the DNAs are drawn apart from each other as the cell grows in size and adds more membrane between the DNAs.

When the cell grows to the size of multiple cells, the cell wall and membrane close off to create two independent cells. The simplicity of prokaryotic cells and the small size of their genome (in comparison to eukaryotes) may be a factor that assists in their rapid rate of reproduction. They are able to divide as rapidly as once every 30 minutes under ideal conditions. Bacteria and other prokaryotes do not reproduce sexually, but they do exchange genetic material with each other in some cases. **Conjugation** is one mechanism used by bacteria to move genes between cells by exchanging circular, extrachromosomal DNA with each other.

## Mitosis

Eukaryotic cells use mitosis to divide into two new daughter cells with the same genome as the parent cell. During what is known as the **cell cycle**, cells grow and divide, creating new cells. The cell cycle is a highly regulated process, linked to the growth and differentiation of tissues. Growth factors can stimulate cells to move through the cell cycle more rapidly; there are also various other factors that can induce cells to differentiate and stop moving forward through the cell cycle. Failure to control the cell cycle properly can result in uncontrolled progression through the cell cycle, which can lead to cancer. Cancer cells contain mutations in genes that regulate the cell cycle. The four stages of the cell cycle are designated as G1, S, G2, and M. The first three stages of this cell cycle are interphase stages—that is, they occur between cell divisions. The fourth stage, mitosis, includes the actual division of the cell.

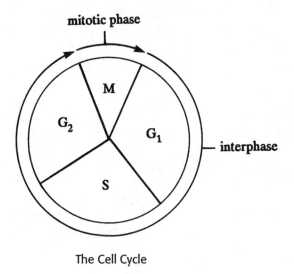

The Cell Cycle

## Cell Cycle Stages

### Stage $G_1$

The $G_1$ stage is characterized by intense growth and activity, both biochemical and biosynthetic. The cell doubles in size, and new organelles such as mitochondria, ribosomes, and centrioles are produced.

### Stage S

This is the stage during which synthesis of DNA takes place (S is for synthesis). Each chromosome is replicated so that during division, a complete copy of the genome can be distributed to both daughter cells.

After replication, the chromosomes each consist of two identical sister **chromatids** held together at a central region called the **centromere**. The ends of the chromosomes are called **telomeres**. Cells entering the $G_2$ stage actually contain twice as much DNA as cells during the $G_1$ stage, since a single cell holds both copies of the replicated genome.

### Stage $G_2$

The cell prepares for mitosis, making any of the components still needed to complete cell division.

### Stage M (Mitosis and Cytokinesis)

During mitosis and cytokinesis, the cell divides to create two similar but smaller daughter cells. Mitosis is further broken down into four stages: **prophase**, **metaphase**, **anaphase**, and **telophase**. Prophase is often further subdivided to create **prometaphase**. Upon completion of mitosis, the cell completes its split into daughter cells via **cytokinesis**.

### Prophase

During interphase, chromosomes in the nucleus are very extended despite their packaging into chromatin; it is not possible to see the chromosomes even under a microscope. **Prophase** begins with the condensation and separation of chromosomes. During that phase, if the chromosomes are stained, they are visible under a microscope as dark solid bands. Cell division cannot occur without this condensation or the chromosomes become tangled with each other.

Another step in prophase is the separation of the **centrioles**, centers of microtubule formation. As the centrioles separate, they nucleate the **spindle apparatus**, a specialized system of microtubules that spans between the centrioles during mitosis. As the centrioles separate toward opposite poles of the cell, the spindle apparatus elongates between them. The nuclear membrane dissolves and the nucleolus becomes indistinct, allowing the spindle fibers access to the chromosomes. The spindle fibers attach themselves to each chromosome with a structure called the **kinetochore**, which attaches in the middle of each chromosome at the centromere, setting the stage for metaphase.

### Metaphase

During **metaphase**, the two centrioles are at opposite poles of the cell. The spindle is fully elongated between the poles, spanning the length of the cell, including the space previously occupied by the nucleus, which has been replaced by the condensed chromosomes. The kinetochore fibers attached to the chromosomes at the centromere align the chromosomes at the metaphase plate, a plane halfway between the two ends of the cell. The alignment of the chromosomes prepares the cell to pull the chromosomes apart toward the two ends of the cell.

### Anaphase

During phase S, each chromosome is replicated; the copies stay bound together. From the S phase through metaphase, each chromosome contains a replicate of itself, and each copy is called a sister chromatid. During **anaphase**, the two sister chromatids in each chromosome are pulled apart by the kinetochore and spindle fibers. The telomeres at the ends of the chromosomes are the last parts of the chromatids to separate. Each chromatid then has its own centromere, by which it is pulled towards opposite poles of the cell through the shortening of the kinetochore fibers. It is crucial that when the sister chromatids separate, each daughter cell receives one of each chromosome. The cell lacking a chromosome or the other cell with an extra chromosome may not function normally because it is lacking a copy of many genes or has an extra copy of genes.

### Telophase

At the beginning of **telophase**, the sister chromatids have been pulled apart so that one copy of each chromosome is at one end of the cell and another copy is at the other end. At this point, the spindle apparatus disappears, a nuclear membrane reforms around each set of chromosomes, and the nucleoli reappear. The chromosomes uncoil, resuming the spread-out form they have during interphase. Each of the two new nuclei contains a complete copy of the genome identical to the original genome and to each other.

### Cytokinesis

After the cell has divided its DNA during **mitosis**, it enters cytokinesis. During cytokinesis, the cytoplasm and all the organelles of the cell are divided as the plasma membrane pinches inward and seals off to complete the separation of the two newly formed daughter cells from each other.

## Asexual Reproduction

**Asexual reproduction** is any method of producing new organisms in which fusion of nuclei from two individuals (fertilization) does not take place. In asexual reproduction, only one parent organism is involved. New organisms produced through asexual reproduction form daughter cells through mitotic cell division and are genetically identical clones of their parents. Asexual reproduction serves primarily as a mechanism for perpetuating primitive organisms and plants, especially in times of low population density. Asexual reproduction can allow more rapid population growth than sexual reproduction, but does not create the great genetic diversity that sexual reproduction does.

## Sexual Reproduction

Most multicellular animals and plants reproduce sexually, as do many protists and fungi. **Sexual reproduction** involves the union of a **haploid cell** from two different parents, producing diploid offspring. These haploid cells are **gametes**—sex cells produced through meiosis in males and females. Gametes have a single copy of the genome (one of each chromosome), and diploid cells have two copies of the genome (two of each chromosome). In humans, all of the cells of the body are diploid, with the exception of the gametes. When the male gamete (the sperm) and the female gamete (the egg) join, a **zygote** is formed that develops into a new organism genetically distinct from both its parents. The zygote is the diploid single-cell offspring, formed from the union of gametes. Sexual reproduction ensures genetic diversity and variability in offspring. Since sexual reproduction is more costly in energy than asexual reproduction, the reason for its overwhelming prevalence must be that genetic diversity is worth the effort. Sexual reproduction does not create new alleles, though. Only mutation can do that. Sexual reproduction increases diversity in populations by creating new combinations of alleles in offspring and therefore new combinations of traits. Genetic diversity is not an advantage to an individual, but allows a population of organisms to adapt and survive in the face of a dynamic and unpredictable environment. The diversity created by sexual reproduction occurs in part during meiotic gamete production and in part through the random matching of gametes to make unique individuals.

### Gamete Formation

Specialized organs called **gonads** produce gametes through meiotic cell division. Male gonads, **testes**, produce male gametes, **spermatozoa**, while female gonads, **ovaries**, produce **ova**. A cell that is committed to the production of gametes, although it is not itself a gamete, is called a **germ cell**. The rest of the cells of the body are called **somatic cells**. Only the genome of germ cells contributes to gametes and offspring. A mutation in a somatic cell, for example, may be harmful to that cell or the organism if it leads to cancer, but a mutation in a somatic cell will not affect offspring since the mutation will not be found in germ cell genomes. Germ cells are themselves diploid and divide to create more germ cells through the process of mitosis, but create the haploid gametes through meiosis. The production of both male and female gametes involves meiotic cell division. Meiosis during both spermatogenesis and oogenesis involves two rounds of cell division in which a single diploid cell first replicates its genome, and then divides into two cells, each with two copies of the genome. Without replicating their DNA, these two cells divide again to produce four haploid gametes. Meiosis in both cases also involves recombination between the homologous copies of chromosomes during the first round of meiotic cell division. This recombination is one of the key sources of genetic diversity provided during sexual reproduction and is discussed in more detail in the section Classical Genetics.

The differences in meiosis as conducted during sperm production and oogenesis are outlined below.

### Human Male Reproductive System

The human male produces sperm in the **testes**, gonads located in an outpocketing of the abdominal wall called the **scrotum**. The sperm develop in a series of small, coiled tubes within the testes called the **seminiferous tubules**. **Sertoli cells** in the seminiferous tubules support the sperm and **Leydig cells** make the **testosterone** that supports male secondary sex characteristics.

The **vas deferens** carries sperm to the urethra that passes through the penis. During ejaculation, the **prostate gland** and **seminal vesicles** along the path add secretions to the sperm that carry and provide nutrients for the sperm as part of **semen**.

As gonads, the testes have a dual function; they produce both sperm and male hormones (such as testosterone). Leydig cells in the testis secrete testosterone beginning in puberty. **Testosterone** and other steroid hormones collectively called **androgens** induce secondary sexual characteristics of the male, such as facial and pubic hair, changes in body shape, and deepening voice changes.

**Spermatogenesis** is the meiotic development of sperm in males. Sperm production occurs throughout adult life in males, and meiosis in sperm production is continuous, proceeding forward without a significant pause. In the testes, diploid germ cells divide mitotically to create primary **spermatocytes**, which continuously undergo meiosis to form four haploid **spermatids** from each primary spermatocyte. The four spermatids are equivalent in size and function, and all four result in viable gametes. Spermatids must mature further to develop the characteristics held by mature sperm: a head containing DNA and a tail that provides motility. A specialized sac at the tip of the sperm called the **acrosome** is full of enzymes that allow the sperm to break through the protective layers around the egg. One birth control strategy has been to inhibit these enzymes so that sperm cannot reach the egg. The testes are located outside the abdominal cavity because they must remain 2–4° cooler than the rest of the body to ensure proper development of sperm.

### Human Female Reproductive System

The **ovum** develops in a discontinuous process called **oogenesis** that is not completed in a single continuous process, unlike spermatogenesis. During development of female children, ova progress to **meiotic prophase I** in the first round of meiotic cell division and then become arrested, stuck at this stage. These ova remain arrested in meiosis throughout the life of a woman, except for the ova that mature during each menstrual cycle and progress through this meiotic block. Women are born with all the **eggs** they will ever have, while males produce fresh sperm daily. This is the reason that genetic anomalies are more common in the eggs of older women; these anomalies have had years to accumulate in ova while sperm have a short life span.

The completion of the first meiotic cell division by maturing ova preparing for ovulation creates one cell with most of the cytoplasm and another smaller cell that has little cytoplasm. This smaller cell may itself divide later to create two smaller cells, but does not create viable ova and is called a **polar body**. The developing ovum becomes a secondary oocyte that pauses again during the second meiotic cell division, even as it is released during ovulation. The ova in humans do not actually complete oogenesis until after fertilization, at which time the ovum releases the last polar body and joins the nuclei of the male and female cells to create the diploid zygote. The unequal distribution of cytoplasm during oogenesis is another feature that is distinct from spermatogenesis.

**Ovaries** are paired structures in the lower portion of the abdominal cavity. As part of the menstrual cycle, one ovum develops each month within a follicle in an ovary. The follicle is a collection of cells around the ova that support its development and secrete hormones. Each ovary is accompanied by a **fallopian tube**, also called an **oviduct**. During ovulation, an ovum leaves the ovary through the follicle and is ejected into the upper end of the oviduct. At birth, all the eggs that a female will ovulate during her lifetime are already present in the ovaries, but these eggs develop and ovulate at a rate of one every 28 days (approximately), starting in puberty.

The ovaries also produce female sex hormones such as **estrogen**. Like male sex hormones, the female sex hormones regulate the secondary sexual characteristics of the female, including the development of the **mammary** (milk) **glands** and wider hip bones (pelvis). They also play an important role in the menstrual cycle, which involves the interaction of the pituitary gland, ovaries, and uterus.

## Embryonic Development

The first step in development is **fertilization**. If sperm are present in the oviduct during ovulation, and a sperm succeeds in encountering the ovum, then fertilization can occur, forming a **zygote**, a single **diploid** cell. During fertilization, the egg nucleus (containing the **haploid number**, or *n* chromosomes) unites with the sperm nucleus (containing *n* **chromosomes**). This union produces a zygote of the original diploid or **2*n*** chromosome number. In this way, the normal somatic number (2*n*) of chromosomes in a diploid cell is restored, and the cell has two homologous copies of each chromosome.

Everything else in development up to adulthood consists of mitotic divisions. If there are two or more eggs released by the ovaries, more than one can be fertilized. The result of several eggs being fertilized is multiple gestation, producing fraternal twins, triplets, quadruplets, etc., which are produced when two or more separate sperm fertilize two or more eggs.

Fraternal twins are related genetically in the same way that any two siblings are. Drugs to treat infertility often induce multiple ovulation and can lead to multiple-birth pregnancies. If there is only one fertilized egg, twins may still result through separation of identical cells during the early stages of cleavage (for example, the two-, four-, or eight-cell stage) into two or more independent embryos. These develop into identical (**monozygotic**) twins, triplets, and so forth, since they all came from the same fertilized egg and have identical genomes. Identical twins are often used in human genetic studies to determine what traits are genetically inherited, since their environment must cause differences between the twins.

When the egg and the sperm join, they trigger a cascade of events that occur as the zygote begins to divide rapidly. These events, which are part of the process of fertilization, may occur either externally or internally.

## Methods of Fertilization

Vertebrates that reproduce in water, including most fish and amphibians, do so through **external reproduction**. Eggs are laid in the water, and sperm are deposited near them. The sperm have flagella, enabling them to swim through the water to the eggs. Since there is no direct passage of sperm from the male to the female, the sperm are likely to be diluted and the chances of fertilization for each ovum are reduced considerably. External fertilization also decreases the probability of survival of the young after fertilization, since the developing animals are easy targets for predators. Vertebrate land animals, such reptiles, birds, and mammals, reproduce through **internal fertilization**. The moist passageway of the female reproductive tract from the vagina through the oviducts provides mobile sperm with a direct route to the egg, increasing the chance of fertilization.

The number of eggs produced depends upon a number of factors. One of these factors is the type of fertilization employed. Because very few sperm actually reach the egg during external fertilization, this process requires large quantities of eggs to ensure success. The type of development practiced by the organism is also significant. If development occurs outside the mother's body from the very beginning, many eggs are required to ensure survival of at least some of the offspring. Finally, the less care the parents provide, the more eggs are required to guarantee survival of enough offspring to continue the species.

## Ingestion and Digestion in Humans

The human digestive system consists of the **alimentary canal** and the associated glands that contribute secretions into this canal. The alimentary canal is the entire path food follows through the body: the **oral cavity, pharynx, esophagus, stomach, small intestine, large intestine,** and **rectum.** Many glands line this canal, such as the gastric glands in the wall of the stomach and intestinal glands in the small intestine. Other glands, such as the pancreas and liver, are outside the canal proper, and deliver their secretions into the canal via ducts.

### Mechanical Digestion

Food is crushed and liquefied by the teeth, tongue, and peristaltic contractions of the stomach and small intestine, increasing the surface area for the digestive enzymes to work upon. **Peristalsis** is a wave-like muscular action conducted by smooth muscle that lines the gut in the esophagus, stomach, small intestine, and large intestine. During this process, rings of muscle encircling the gut contract, which moves food through the gut.

### Chemical Digestion

Several exocrine glands associated with the digestive system produce secretions involved in breaking food molecules into simple molecules that can be absorbed. Polysaccharides are broken down into glucose, triglycerides are hydrolyzed into fatty acids and glycerol, and proteins are broken down into amino acids.

Chemical digestion begins in the mouth. In the mouth, the **salivary glands** produce saliva, which lubricates food and begins starch digestion. **Saliva** contains **salivary amylase** (ptyalin), an enzyme that breaks the complex starch polysaccharide into maltose (a disaccharide). As food leaves the mouth, the **esophagus** conducts it to the stomach by means of peristaltic waves of smooth muscle contraction.

There are several more detailed steps involved in the human digestive system, but for now it should suffice to know the basics of mechanical and chemical digestion.

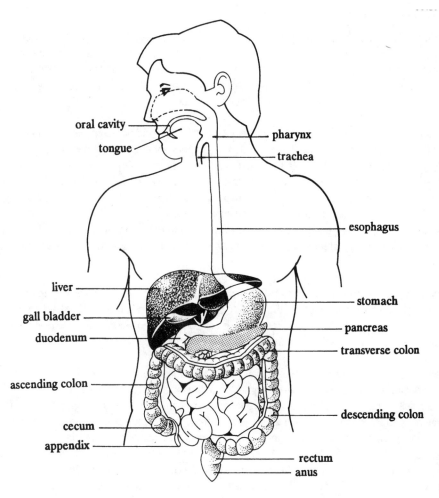

Human Digestive System

## Circulation

Through ingestion and digestion, organisms make nutrients available to cells through absorption. These nutrients, along with gases and wastes, must also be transported throughout the body to be used. The system involved in transport of these materials to different parts of the body is called the **circulatory system**. Small animals have their cells either directly in contact with the environment or in close enough proximity that diffusion alone provides for the movement of gases, wastes, and nutrients making a specialized system for circulation unnecessary. Larger, more complex organisms require circulatory systems to move material within the body.

### Circulation in Vertebrates

Vertebrates have closed circulatory systems, with a chambered heart that pumps blood through arteries into tiny capillaries in the tissues. Blood passing through capillaries is led into veins that connect to the heart. The chambers of vertebrate hearts include atria and ventricles. **Atria** are chambers where blood from veins collects and is pumped into ventricles, while **ventricles** are larger, more muscular chambers that pump blood through the body.

Birds and mammals have four-chambered hearts, with two atria and two ventricles. The right ventricle pumps deoxygenated blood to the lungs through the pulmonary artery. Oxygenated blood returns through the pulmonary vein to the left atrium. From there it passes to the left ventricle and is pumped through the aorta and arteries to the rest of the body. Valves in the chambers of the heart keep blood from moving backward. There are two separate circulatory systems: one for the lungs, called pulmonary circulation, and systemic circulation for the rest of the body. A four-chambered heart splits the blood that is pumped through the lungs and the blood that travels through the rest of the body, which allows much greater pressure in the systemic circulatory system than is possible with a two-chambered heart.

The heartbeat a doctor hears through a stethoscope is the sound of the chambers of the heart contracting in a regular pattern called the **cardiac cycle**. The heart is composed of specialized muscle tissue called **cardiac muscle**. Cardiac muscle cells are connected together in an electrical network that transmits nervous impulses throughout the muscle to stimulate contraction.

The transmission and spreading of the signal is highly controlled to coordinate the beating of the chambers. During each cardiac cycle, the signal to contract initiates on its own in a special part of the heart called the **sinoatrial node**, or the pacemaker region. Cells from this region fire impulses in regular intervals all on their own, without stimulation from the nervous system. Once the signals start, they spread through both atria, which then contract, forcing blood into the ventricles. The signal then passes into the ventricles and spreads throughout their walls, causing the ventricles to contract and move blood into the major arteries. Ventricular contraction occurs during the **systole** part of the cardiac cycle, and the atria contract during the **diastole** part of the cardiac cycle. The signal that causes the beating of the heart originates spontaneously within the heart without nervous stimulation, but the heart rate can be altered by nervous stimulation. The most important nervous stimulation of the heart is induced by the vagus nerve of the parasympathetic nervous system, which acts to slow the heart rate. The vagus nerve is more or less always stimulating the heart, and can increase the heart rate simply by stimulating the heart less than usual. The sympathetic nervous system and epinephrine increase the heart rate.

### Arteries

The **arteries** carry blood from the heart to the tissue of the body. They repeatedly branch into smaller arteries (arterioles) until they reach capillaries, where exchange with tissues occurs. Arteries are thick-walled, muscular, and elastic; they conduct blood at high pressure and have a pulse caused by periodic surges of blood from the heart. Arterial blood is oxygenated; however, blood in the pulmonary artery is not, as it carries deoxygenated blood from the heart to the lungs to renew the oxygen supply.

### Veins

**Veins** carry blood back to the heart from the capillaries. Veins are relatively thin-walled, conduct at low pressure because they are at some distance from the pumping heart, and contain many valves to prevent backflow. Veins have no pulse; they usually carry dark red, deoxygenated blood (except for the pulmonary vein, which carries recently oxygenated blood from the lungs). The movement of blood through veins is assisted by the contraction of skeletal muscle around the veins, squeezing blood forward. Once it moves forward in this way, valves keep the blood from going back.

### Capillaries

**Capillaries** are thin-walled vessels that are very small in diameter. In fact, their walls are made of only one layer of endothelial cell; as such, red blood cells must pass through capillaries in single file. Capillaries, not arteries or veins, permit the exchange of materials between the blood and the body's cells. Their small size and thinness of the endothelium assist in the diffusion of material through the walls. Also, some of the liquid component of blood seeps from capillaries, bathing cells with nutrients. Proteins and cells are too large to pass into tissue and stay in the blood within the capillary walls. Some of the fluid that enters tissues passes directly into the blood at the other end of the capillary, and the rest circulates in the lymphatic system. If the capillaries are too permeable or too much liquid stays in the tissues, swelling results.

At times, diverse tissues require differing blood flow. The body regulates much blood flow in tissues locally. Arterioles that feed capillaries in tissue have smooth muscle in their walls that can relax or constrict to allow more or less blood into a specific area. Factors like the level of oxygen and carbon dioxide in blood that are affected by metabolic activity also act on the arteriole smooth muscle, matching blood flow to the metabolic needs of the tissue.

### Lymphatic System

**Lymph vessels** are the foundation for the lymphatic system, which is independent of the circulatory system. This system carries extracellular fluid (at this stage known as **lymph**) at very low pressure, without cells. The **lymph nodes** are responsible for filtering lymph to rid it of foreign particles, maintaining the proper balance of fluids in tissues of the body, and transporting chylomicrons as part of fat metabolism. The system ultimately returns lymph to the blood system via the largest lymph vessel, the thoracic duct, which empties lymph back into circulation shortly before it enters the heart.

## Blood

The fluid moved through the body by the circulatory system is blood, which is composed of a liquid component, plasma, and cells. The cells include red blood cells (**erythrocytes**), **platelets**, and white blood cells (**lymphocytes**). Each of these types of cells has specific functions. **Plasma** is composed of water, salts, proteins, glucose, hormones, lipids, and other soluble factors. The main salts in plasma are sodium chloride and potassium chloride; because of this, it has been noted that plasma is similar in composition to seawater, our evolutionary origin. Calcium is another important element in extracellular fluid, including blood. The body regulates the blood volume and salt content through water intake and through excretion of urine.

Oxygen is dissolved as a gas to a small extent in blood, although most oxygen is transported bound to hemoglobin in red blood cells. Carbon dioxide is converted to carbonic acid in the blood. Glucose present in blood is transported as dissolved sugar for cells to uptake as needed. Hormones are transported through blood from the tissue from which they are secreted to the tissues where they exert their actions. The protein component of plasma consists of antibodies for immune responses, fibrinogen for clotting, and serum albumin. The protein component of blood helps draw water into blood in the capillaries, preventing loss of fluid from the blood into the tissues, which would cause swelling.

**Red blood cells** are the most abundant cells present in blood, and their primary function is to transport oxygen. After they are formed in the bone marrow, mature red blood cells (**erythrocytes**) lose their nuclei and become biconcave discs. They live for about four months in the circulatory system before they are worn out and destroyed in the spleen. Without a nucleus, mature red blood cells cannot make new proteins to repair themselves. Red blood cells also lose mitochondria, which renders them incapable of performing aerobic respiration. If they were able to carry on this form of respiration, they would use up the oxygen they carry to the tissues of the body. Instead, they produce energy in the form of ATP without using oxygen, through the process of glycolysis.

The oxygen-carrying component of red blood cells is the protein **hemoglobin**. In the lungs, where the partial pressure of oxygen is high, hemoglobin readily picks up oxygen. In the tissues, where the partial pressure of oxygen is low, oxygen leaves hemoglobin to diffuse into tissues. The hemoglobin molecule has evolved to deliver oxygen more efficiently in response to changes in tissues. During periods of great metabolic activity in muscle, the pH of the blood can decrease and carbon dioxide increase, both of which tend to reduce the affinity of hemoglobin for oxygen and cause it to leave more oxygen in the tissue.

### Blood Types

Red blood cells manufacture two prominent types of antigens, antigen A (associated with blood type A) and antigen B (blood type B). In any given individual, one, both, or neither antigen may be present.

The plasma of every individual also contains antibodies for the antigens that are not present in the individual's red blood cells (if an individual were to produce antibodies against his or her own red cells, they would agglutinate and the blood would clump). People with type A blood have anti-B antibodies, and individuals with type B blood produce anti-A antibodies. Those with type O blood have neither A nor B antigens; rather, they have both anti-A and anti-B antibodies. People with type AB blood have neither type of antibody.

### Immune System

The interior of the body is an ideal growth medium for some pathogenic organisms, such as disease-causing bacteria and viruses. To prevent this, the body has defenses that either prevent organisms from getting into the interior of the body or stop them from proliferating if they are within the body. The system that plays this protective role is called the **immune system**. The trick for the immune system is to be able to mount aggressive defenses, and, at the same time, to distinguish foreign bodies to avoid attacking one's own tissues and causing disease. Autoimmune disorders cause the body's immune system to assault its own tissue as if it were a foreign invader.

**Passive immune** defenses are barriers to entry. These include the skin, the lining of the lungs, the mouth, and stomach. The skin is a very effective barrier to most potential pathogens, but if wounded, the barrier function of skin is lost. This is why burn patients are very susceptible to infection. The lungs are a potential route of entry, but are patrolled by immune cells, and have mucus to trap invaders; the cilia lining the respiratory tract removes trapped invaders.

**Active immunity** is conferred by the cellular part of the immune system. White blood cells are actually several different cell types that are involved in the defense of the body against foreign organisms in different ways. White blood cells include **phagocytes**, which engulf bacteria with amoeboid motion, and **lymphocytes**. There are several types of lymphocytes, but the most abundant are B and T cells, which are involved in immune responses. B cells produce **antibodies**, or **immunoglobins**, which are secreted proteins specific to foreign molecules such as viral or bacterial proteins. T cells, often referred to as helper cells, coordinate immune responses, while "killer" T cells directly dispose of cells that are infected with intracellular pathogens, such as viruses, or cells that are aberrant, such as malignant cells. These lymphocytes respond to a specific antigen. Since the body does not know what antigens or pathogens may attack it, the immune system creates a varied population of B and T cells in which each cell recognizes only one antigen, but the population of cells contains a huge range of specificities. If a B cell or T cell encounters an antigen that matches its specificity, then it is stimulated to proliferate and create more cells with the same specificity. This amplification of a clone of cells that respond to the invading antigen helps the body respond and remain immune from future infections by the same pathogen. When a B cell encounters an antigen it recognizes, it proliferates to make more B cells that produce antibody. The stimulated B cells also produce memory cells that do not make antibody, but have the same specificity and will lie dormant for many years, ready to respond if the body is challenged again with the same antigen.

## Respiration

Cells performing aerobic respiration require oxygen and need to eliminate carbon dioxide. To do this, organisms must exchange gases with the environment. The respiratory system provides oxygen and removes $CO_2$. The oxygen is used to drive electron transport and ATP production, and $CO_2$ is produced from burning glucose. No human can live without breathing for more than a few minutes.

### Respiration in Humans

Humans have developed a complex system of respiration to transport oxygen to their cells and rid their bodies of waste products like carbon dioxide. The **lungs** are designed to move air between the exterior atmosphere and an interior air space that is in close contact with capillaries. Here, oxygen and carbon dioxide diffuse between the blood and air; blood circulates through the body to exchange gases with the tissues, and then returns to the lungs. The lungs are found in a sealed cavity in the chest, bound by the ribs, chest wall, and the muscular **diaphragm** on the bottom. The diaphragm is curved upward when released, and flattens when contracted, expanding the chest cavity. During inhalation, chest muscles move the ribs up and out as the diaphragm moves down; this creates both a larger chest cavity and a vacuum that draws air into the respiratory passages. The reverse process decreases the size of the chest cavity and forces air out of the lungs (exhalation). Exhalation is largely a passive process that does not require muscle contraction. During exhalation the elasticity of the lungs draws the chest and diaphragm inward when the muscles relax, decreasing the volume of the lungs and causing air to be forced out. The breathing rate is controlled by the **medulla oblongata**, the part of the brain that monitors carbon dioxide content in the blood. Excess $CO_2$ in the blood stimulates the medulla to send messages to the rib muscles and the diaphragm to increase the frequency of respiration.

The air passages involved in respiration consist of the **nose, pharynx, larynx, trachea, bronchi, bronchioles,** and the **alveoli**. The **nose** adds moisture and warmth to inhaled air, and helps to filter it, removing particulates and organisms before the air passes to the next air passage. The **pharynx** is involved in diverting ingested material into the esophagus and away from the lungs to prevent choking. The **larynx** contains a membrane that vibrates in a controlled manner with the passage of air to create the voice. The **trachea** carries air through the vulnerable throat protected by flexible but strong rings of cartilage. At the end of the trachea the respiratory passage splits into the two lungs and into smaller and smaller passages that terminate in the **alveoli**, tiny air sacs that are the site of gas exchange in the lungs.

The alveoli have thin, moist walls and are surrounded by thin-walled capillaries. Oxygen passes into the blood by diffusion through the alveolar and capillary walls; $CO_2$ and $H_2O$ pass out in the same manner. Note that all exchanges at the alveoli involve passive diffusion. Since passive diffusion drives gas exchange, both in the lungs as well as the tissues, gases always diffuse from higher to lower concentration. In the tissues, $O_2$ diffuses into tissues and $CO_2$ leaves, while in the lungs this is reversed due to high oxygen pressure and low $CO_2$ levels. $CO_2$ is carried in blood mainly as dissolved carbonate ions.

## Thermoregulation and the Skin

In humans, the **skin** protects the body from microbial invasion and environmental stresses like dry weather and wind. Specialized epidermal cells called **melanocytes** synthesize the pigment **melanin**, which protects the body from ultraviolet light. The skin is a receptor of stimuli, such as pressure and temperature, is an excretory organ (removing excess water and salts from the body), and also a thermoregulatory organ (helping control both the conservation and release of heat). **Sweat glands** secrete a mixture of water, dissolved salts, and urea via sweat pores. As sweat evaporates, the skin is cooled. Thus, sweating has both an excretory and thermoregulatory function. Sweating is under autonomic (involuntary) nervous control.

Subcutaneous fat in the **hypodermis** insulates the body. Hair entraps and retains warm air at the skin's surface. Hormones such as epinephrine can increase the metabolic rate, thereby increasing heat production. In addition, muscles can generate heat by contracting rapidly (shivering). Heat loss can be inhibited through the constriction of blood vessels (**vasoconstriction**) in the **dermis**, moving blood away from the cooling atmosphere. Likewise, dilation of these same blood vessels (**vasodilation**) dissipates heat.

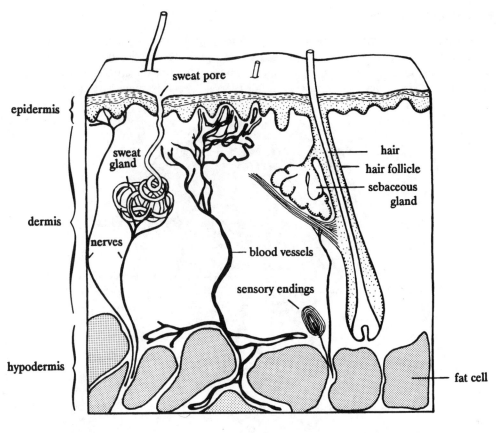

Human Skin

## Excretion

Excretion is the term given to the removal of metabolic wastes produced in the body. (Note that it is to be distinguished from elimination, which is the removal of indigestible materials.) Sources of metabolic waste are listed in the table below.

| Waste | Metabolic Activity Producing the Waste |
|---|---|
| Carbon dioxide | Aerobic respiration |
| Water | Aerobic respiration, dehydration synthesis |
| Nitrogenous wastes (urea, ammonia, uric acid) | Deamination of amino acids |
| Mineral salts | All metabolic processes |

## Human Excretory System

The principle organs of excretion in humans are the **kidneys**. The kidneys form urine to remove nitrogenous wastes in the form of urea; they also regulate the volume and salt content of the extracellular fluids. From the kidney the urine passes into a **ureter tube** leading to the **urinary bladder**, where urine is stored until urination occurs. During urination, the urine leaves the bladder through the **urethra**.

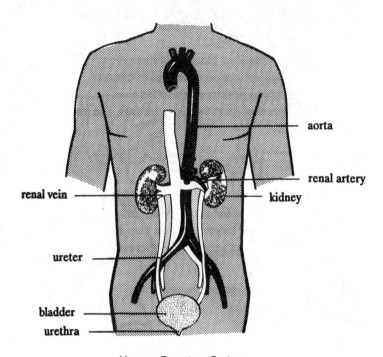

Human Excretory System

## Endocrine System

The body has two communication systems to coordinate the activities of different tissues and organs, the nervous system and the **endocrine system**. The endocrine system is the network of glands and tissues that secrete **hormones**, chemical messengers produced in one tissue and carried by the blood to act on other parts of the body. Compared to the nervous system, the signals conveyed by the endocrine system take much more time to take effect. A nervous impulse is produced in a millisecond and travels anywhere in the body in less than a second. Hormones require time to be synthesized, can travel no more quickly than the blood can carry them, and often cause actions through inducing protein synthesis or transcription, activities that require time. However, hormone signals tend to be more long lasting than nerve impulses. When the nerve impulse ends, a target such as skeletal muscle usually returns quickly to its starting state. When a hormone induces protein synthesis, the proteins remain long after the hormone is gone. Often the two systems work together. The **endocrine glands**, such as the pancreas or the adrenal cortex, can be the direct targets (effectors) of the autonomic nervous system. The hormone adrenaline acts in concert with the sympathetic nervous system to produce a set of results similar to those produced by sympathetic neurons.

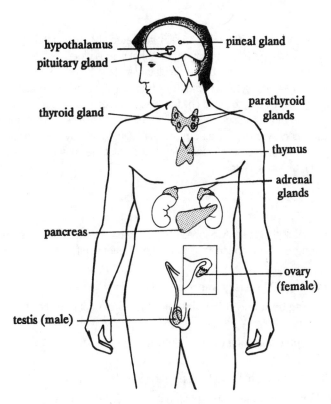

hypothalamus

pineal gland

pituitary gland

thyroid gland

parathyroid glands

thymus

adrenal glands

pancreas

ovary (female)

testis (male)

**Human Endocrine System**

Endocrine glands secrete hormones directly into the bloodstream. This is in contrast to **exocrine secretions** that do not contain hormones and are released through ducts into a body compartment. An example of exocrine secretion is the release of digestive enzymes by the pancreas into the small intestine through the pancreatic duct. Both endocrine and exocrine functions can be found in the same organ. The pancreas simultaneously produces exocrine secretions, such as digestive enzymes, and endocrine secretions, such as insulin and glucagon, which are released into the blood to exert their effects throughout the body.

Hormones are secreted by a variety of tissues, including the **hypothalamus, pituitary, thyroid, parathyroids, adrenals, pancreas, testes, ovaries, pineal, kidneys, heart,** and **thymus**. It is likely that additional tissues like skin and fat, though not traditionally considered glands, also have endocrine functions. Some hormones regulate a single type of cell or organ, while others have more widespread actions. The specificity of hormonal action is determined by the presence of specific receptors on or in the target cells. A common principle that regulates the production and secretion of many hormones is the **feedback loop**. Often several hormones regulate each other in a chain.

### Hypothalamus

The **hypothalamus**, a section of the posterior forebrain, is located above the pituitary gland and is intimately associated with it via a portal circulatory system that carries blood directly from the hypothalamus to the pituitary. In most parts of the circulatory system, blood flows directly back to the heart from capillaries, but in a portal system blood flows from capillaries in one organ to capillaries in another. When the hypothalamus is stimulated (by feedback from endocrine glands or by neurons innervating it), it releases hormone-like substances called **releasing factors** into the anterior pituitary-hypothalamic portal circulatory system. These hormones are carried directly to the pituitary by the portal system. In their turn, these releasing factors stimulate cells of the anterior pituitary to secrete the hormone indicated by the releasing factor.

### Pituitary

The **pituitary gland** is a small gland with two lobes lying at the base of the brain. The two lobes, anterior and posterior, function as independent glands. The anterior pituitary secretes several hormones.

- **Growth hormone** (GH) fosters growth in a variety of body tissues.
- **Thyroid stimulating hormone** (TSH) stimulates the thyroid gland to secrete its own hormone, thyroxine.
- **Adrenocorticotrophic hormone** (ACTH) stimulates the adrenal cortex to secrete its corticoids.
- **Prolactin** is responsible for milk production by the female mammary glands.
- **Follicle-stimulating hormone** (FSH) spurs maturation of seminiferous tubules in males and causes maturation of ovaries in females. It also encourages maturation of follicles in the ovaries.
- **Luteinizing hormone** (LH) induces interstitial cells of the testes to mature by beginning to secrete the male sex hormone testosterone. In females, a surge of LH stimulates ovulation of the primary oocyte from the follicle. LH then induces changes in the follicular cells and converts an old follicle into a yellowish mass of cells rich in blood vessels. This new structure is the **corpus luteum**, which subsequently secretes progesterone and estrogen.

The **posterior pituitary** is a direct extension of nervous tissue from the hypothalamus. Nerve signals cause direct hormone release. The two hormones secreted by the posterior pituitary are ADH and oxytocin.

- **Antidiuretic hormone** (ADH), also known as vasopressin, acts on the kidney to reduce water loss.
- **Oxytocin** acts on the uterus during birth to cause uterine contraction.

### Thyroid

The thyroid hormone, **thyroxine**, is a modified amino acid that contains four atoms of iodine. It accelerates oxidative metabolism throughout the body. An abnormal deficiency of thyroxine causes goiter, decreased heart rate, lethargy, obesity, and decreased mental alertness. In contrast, hyperthyroidism (too much thyroxine) is characterized by profuse perspiration, high body temperature, increased basal metabolic rate, high blood pressure, loss of weight, and irritability.

### Parathyroid Glands

The parathyroid glands are small pea-like organs located on the posterior surface of the thyroid. They secrete parathyroid hormone, which regulates calcium and phosphate balance in blood, bones, and other tissues. Increased parathyroid hormone increases bone formation. Plasma calcium must be maintained at a constant level for the function of muscles and neurons.

### Pancreas

The pancreas is a multifunctional organ. It has both an **exocrine** and an **endocrine function**. The exocrine function of the pancreas secretes enzymes through ducts into the small intestine. The endocrine function, on the other hand, secretes hormones directly into the bloodstream. The endocrine function of the pancreas is centered in the **islets of Langerhans**, localized collections of endocrine alpha and beta cells that secrete glucagon and insulin respectively. **Insulin** stimulates the muscles to remove glucose from the blood when glucose concentrations are high, such as after a meal. Insulin is also responsible for spurring muscles and the liver to convert glucose to glycogen, the stored form of glucose. The islets of Langerhans also secrete **glucagon**, which responds to low concentrations of blood glucose by stimulating the breakdown of glycogen into glucose, keeping the level of glucose in blood high enough to supply tissues.

### Adrenal Glands

The adrenal glands are situated on top of the kidneys and consist of the **adrenal cortex** and the **adrenal medulla**.

In response to stress, ACTH stimulates the adrenal cortex to synthesize and secrete the steroid hormones collectively known as **corticosteroids**. Corticosteroids are effective anti-inflammatory medicines, but their use is limited by their alterations of fat metabolism and their suppression of the immune system. The adrenal cortex also secretes small quantities of androgens (male sex hormones) in both males and females. Since, in males, testes produce most of the androgens, the physiologic effect of the adrenal androgens is quite small. In females, however, overproduction of the adrenal androgens may have masculinizing effects, such as excessive facial hair.

The secretory cells of the adrenal medulla can be viewed as specialized sympathetic nerve cells that secrete hormones into the circulatory system. This organ produces **epinephrine** (adrenaline) and **norepinephrine** (noradrenaline).

Epinephrine increases the conversion of glycogen to glucose in liver and muscle tissue, causing a rise in blood glucose levels and an increase in the basal metabolic rate. Both epinephrine and norepinephrine increase the rate and strength of the heartbeat, as well as dilate and constrict blood vessels. These in turn increase the blood supply to skeletal muscles, the heart, and the brain, while decreasing the blood supply to the kidneys, skin, and digestive tract. These effects are known as the "**fight-or-flight response**," and are elicited by sympathetic nervous stimulation in response to stress. Both of these hormones are also neurotransmitters.

### Ovaries and Testes

The gonads are important endocrine glands, with testes producing testosterone in males and ovaries producing estrogen in females. See the section on reproduction earlier in this lesson for more details.

## Nervous System

The nervous system enables organisms to receive and respond to stimuli from their external and internal environments. Your brain and spinal column regulate your breathing, your movement, and your perception of sight, sound, touch, smell, and taste. They allow organisms to not only perceive their environment but to respond to their experience, and alter their behavior over time through learning.

### Functional Units of the Nervous System

To understand the nervous system, it is best to start with the basic functional unit of the nervous system—the **neuron**. Neurons are specialized cells designed to transmit information in the form of electrochemical signals called **action potentials**. These signals are generated when neurons alter the voltage found across their plasma membrane. The excitable membrane is the property that allows neurons to carry an action potential.

### Synapses

The nervous system is not simply a network of electrical wires with the brain as the switchboard. There is a strong chemical component to the signals that neurons convey. Neurons do not usually carry the action potential all the way to the membrane of the target cell. When a neuron reaches a target cell, the **axon** ends in a synaptic terminal, with a gap called the **synapse** between the neuron and the target cell. The membrane potential is then converted to a chemical signal, or **neurotransmitter**, that is released across a small gap between the neuron and the target cell. This gap between the neuron and the target cell is called the **synaptic cleft**. The target cell in communication with the neuron then receives the chemical signal by binding the neurotransmitter and starting a signal of its own. There are many types of synapses of neurons with other neurons. For motor neurons in the somatic nervous system, a specialized synapse of motor neurons with skeletal muscle cells is called the **neuromuscular junction**.

### Organization of the Nervous System

As organisms evolve and become more complex, their nervous systems undergo corresponding increases in complexity. Simple organisms can only respond to simple stimuli, while complex organisms like humans can discern subtle variations of a stimulus, such as a particular shade of color.

### Vertebrate Nervous System

Vertebrates have a **brain** enclosed within the **cranium** and a **spinal cord;** together these form the **central nervous system** (CNS) that processes and stores information. Throughout the rest of the body is the **peripheral nervous system**, containing motor or efferent neurons that carry signals to effector organs, such as muscles and glands, to take actions in response to nervous impulses. Sensory neurons in the peripheral nervous system convey information back to the CNS for processing and storage. Another division of the nervous system is between the autonomic and voluntary components of efferent pathways.

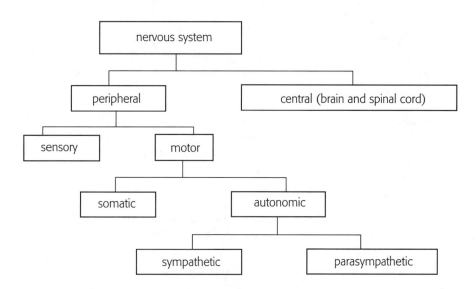

**Organization of the Vertebrate Nervous System**

### Peripheral Nervous System

The peripheral nervous system carries nerves from the CNS to target tissues of the body and includes all neurons that are not part of the CNS. The peripheral nervous system consists of 12 pairs of cranial nerves, which primarily innervate the head and shoulders, and 31 pairs of spinal nerves, which innervate the rest of the body. Cranial nerves exit from the brainstem and spinal nerves exit from the spinal cord. The peripheral nervous system has two primary divisions, the somatic and the autonomic nervous systems.

### Somatic Motor Nervous System

This system innervates skeletal muscle and is responsible for voluntary movement, generally subject to conscious control. Motor neurons release the neurotransmitter acetylcholine (ACh) onto ACh receptors located on skeletal muscle. This causes depolarization of the skeletal muscle, leading to muscle contraction. In addition to voluntary movement, the somatic nervous system is also important for reflex action.

### Autonomic Nervous System

The autonomic nervous system is neither structurally nor functionally isolated from the CNS or the peripheral system. Its function is to regulate the involuntary functions of the body, including the heart and blood vessels, the gastrointestinal tract, urogenital organs, structures involved in respiration, and the intrinsic muscles of the eye. In general, the autonomic system innervates glands and smooth muscle, but not skeletal muscles. It is made up of the sympathetic nervous system and the parasympathetic nervous system.

### Sympathetic Nervous System

This system utilizes norepinephrine as its primary neurotransmitter. It is responsible for activating the body during emergency situations and actions (the fight-or-flight response), including strengthening of heart contractions, increases in heart rate, dilation of the pupils, bronchodilation, and vasoconstriction of vessels feeding the digestive tract.

One tissue regulated by the sympathetic system is the adrenal gland, which produces adrenaline in response to stimulation. Adrenaline produces many of the same fight-or-flight responses as the sympathetic system alone.

### Parasympathetic Nervous System

Acetylcholine serves as the primary neurotransmitter for the parasympathetic nervous system. One of this system's main functions is to deactivate or slow down the activities of muscles and glands (the rest-and-digest response). These activities include pupillary constriction, slowing down of the heart rate, bronchoconstriction, and vasodilation of vessels feeding the digestive tract. The principal nerve of the parasympathetic system is the vagus nerve. Most of the organs innervated by the autonomic system receive both sympathetic and parasympathetic fibers, the two systems being antagonistic to one another.

## The Human Brain

The human brain is divided into several anatomical regions with different functions.

- **Cerebral cortex.** The cerebral cortex controls all voluntary motor activity by initiating the responses of motor neurons present within the spinal cord. It also controls higher functions, such as memory and creative thought. The cortex is divided into hemispheres, left and right, with some specialization of function between them ("left-brain, right-brain"). The cortex consists of an outer portion containing neuronal cell bodies (gray matter) and an inner portion containing axons (white matter).

- **Olfactory lobe.** This serves as the center for reception and integration of olfactory input.

- **Thalamus.** Nervous impulses and sensory information are relayed and integrated en route to and from the cerebral cortex by this region.

- **Hypothalamus.** Hunger, thirst, pain, temperature regulation, and water balance are visceral and homeostatic functions controlled by this center.

- **Cerebellum.** Muscle activity is coordinated and modulated here.

- **Pons.** This serves as the relay center for cerebral cortical fibers en route to the cerebellum.

- **Medulla oblongata.** This influential region controls vital functions like breathing, heart rate, and gastrointestinal activity. It has receptors to detect carbon dioxide. When carbon dioxide levels become too high, the medulla oblongata forces you to breathe. When you hold your breath for too long and carbon dioxide levels rise in your body, you pass out. The medulla oblongata makes you breathe involuntarily to bring an influx of oxygen into your body.

- **Reticular Activating System.** This network of neurons in the brain stem is involved in processing signals from sensory inputs and transmitting them to the cortex and other regions. This system is also involved in regulating the activity of other brain regions, such as the cortex, in order to alter levels of alertness and attention.

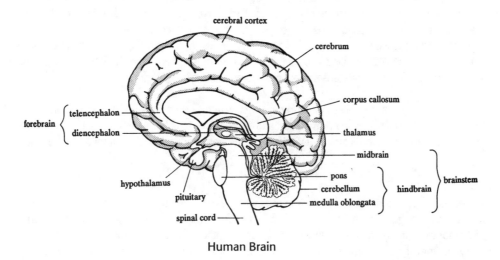

**Human Brain**

The **spinal cord** is also part of the CNS. The spinal cord acts as a route for axons to travel out of the brain. It also serves as a center for many reflex actions that do not involve the brain, such as the **knee-jerk reflex.**

## Sensory Systems of the Nervous System

All complicated nervous systems are made more useful through input mechanisms that we know as our senses. Sight, hearing, balance, taste, smell, and touch provide an influx of data for the nervous system to assimilate. Other sensory information that we are not consciously aware of is also provided to the CNS, including internal conditions such as the management of temperature and carbon dioxide levels. All of these sensory detection systems use cells that are usually specialized, modified neurons to receive information and alter their membrane potential in response to information. This altered membrane potential can then trigger an action potential to carry information back to the CNS. Some sensory cells detect chemical information (taste and smell), some detect electromagnetic energy (vision), and others detect mechanical information (sound, pressure). All sensation is caused by action potentials that are sent to the CNS by sensory cells. An action potential from the eye is the same as an action potential from the ear. The difference in perception, how we experience the information, is determined by how the information is received and processed by the CNS. An action potential from the eye is perceived as sight because it passes to the visual center of the brain for processing.

### Sight

The eye detects light energy and transmits information about intensity, color, and shape to the brain. The transparent **cornea** at the front of the eye bends and focuses light rays. These rays then travel through an opening called the **pupil**, whose diameter is controlled by the pigmented, muscular **iris.**

The iris responds to the intensity of light in the surroundings (light makes the pupil constrict). Light continues through the **lens**, which is suspended behind the pupil. This lens focuses the image onto the **retina**, which contains photoreceptors that transduce light into action potentials. The image on the retina is actually upside down but revision and interpretation in the cerebral cortex result in the perception of the image right-side up. The image from both eyes is also integrated in the cortex to produce the binocular vision with depth perception that allows us to throw, catch, and drive with improved ability. The shape of the lens is changed to focus images from nearby or far objects. To see nearby objects, the muscles attached to the lens are relaxed and the lens rounds up, focusing light more sharply. If the shape of the eye is either too short or too long, or if the lens becomes stiff with age, then the eye is unable to focus the image and corrective lenses may be required to bring images into focus.

There are two types of specialized **photoreceptor cells** in the eye that respond to light: cones and rods. **Cones** respond to high-intensity illumination and are sensitive to color, while **rods** detect low-intensity illumination and are important in night vision. **Optic nerves** conduct visual information to the brain.

### Hearing and Balance

The ear transduces sound energy into impulses that are perceived by the brain as sound. Sound waves pass through three regions as they enter the ear. First, they enter the outer ear, which consists of the **auricle** (pinna) and the **auditory canal**. Located at the end of the auditory canal is the **tympanic membrane** (eardrum) of the middle ear, which vibrates at the same frequency as the incoming sound. Next, three bones, or **ossicles** (malleus, incus, and stapes), amplify the stimulus, and transmit it through an oval window leading to the fluid-filled inner ear.

### Taste and Smell

**Taste buds** are chemical sensory cells located on the tongue, the soft palate, and the epiglottis. The outer surface of a taste bud contains a taste pore, from which microvilli, or taste hairs, protrude. Interwoven around taste buds is a network of nerve fibers that are stimulated by the taste buds, and these neurons transmit impulses to the brainstem. There are four main kinds of taste sensations: sour, salty, sweet, and bitter.

**Olfactory receptors** are chemical sensors found in the olfactory membrane, which lies in the upper part of the nostrils over a total area of about 5 cm$^2$. The receptors are specialized neurons from which olfactory hairs project. When odorous substances enter the nasal cavity, they bind to receptors in the cilia, depolarizing the olfactory receptors. Axons from the olfactory receptors join to form the olfactory nerves, which project to the olfactory bulbs in the base of the brain.

## Motor Systems

One of the key systems of the body is the system of muscles that are effectors for the CNS. To exert an effect muscles also require something to act against, which is the skeletal system.

Vertebrates have an **endoskeleton** as a framework for the attachment of skeletal muscles, permitting movement when a muscle contracts by bringing two bones together—which is the basis for all voluntary movement. The endoskeleton also provides protection, since bones surround delicate, vital organs. For example, the rib cage protects the thoracic organs (heart and lungs), while the skull and vertebral column protect the brain and spinal cord. The vertebrate skeleton contains **cartilage** and **bone**, both formed from connective tissue.

**Cartilage**, although firm, is also flexible and is not as hard or as brittle as bone. It makes up the skeletons of lower vertebrates, such as sharks and rays. In higher animals, cartilage is the principal component of embryonic skeletons, and is replaced during development by the aptly termed replacement bone. Because cartilage has no vessels or nerves, it takes longer to heal than bone.

**Bone** makes up most of the skeleton of mature higher vertebrates, including humans; it is made of calcium, phosphate salts, and strands of the protein collagen. A hollow cavity within each long bone is filled with **bone marrow**, the site where the formation of blood cells takes place. Bones are connected at joints, either immovable, as in the skull, or movable like the hip. In the latter type, ligaments serve as bone-to-bone connectors, while tendons attach skeletal muscle to bones and bend the skeleton at the site of movable joints. In the vertebrate skeleton, the **axial skeleton** is the midline basic framework of the body, consisting of the skull, vertebral column, and the rib cage. The **appendicular skeleton**, on the other hand, includes the bones of the appendages, as well as the pectoral and pelvic girdles.

## Muscle System

The muscle system serves as an effector of the nervous system. Muscles contract to implement actions after they receive nervous stimuli. For example, your arm muscles will automatically contract if you touch a hot stove. A skeletal muscle originates at a point of attachment to a stationary bone. It is this point that moves during contraction. An **extensor** extends or straightens the bones at a joint—for example, straightening out a limb. A **flexor** is a muscle that serves to bend a joint to an acute angle, as in bending the elbow to bring the forearm and upper arm together. Bones and muscles work together like a lever system.

### Types of Muscles

Vertebrates possess three different types of muscle tissues: **smooth**, **skeletal**, and **cardiac**. In all three types, muscles cause movement by contraction, and the sliding of actin and myosin filaments past each other within cells causes the contraction. The differences between the types of muscle include where they are located, what they do, and what the cells look like.

Also known as involuntary muscle, **smooth muscle** is generally found in visceral systems and is innervated by the autonomic nervous system. Each muscle fiber consists of a single cell with one centrally located nucleus. Smooth muscle is nonstriated, meaning it does not have clearly organized arrays of actin and myosin filaments. Smooth muscle is present in the walls of arteries and veins, the walls of the digestive tract, bladder, and uterus. Smooth muscle contracts in response to action potentials, and the contraction is mediated by actin-myosin fibers like in other muscle, although the fibers do not have the clear organization displayed in other muscle types. Smooth muscle cells in tissue are connected to each other through junctions that allow electrical impulses to pass directly from one cell to the next without passing through chemical synapses.

**Skeletal muscles** are also known as voluntary muscles; they produce intentional physical movement. A skeletal muscle cell is a single, large multinucleated fiber containing alternating light and dark bands called **striations**. Overlapping strands of thick myosin protein filaments that slide past thin actin protein filaments during muscle contraction cause these bands. The actin and myosin filaments in skeletal muscle are organized into sections called **sarcomeres** that form contractile units within each muscle cell. The somatic nervous system innervates skeletal muscle. Each skeletal muscle fiber is stimulated by nerves through neuromuscular synapses. When a nerve stimulates a muscle cell, an action potential moves over the whole muscle fiber, releasing calcium in the cytoplasm of the cell. This calcium causes the actin and myosin to slide over each other, shortening the fibers and the cell. Many muscle cells are bundled together to create muscles.

The tissue that makes up the heart is known as cardiac muscle. It has characteristics of both skeletal and smooth muscle. **Cardiac muscle** cells have a single nucleus, like smooth muscle, and are striated like skeletal muscle. Cardiac muscle cells are connected by gap junctions just like smooth muscles are, so cells can pass action potentials directly throughout the heart and do not require chemical synapses. Cardiac muscle contraction is regulated by the autonomic nervous system, which increases the rate and strength of contractions through sympathetic stimulation and decreases their rate through the parasympathetic system. Cardiac muscle has an internal pacemaker responsible for the heartbeat that is modified by the nervous system but does not require the nervous system to maintain a regular heartbeat.

## Plants

Plants are so distinct in their body form and so important to life on Earth that we present their physiology separately. Plants are multicellular autotrophs that use the energy of the sun, carbon dioxide, water, and minerals to manufacture carbohydrates through photosynthesis. The chemical energy plants produce is used for respiration by the plants themselves and is the source of all chemical energy in most ecosystems. The life cycle of vascular plants is distinct from that of animals, alternating between diploid and haploid forms in each generation.

### Plant Organs

Although we may not usually think of plants as having organs, the fact is that roots, stems, and leaves each have a defined function and are composed of tissues that perform distinct functions, in the same manner as animal organs. Stems provide support against gravity and allow for the transport of fluid through vascular tissue. Water travels upward from the roots to the leaves and nutrients travel from the leaves down through the rest of the plant. The roots provide anchoring support, and also remove water and essential minerals from the soil. Another important plant tissue is the **phloem**. The phloem transports nutrients from the leaves to the rest of the plant. This nutrient liquid is commonly called sap. Cells present in the phloem are alive when they perform their transport function. The phloem cells are tube-shaped; liquid sap moves through the tube-shaped cells. Like terrestrial animals, plants need a protective coating. For plants, an external layer of epidermis cells provides this. Another plant tissue is the **ground tissue**, involved in storage and support.

### Plant Cells

Plant cells have all of the same essential organelles as other eukaryotic cells, including mitochondria, ER, Golgi, and nucleus. A major distinction of plant cells is the presence of the photosynthetic organelle known as the **chloroplast**. Some plant cells contain large storage vacuoles not found in animal cells. Another distinct feature of plant cells is their cell wall. On the outside of its plasma membrane, each plant cell is surrounded by a stiff cell wall made of **cellulose**. The cellulose cell wall helps to provide structure and support for the plant. From grasses to trees, plants rely on the cellulose present in cell walls to help provide support against gravity.

### Phyla

Within the plant kingdom there are several major phyla. One of the major distinctions for these plant groups is whether or not a plant has vascular tissue for the transport of fluids. Plants without vascular tissue are small, simple plants called **nontracheophytes**; mosses are an example of this group. The rest of plants—including pines, ferns, and flowering plants—are known as **tracheophytes**. The evolution of vascular tissue was an important step in the colonization of land by plants, since it increases the support of plants against gravity, and increases their ability to survive dry conditions. Ferns are a phylum of tracheophytes that do not produce seeds for reproduction—they employ spores instead.

### Asexual Reproduction in Plants

Many plants utilize asexual reproduction, such as **vegetative propagation**, to increase their numbers. Vegetative propagation offers a number of advantages to plants, including speed of reproduction, lack of genetic variation, and the ability to produce seedless fruit. This process can occur either naturally or artificially.

### Sexual Reproduction in Plants

Most plants are able to reproduce both sexually and asexually; some do both in the course of their life cycles, while others do one or the other. In the life cycles of mosses, ferns, and other vascular plants, there are two stages associated with life cycles: **diploid** and **haploid**.

### Diploid and Haploid Generations

In the diploid or **sporophyte** generation, the asexual stage of a plant's life cycle, diploid nuclei divide meiotically to form haploid spores (not gametes) and the spores germinate to produce the haploid (or gametophyte) generation. The **gametophyte** generation is a separate haploid form of the plant concerned with the production of male and female gametes. Union of the gametes at fertilization restores the diploid sporophyte generation. Since there are two distinct generations, one haploid and the other diploid, this cycle is sometimes referred to as the **alternation of generations**. The relative lengths of the two stages vary with the plant type. In general, the evolutionary trend has been toward a reduction of the gametophyte generation, and increasing importance of the sporophyte generation.

### Sexual Reproduction in Flowering Plants

In flowering plants, also known as angiosperms, the evolutionary trend mentioned above continues; the gametophyte consists of only a few cells and survives for a very short time.

### Flowers

The flower is the organ for sexual reproduction present in angiosperms; it consists of male and female organs. The flower's male organ is known as the **stamen**. It consists of a thin, stalk-like filament with a sac at the top. This structure is called the **anther**, and it produces haploid spores. The haploid spores develop into pollen grains. The haploid nuclei within the spores become sperm nuclei, which fertilize the ovum. Meanwhile, the flower's female organ is termed a **pistil**. It consists of three parts: the **stigma**, the **style**, and the **ovary**. The stigma is the sticky top part of the flower, protruding beyond the flower, which catches pollen. The tube-like structure connecting the stigma to the ovary at the base of the pistil is known as the style; this organ permits the sperm to reach the ovules. And the ovary, the enlarged base of the pistil, contains one or more ovules. Each ovule contains the monoploid egg nucleus.

**Petals** are specialized leaves that surround and protect the pistil. They attract insects with their characteristic colors and odors. This attraction is essential for cross-pollination—that is, the transfer of pollen from the anther of one flower to the stigma of another (introducing genetic variability). Note that some species of plants have flowers that contain only stamens (these plants are known as male plants) while others contain only pistils (these are known as female plants).

**Male gametophytes** (pollen grains) develop from the spores made by the sporophyte (for example, a rose bush). Pollen grains are transferred from the anther to the stigma. Agents of cross-pollination include insects, wind, and water. The flower's reproductive organ is brightly colored and fragrant in order to attract insects and birds, which help to spread male gametophytes. Pollen being carried directly from plant to plant is more efficient than relying on wind to do so; it also helps to prevent self-pollination, which does not create diversity. When the pollen grain reaches the stigma (pollination), it releases enzymes that enable it to absorb and utilize both food and water from the stigma, as well as to germinate a pollen tube. The pollen tube is what remains of the evolutionary gametophyte. The pollen's enzymes proceed to digest a path down the pistil to the ovary. Within the pollen tube are the haploid tube nucleus and two sperm nuclei. **Female gametophytes** develop in the ovule from one of four spores. This embryo sac contains nuclei, including the two polar (**endosperm**) nuclei and an egg nucleus.

The gametes involved in fertilization are nuclei, not complete cells. The sperm nucleus of the male gametophyte (pollen tube) enters the female gametophyte (embryo sac), and double fertilization occurs. One sperm nucleus fuses with the egg nucleus to form the diploid zygote, which develops into the embryo. The other sperm nucleus fuses with the two polar bodies to form the **endosperm** (**triploid** or **3n**). The endosperm provides food for the embryonic plant. In dicotyledonous plants, the endosperm is absorbed by the seed leaves (**cotyledons**).

There is definitely more to know about flowers, but for now, this should cover the topics you might face on your nursing school entrance exam.

## Classical Genetics

The study of patterns and mechanisms in the transmission of inherited traits from one generation to another is known as classical genetics. The foundations for this field were laid by the monk Gregor Mendel, who in the mid-nineteenth century performed a series of experiments to determine the rules of inheritance in garden pea plants.

The study of classical genetics requires an understanding of **meiosis**, the mechanism of gamete formation. Mendel knew that alleles are inherited from each parent, and that these alleles were somehow linked to the various characteristics he studied in peas, but it was not until meiosis was truly elucidated that the mechanisms behind heredity were understood.

## Meiosis

During asexual reproduction, a single diploid cell is used to create new identical copies of an organism. Two parents contributing to the genome of offspring characterize sexual reproduction, the end result being offspring that are genetically unique. This process requires that each parent contribute a cell with one copy of the genome. **Meiosis** is the process whereby these sex cells are produced.

As in mitosis, the gametocyte's chromosomes are replicated during the **S phase** of the cell cycle. The first round of division (**meiosis I**) produces two intermediate daughter cells. The second round of division (**meiosis II**) involves the separation of the sister chromatids, resulting in four genetically distinct haploid gametes. In this way, a diploid cell produces haploid daughter cells. Since meiosis reduces the number of chromosomes in each cell from $2n$ to $1n$, it is sometimes called **reductive division**. Each meiotic division has the same four stages as mitosis, although it goes through each of them twice (except for DNA replication). The stages of meiosis are detailed in the following paragraphs.

### Interphase I

Gametocyte chromosomes are replicated during the S phase of the cell cycle, while the centrioles replicate at some point during interphase.

### Prophase I

During this stage, chromatin condenses into chromosomes, the spindle apparatus forms, and both the nucleolus and nuclear membrane disappear. Homologous chromosomes (matching chromosomes that code for the same traits, one inherited from each parent) come together and intertwine during a process called **synapsis**. At this stage each chromosome consists of two sister chromatids, and each synaptic pair of homologous chromosomes contains four chromatids—which is why the pairs are often called **tetrads**.

Sometimes chromatids of homologous chromosomes break at corresponding points and exchange equivalent pieces of DNA; this process is called **crossing over** or **recombination**. Note that crossing over occurs between homologous chromosomes and not between sister chromatids of the same chromosomes. The chromatids involved are left with an altered but structurally complete set of genes. The chromosomes remain joined at the points where crossing over occurred, known as chiasmata. Such genetic recombination can "unlink" linked genes, thereby increasing the variety of genetic combinations that can be produced via gametogenesis. Recombination among chromosomes results in increased genetic diversity within a species. Note that sister chromatids are no longer identical after recombination has occurred.

### Metaphase I

Homologous pairs (tetrads) align at the equatorial plane of dividing cells, and each pair attaches to a separate spindle fiber by its kinetochore.

### Anaphase I

Homologous pairs separate and are pulled to opposite poles of the cell. This process is called **disjunction**, and it accounts for a fundamental Mendelian law. During disjunction, each chromosome of paternal origin separates (or disjoins) from its homologue of maternal origin, and either chromosome can end up in either daughter cell. Thus, the distribution of homologous chromosomes to the two intermediate daughter cells is random with respect to parental origin. Each daughter cell will have a unique pool of alleles provided by a random mixture of maternal and paternal origin. These genes may code for alternative forms of a given trait.

### Telophase I and Cytokinesis

A nuclear membrane forms around each new nucleus. At this point, each chromosome still consists of sister chromatids joined at the centromere. Next, the cell divides into two daughter cells through the process of cytokinesis. Each daughter receives a nucleus containing the haploid number of chromosomes. Between cell divisions there may be a short rest period, or interkinesis, during which the chromosomes partially uncoil.

### Prophase II

The centrioles migrate to opposite poles and the spindle apparatus forms.

### Metaphase II

The chromosomes line up along the equatorial plane once again. The centromeres divide, separating the chromosomes into pairs of sister chromatids.

### Anaphase II

The sister chromatids are pulled to opposite poles by spindle fibers.

### Telophase II

Finally, a nuclear membrane forms around each new haploid nucleus. Cytokinesis follows and two daughter cells are formed. Thus, by the time meiosis is completed, four haploid daughter cells are produced per gametocyte. In females, only one of these becomes a functional gamete.

The diagram on the following page summarizes the various stages of meiosis I and meiosis II. Notice that the random distribution of homologous chromosomes in meiosis, coupled with crossing over in prophase I, enables an individual to produce gametes with many different genetic combinations. Every gamete gets one copy of each chromosome, but the copy of each chromosome found in a gamete is random. For example, each gamete has a chromosome #9, but this chromosome can be either of the two copies of this chromosome. With 22 autosomal chromosomes, this factor alone allows for $2^{22}$ possible gametes, not including the additional genetic diversity created by recombination. This is why sexual reproduction produces genetic variability in offspring, as opposed to asexual reproduction, which produces identical offspring. The possibility of so many different genetic combinations is believed to increase the capability of a species to evolve and adapt to a changing environment.

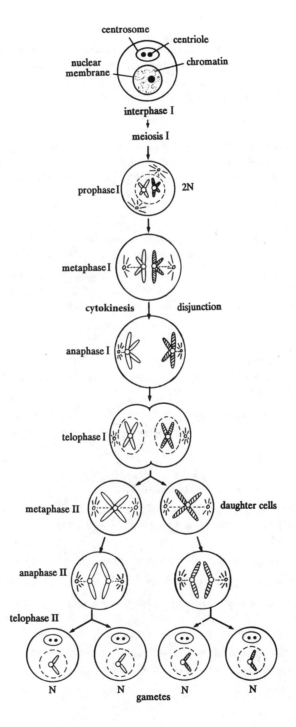

centrosome
centriole
nuclear membrane
chromatin
interphase I
meiosis I
prophase I — 2N
metaphase I
cytokinesis — disjunction
anaphase I
telophase I
metaphase II — daughter cells
anaphase II
telophase II
N — N — N — N
gametes

Meiosis

## Mendelian Genetics

Around 1865, based on his observations of seven characteristics of the garden pea, Gregor Mendel developed the basic principles of genetics—**dominance, segregation**, and **independent assortment**. Although Mendel formulated these principles, he was unable to propose any mechanism for hereditary patterns, since he knew nothing about chromosomes or genes. Hence his work was largely ignored until the early 1900s.

After Mendel's work was rediscovered, Thomas H. Morgan tied the principles of genetics to the chromosome theory. He linked particular traits to regions of specific chromosomes visible in the salivary glands of the fruit fly *Drosophila melanogaster*. Morgan brought to light the giant chromosomes that are found in the fruit fly's salivary glands—they are at least 100 times the size of normal chromosomes. These chromosomes are banded, and the bands coincide with gene locations, allowing geneticists to see major changes in the fly genome. Morgan also described sex-linked genes. The fruit fly is a highly suitable organism for genetic research. With its short life cycle, it reproduces often and in large numbers, providing large sample sizes. It is easy to breed in a laboratory, and has a fairly complex body structure. Its chromosomes are large and easily recognizable in both size and shape, but few in number (eight chromosomes and four pairs of chromosomes). Finally, mutations occur relatively frequently in this organism, allowing genes of affected traits to be studied.

There are several basic rules of gene transmission and expression.

- **Genes** are elements of DNA that are responsible for observed traits.
- In eukaryotes, genes are found in large, linear chromosomes, and each chromosome is a very long, continuous DNA double helix.
- Humans have 23 different chromosomes, with two copies of each chromosome in most cells.
- Each chromosome contains a specific sequence and arrangement of genes.
- Each gene has a specific location on a chromosome.
- Diploid organisms have two copies of each chromosome and therefore two copies of each gene (except for the **X** and **Y** chromosomes in males).
- The two copies of each gene can have a different sequence in an organism and a gene can have several different sequences in a population. These different versions of a gene are called **alleles**.
- The type of alleles an organism has—that is, its genetic composition—is called the **genotype**.
- The appearance and physical expression of genes in an organism is called the **phenotype**.
- Types of alleles include dominant and recessive alleles. A dominant allele is expressed in an organism regardless of the second allele in the organism. A recessive allele will not be expressed if the other allele an organism carries is a dominant one.
- A **homozygous** individual has two copies (two alleles) of a gene that are identical and a **heterozygous** individual has two different alleles for a gene.
- The phenotype of an individual is determined by the genotype.

## Dominant Versus Recessive

If two members of a pure-breeding strain are mated, their offspring will always have the same phenotype as their parents because they are all homozygous for the same allele. What happens if two different pure-breeding strains that are homozygous for two different alleles are crossed? A good example is a flower that has its color determined by two different alleles. All of the offspring of the cross match utilize the phenotype of one parent and not the other. For example, if a pure-breeding red strain is crossed with a pure-breeding white one, the offspring may all be red. Where did the allele coding for the white trait go? Did it disappear from the offspring? If it is true that both parents contribute one copy of a gene to each of their offspring, then the allele cannot disappear. The offspring must all contain both a white allele and a red allele. Despite having both alleles, they only express one. To continue the example, the red allele would be considered the dominant allele and white a recessive allele.

Every human has two copies of each of their 23 chromosomes, with the exception of the **X** and **Y** chromosome in men. Thus, each gene is present in two copies that can either be the same, or different. For example, a gene for eye color could have two alleles: **B** or **b**. **B** is a **dominant allele** for brown eye color and **b** is a **recessive allele** for blue eye color. There are three potential genotypes: **BB**, **Bb**, or **bb**. Individuals with the BB or Bb genotype have brown eyes. Because the **B** allele is dominant and the recessive **b** allele is not expressed in the heterozygote. Only people with the homozygous **bb** genotype have blue eyes.

## Test Crosses

Often, a geneticist will study the transmission of a trait in a species by performing crosses (matings) between organisms with defined traits. For example, an investigator may identify two possible phenotypes for flower color in pea plants: pink and white. Pink plants bred together always produce pink offspring and white plants bred together always produce offspring with white flowers. It is likely that the differences in flower color are caused by different alleles in a gene that controls flower color. Which of these traits is determined by a recessive or dominant allele? You cannot tell based on the color alone which trait will be dominant or recessive. Either pink or white could be dominant—or neither. The way to determine the dominant or recessive nature of each allele is by performing a test cross. Since the pink plants always produce pink plants and the white plants always produce white plants, these are both termed **pure-breeding** plants and are each homozygous for either the **P** allele (**PP** genotype has a pink phenotype) or for the **p** allele (**pp** genotype has a white phenotype). What will be the phenotype of a plant with the **Pp** genotype?

## Punnett Square

When performing a test cross, a useful tool is called a **Punnett Square**. To perform a Punnett Square, first determine the possible gametes each parent in the cross can produce. In the example above, a **PP** parent can only make gametes with the **P** allele and the **pp** parent can only make gametes with the **p** allele:

- **PP** parent: Gametes have either one **P** allele or the other **P** allele.
- **pp** parent: Gametes have either one **p** allele or the other **p** allele.

The next step is to examine all of the ways these gametes could combine if these two parents were mated together in a test cross. This is where the Punnett Square comes in. On one side of the square, align the gametes from one parent, and on the other side of the square align the gametes from the other parent. At the intersection of each potential gamete pairing, fill in the square with the diploid zygote produced by matching the alleles. In this example, all of the offspring of this cross are going to be heterozygous.

If all of the offspring are pink, what does this reveal about the nature of these alleles? If the heterozygous **Pp** plant has the same phenotype as the homozygous **PP** plant, then the **P** allele is dominant over the **p** allele. The offspring of this cross (shown within the box) can be called the $F_1$ generation.

A Cross Between Two Pure-Breeding Strains ($F_1$ generation):

|      | *P*  | *P*  |
|------|------|------|
| *p*  | *Pp* | *Pp* |
| *p*  | *Pp* | *Pp* |

The $F_1$ offspring all have the **Pp** genotype and the pink phenotype. What will occur if two of these $F_1$ plants are crossed? A Punnett Square can be used again to predict the genotypes in the $F_2$ generation.

- Parent 1: **P** and **p** gametes are produced.
- Parent 2: **P** and **p** gametes are produced.

$F_2$ Generation Punnett Square:

|      | *P*  | *p*  |
|------|------|------|
| *P*  | *PP* | *Pp* |
| *p*  | *Pp* | *pp* |

Since we know the **P** allele for pink is dominant, we can use the genotypes to predict phenotypes of the $F_2$ generation. **PP** homozygotes will be pink, and **Pp** heterozygotes will also be pink since **P** is dominant. Like the original pure-breeding white plants, **pp** plants will be white.

|      | *P*          | *p*           |
|------|--------------|---------------|
| *P*  | *PP* (pink)  | *Pp* (pink)   |
| *p*  | *Pp* (pink)  | *pp* (white)  |

The ratios of the different genotypes and phenotypes in the Punnett Square should match the statistical probability of what would be produced by such a cross. For example, if two heterozygous **Pp** plants are crossed, 75% of the offspring will be pink and 25% white. This prediction from the Punnett Square is based on the ratio of 3:1 for phenotypes that will produce pink (3) to white (1).

The different pea plant traits helped Mendel formulate the two fundamental rules of Mendelian genetics, the Law of Segregation and the Law of Independent Assortment. Mendel derived these rules based purely on his knowledge of the transmission of traits, without knowing anything about the molecular basis for his observations or the mechanisms of meiosis.

### Laws of Segregation

The Law of Segregation states that if there are two alleles in an individual that determine a trait, these two alleles will separate during gamete formation and act independently. For example, when a heterozygous **Pp** plant is forming gametes, the **P** and the **p** alleles can separate into different gametes and act independently during a cross. If this were not the case, and the **P** and **p** alleles could not separate, then all of the offspring would remain **Pp** and all of the $F_2$ would be pink. The fact that white offspring are produced indicates that alleles do indeed segregate into gametes independently. The molecular basis for this observation is that during meiosis, each homologous chromosome carrying two different alleles will end up in a different haploid gamete.

### Law of Independent Assortment

The Law of Independent Assortment describes the relationship between different genes. If the gene that determines plant height is on a different chromosome than the gene for flower color, then these traits will act independently during test crosses.

### Linkage

There is a significant exception to the law of independent assortment. For genes to assort independently into gametes during meiosis, they must be on different chromosomes. If two genes are located near each other on the same chromosome, then the alleles for these genes will stay together during meiosis. The phenomenon in which alleles fail to assort independently because they are on the same chromosome is called **linkage**.

### Inheritance Patterns

Ethical restraints forbid geneticists from performing test crosses in human populations. Instead, they must rely on examining matings that have already occurred, using tools such as pedigrees. A **pedigree** is a family tree depicting the inheritance of a particular genetic trait over several generations. By convention, males are indicated by squares, and females by circles. Matings are indicated by horizontal lines, and descendants are listed below matings, connected by a vertical line. Individuals affected by a particular trait are generally shaded, while the symbols for unaffected individuals are left unshaded. When carriers of sex-linked traits have been identified (typically, female heterozygotes), they are usually half shaded.

The sample pedigrees illustrate two types of heritable traits: recessive disorders and sex-linked disorders. When analyzing a pedigree, look for individuals with the recessive phenotype. Such individuals have only one possible genotype—homozygous recessive. Matings between them and the dominant phenotype behave as test crosses; the ratio of phenotypes among the offspring allows deduction of the dominant genotype. In any case where only males are affected, sex linkage should be suspected.

### Recessive Disorders

Note how the autonomal recessive disorder presented in the following figure has skipped a generation. Albinism is an example of this form of disorder.

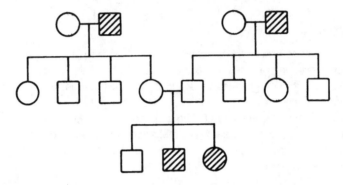

**Recessive Disorder**

### Sex-Linked Disorders

Gender skewing is evident in this type of disorder, which includes traits such as hemophilia. Sex-linked recessive alleles are almost always expressed only by males and transmitted from one generation to another by female carriers.

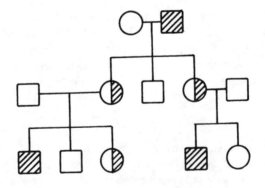

**Sex-Linked Disorder**

### Non-Mendelian Inheritance Patterns

While Mendel's laws hold true in many cases, these laws cannot explain the results of certain crosses. Sometimes an allele is only incompletely dominant or, perhaps, codominant. The genetics that enable the human species to have two genders would also not be possible under Mendel's laws.

## Incomplete Dominance

Incomplete dominance is a blending of the effects of contrasting alleles. Both alleles are expressed partially, neither dominating the other. An example of incomplete dominance is found in the four o'clock plant and the snapdragon flower. When a red flower (**RR**) is crossed with a white flower (**WW**), a pink blend (**RW**) is created. When two pink flowers are crossed, the yield is 25% red, 50% pink, and 25% white (phenotypic and genotypic ratio 1:2:1).

## Codominance

In a pattern of codominance, both alleles are fully expressed without one allele being dominant over the other. An example is blood types. Blood type is determined by the expression of antigen proteins on the surface of red blood cells. The **A** allele and the **B** allele are codominant if both are present, combining to produce AB blood.

## Sex Determination

Most organisms have two types of chromosomes: **autosomes**, which determine most of an organism's body characteristics, and **sex chromosomes**, which determine the sex of an organism. Humans have 22 pairs of autosomes and one pair of sex chromosomes. The sex chromosomes are known as **X** and **Y**. In humans, **XX** is present in females and **XY** in males. The Y chromosome carries very few genes. As all eggs contain X chromosomes only, sex is determined at the time of fertilization by the type of sperm fertilizing the egg. If the sperm carries an X chromosome, the offspring will be female (**XX**); if the sperm carries a Y chromosome, the offspring will be male (**XY**).

This process is illustrated in the Punnett Square that follows.

|  | X | Y | (From the father) |
|---|---|---|---|
| X | XX | XY |  |
| (From the mother) X | XX | XY |  |

The ratio of the sex of the offspring is 1:1.

## Sex Linkage

Genes for certain traits, such as color blindness or hemophilia, are located on the X chromosomes. Hence these genes are linked with the genes controlling sex determination. These genes seem to have no corresponding allele on the Y chromosome; with the result that the X chromosome contributed by the mother is the sole determinant of these traits in males.

## Mutations

Mutations can create new alleles, the raw material that drives evolution via natural selection. Mutations are changes in the genes that are inherited. To be transmitted to the succeeding generation, mutations must occur in sex cells—eggs and sperm—rather than somatic cells (body cells). Mutations in non-sex cells are called somatic cell mutations and affect only the individual involved, not subsequent generations. A somatic mutation can cause cancer, but will have no affect on offspring since it is not present in gametes. Many mutations are recessive and harmful. Because they are recessive, these mutations can be masked or hidden by the dominant normal genes.

### Chromosomal Mutations

These mutations result in changes in chromosomal structure or abnormal chromosome duplication. In crossing over, segments of chromosomes switch positions during meiotic synapsis. This process breaks linkage patterns normally observed when the genes are on the same chromosome. A translocation is an event in which a piece of a chromosome breaks off and rejoins a different chromosome.

# ECOLOGY

To understand how organisms live, biologists study molecules, cells, tissues, and organs, breaking organisms down into their fundamental units. Organisms from bacteria to humans do not live on Earth in an isolated state, however. All organisms, including humans, live by interacting with other organisms and with the nonliving (**abiotic**) environment. Life on Earth is a network of interacting organisms that depend on each other for survival. Ecology is the study of the interactions between organisms and their environment, and how these shape both the organisms and the environments they live in.

## Populations in the Environment

Since ecology seeks to understand life at a broader level than the organism, it is the population rather than the individual that is the basic unit of study in this discipline. A species comprises individuals that can mate to produce fertile offspring. A **population** is a group of individual members of a species that interbreed and share the same gene pool, the same definition used in population genetics. Every environment will include many different interacting populations. Properties such as population growth and maximal population size do not pertain to properties displayed by individuals. The distinct properties of populations are important for ecosystems.

## Populations in Communities and Ecosystems

The next level of biological organization beyond a population is a **community**, which is all the interacting populations living together in an environment. The populations within a community interact with each other in a variety of ways, including **predation** (the consumption of one organism by another, usually resulting in the death of the organism that is eaten); **competition** (a competitive relationship between populations in a community that exists when different populations in the same location use a limited resource); and **symbiosis** (symbionts live together in an intimate, often permanent association that may or may not be beneficial or harmful to either group). These interactions affect the number of individuals in each population within a community and the number of different species in a community. An **ecosystem** is defined by several different conditions: a living community that is within an abiotic (nonliving) environment; the interactions between populations; as well as the flow of energy and molecules within the system.

### The Food Web

The term **food chain** is often used to describe a community with a simple linear relationship between a series of species in which one group eats another. For example, a food chain might contain grass as the producer, mice as the primary consumer, snakes as the secondary consumer, and hawks as the tertiary consumer. The different levels in the food chain, such as producers and primary consumers, are sometimes called **trophic levels**. A more realistic depiction of the relationships within the community is a **food web**, in which every population interacts not with one other population, but several other populations. An animal in an ecosystem is often preyed on by several different predators, and predators commonly have a diet of several different prey, not just one. The greater the number of potential interactions in a community food web, the more stable the system will be, and the better able it will be to withstand and rebound from external pressures such as disease or extreme weather.

## Biomes

The plant and animal life that can inhabit a region is determined by the terrestrial and climatic conditions in a particular region. If an organism does not have the suitable adaptations for an area, it will not be able to survive. A distinct community inhabits each geographic region, known as a biome.

### Terrestrial Biomes

Land biomes are characterized and named according to the climax vegetation present in a region. Climax vegetation is the vegetation that becomes dominant and stable after years of evolutionary development. Since plants are important as food producers, they determine the nature of the inhabiting animal population; hence the climax vegetation determines the climax animal population. There are eight types of terrestrial biomes that result from all these factors.

- Tropical Forest
- Savanna
- Desert
- Temperate Deciduous Forest
- Northern Coniferous Forest
- Taiga
- Tundra
- Polar Region

### Aquatic Biomes

In addition to the eight terrestrial biomes, there are aquatic biomes, each with its own characteristic plants and animals. More than 70% of the Earth's surface is covered by water, and most of the Earth's plant and animal life is found there. As much as 90% of the Earth's food and oxygen production (photosynthesis) takes place in water. Aquatic biomes are classified according to criteria quite different from the criteria used to classify terrestrial biomes. Plants have little controlling influence in communities of aquatic biomes, as compared to their role in terrestrial biomes. Aquatic areas are also the most stable ecosystems on Earth. Conditions affecting temperature, amount of available oxygen and carbon dioxide, and amount of suspended or dissolved materials are stable over very large areas, and show little tendency to change. For these reasons, aquatic food webs and aquatic communities tend to be balanced. There are two types of major aquatic biomes.

- Marine
- Freshwater

# EVOLUTION AND DIVERSITY

In this section, we'll be covering topics ranging from types of evidence for evolution to the taxonomic classification of various common species.

## Evidence of Evolution

Evolution provides a sweeping framework for the understanding of the diversity of life on Earth. Living systems—which include cells, organisms, and ecosystems—arose through geologic time, selected out of diverse possibilities. What is the evidence that supports the evolutionary view of life? The evidence takes several forms.

### The Fossil Record

Fossils are preserved impressions or remains in rocks of living organisms from the past. Fossils provide some of the most direct and compelling evidence of evolutionary change and are generally found in sedimentary rock. When animals settle in sediments after death, their remains can be embedded in the sediment. These sediments then might be covered over with additional layers of sediment that turn to rock through exposure to heat and pressure over many millions of years. The embedded remains turn to stone, replaced with minerals that preserve an impression of the form of the organism, often in a quite detailed state. Most fossils are of the hard, bony parts of animals, since these are preserved the most easily. Fossils of soft body parts or of invertebrates are much more unusual, more than likely because these parts usually decay before fossil formation can occur. In some cases, however, animals that died in anaerobic sediments have resisted decay and have provided soft-body fossils.

When a fossil is discovered, its age must be determined in order to place it correctly in the timeline of life on Earth. One way to place the date is to compare the location of the fossil sediment to other sedimentary rock formations in which the age is already known. Dating using **radioactive decay** is also very useful. Carbon dating is frequently used for material that is only a few thousand years old, but cannot be used for older material since the decay rate of carbon is too rapid.

The conditions for fossil formation are relatively particular, especially for the preservation of invertebrates or soft body parts. Scientists locate fossils by luck, and can only look at a tiny percentage of possible fossil locations. A great variety of fossils have been located, including fossils that provide a clear story of the evolution of modern species.

Fossils have revealed that the archaeopteryx is an example of a feathered dinosaur that was probably an intermediate species in the evolution of birds. Changes that have appeared in fossils created during various frames of time have provided a great deal of insight into the evolutionary paths that resulted in modern species including horses, whales, and humans. Any of the so-called "gaps" in the fossil record is probably the result of the scarcity of fossils and difficulty in finding them, and is not evidence that evolution did not occur.

## Comparative Anatomy

One way to find an evolutionary relationship between organisms is by examining their external and internal anatomy. Animals that evolved from a common ancestor might have anatomical features in common with a common ancestor. Alternatively, two organisms might share features that look the same but evolved from different ancestors and resulted in similar structures as a result of similar functions. When we compare the anatomies of two or more living organisms, not only can we form hypotheses about their common ancestors, but we can also glean clues that shed light upon the selective pressures that led to the development of certain adaptations, such as the ability to fly. Comparative anatomists study **homologous** and **analogous structures** in organisms.

## Homologous Structures

Homologous structures have the same basic anatomical features and evolutionary origins. They demonstrate similar evolutionary patterns with late divergence of form due to differences in exposure to evolutionary forces. Examples of homologous structures include the wings of bats, the flippers of whales, the forelegs of horses, and the arms of humans. These structures were all derived from a common ancestor but diverged to perform different functions in what is termed **divergent evolution**.

## Analogous Structures

Analogous structures have similar functions but may have different evolutionary origins and entirely different patterns of development. The wings of a fly (membranous) and the wings of a bird (bony and covered in feathers) are analogous structures that have evolved to perform a similar function—to fly. The wings of flies and birds might look the same but this does not indicate that they share a winged ancestor. When structures look the same and share a common function but are not derived from a common ancestor, it is called **convergent evolution**. Analogous organs demonstrate superficial resemblances that cannot be used as a basis for classification.

## Comparative Embryology

Comparison of embryonic structures and routes of embryo development is another way to derive evolutionary relationships. The development of the human embryo is very similar to the development of other vertebrate embryos. Adult tunicates (sea squirts) and amphibians lack a notochord (a stiff, solid dorsal rod), one of the key traits of the chordate phylum, but their embryos both possess notochords during development. This indicates these animals are in fact vertebrates with a common evolutionary ancestor even though the adults do not resemble each other. The earlier that embryonic development diverges, the more dissimilar the mature organisms are. Thus, it is difficult to differentiate between the embryo of a human and that of an ape until relatively late in the development of each embryo, while human and sea urchin embryos diverge much earlier.

Other embryonic evidence of evolution includes characteristics such as the teeth that appear in an avian embryo (recalling the reptile stage); the resemblance of larval mollusks (shellfish) to annelids (segmented worms); and the tail that is present on the human embryo for a period of time (indicating relationships to other mammals).

### Molecular Evolution

If organisms are derived from a common ancestor, this should be evident not just at the anatomical level but also the molecular level. The traits that distinguish one organism from another are ultimately derived from differences in genes. With the advent of molecular biology, the genes and proteins of organisms can be compared to determine their evolutionary relationship. The closer the genetic sequences of organisms are to each other, the more closely their evolutionary progression has been related and the more recently they diverged from a common ancestor. Some genes change rapidly during evolution while others have changed extremely slowly. The rate of change in a gene over time is called the **molecular clock**. The rate of change in a gene's sequence is probably a function of the level of resistance a gene has to changes.

Genes that change very slowly over extremely long periods of time do not tolerate change very well and play key roles in the life of cells and organisms. Ribosomal RNA has changed slowly enough that it can be used to compare organisms all the way back to the divergence of eukaryotes, bacteria, and archaebacteria. The enzymes involved in glycolysis play an essential role in energy production for all life; they also evolve very slowly, allowing comparison of their genetic sequences and illuminating evolutionary relationships over billions of years. Computers can be used to compare the gene sequences of many organisms, allowing researchers to determine how long ago organisms evolved from a common ancestor. Genes that have evolved over a more recent period of time and genes that evolve more rapidly can be used to analyze recent evolutionary events.

### Vestigial Structures

**Vestigial structures** are structures that appear to be useless in the context of a particular modern-day organism's behavior and environment. It is apparent, however, that these structures had some function in an earlier stage of a particular organism's evolution. They serve as evidence of an organism's evolution over time, and can help scientists to trace its evolutionary path. There are many examples of vestigial structures in humans, other animals, and plants. The appendix—small and useless in humans—assists digestion of cellulose in herbivores, indicating a vegetarian ancestry in humans.

## Mechanisms of Evolution

### The Population as the Basic Unit of Evolution

Evolution is the change a species undergoes over time. These changes are the result of modifications in the gene pool of a population of organisms. Evolution does not happen in one individual, but in a population of organisms. What is a population? A **population** is a group of individuals in a particular species that interbreed.

In classical genetics, it is observed that a genotype of organisms produces their phenotype, the physical expression of inherited traits. A population of organisms includes individuals with a range of phenotypes and genotypes. However it is possible to describe a population by certain traits exhibited by the group as a whole, such as the abundance of particular alleles. The sum total of all alleles in a population is called the **gene pool** and the frequency with which a specific allele appears in a gene pool is called the **allele frequency**. Each individual receives its specific set of alleles from the gene pool, and not every individual receives the same alleles, leading to individual variation in genotypes and phenotypes. All of these allow for mixing of alleles in a population to create variation in individual genotypes and phenotypes. Mutation in a population can create new alleles. Evolution is caused by changes in the gene pool of a population over time, as a result of changes to individuals in a population caused by the alleles they carry.

## Speciation

A **species** is a group of organisms that is able to successfully interbreed with each other to produce fertile offspring and not with other organisms. The key to defining a species is not external appearance. Within a species, there can be great phenotypic variation, as in domesticated dogs. What defines a species is reproductive isolation, an inability to interbreed and create fertile offspring. Horses and donkeys can interbreed and create offspring, mules. However, mules are sterile, meaning the horses and donkeys are two different species.

## Classification and Taxonomy

Evolution has created a great diversity of organisms on Earth, but these organisms are related to each other through common ancestors they shared in the history of life. By examining organisms for common features and common ancestors, it should be possible to make sense of the diversity of life by grouping organisms into categories. The science of classifying living things and using a system of nomenclature to name them is called **taxonomy**. Carolus Linnaeus invented modern taxonomy in the 1700s, grouping organisms and naming them according to a hierarchical system.

Modern classification systems seek to group organisms on the basis of evolutionary relationships. The bat, whale, horse, and human are placed in the same class of animals (mammals) because they are believed to have descended from a common ancestor. The taxonomist classifies all species known to have descended from the same common ancestor within the same broad taxonomic group.

Since much about early evolutionary history is not understood, there is some disagreement among biologists as to the best classification system to employ, particularly with regard to groups of unicellular organisms. Taxonomic organization proceeds from the largest, broadest group to the smaller, more specific subgroups. The largest group, known as a kingdom, is broken down into smaller and smaller subdivisions. Members of each smaller group have more specific characteristics in common. Furthermore, each subgroup is distinguishable from the next. The names used to classify these systems are subject to discussion and revision as time and research yields new insights into the relationships between organisms.

Some classifications are clearer than others. Viruses are obligate intracellular parasites that cannot conduct metabolic activities or replicate on their own. As such, they are not generally considered living, although they are certainly important to living systems. They are not classified within taxonomic systems, however.

## Classification and Subdivisions

Each **kingdom** has several major divisions known as phyla. A **phylum** has several **subphyla**, which are further divided into **classes**. Each class consists of many **orders**, and these orders are subdivided into **families**. Each family is made up of a **genus** or many **genera**. Finally, the **species** is the smallest subdivision.

Hence, the order of classificatory divisions is as follows:

KINGDOM → PHYLUM → SUBPHYLUM → CLASS → ORDER → FAMILY → GENUS → SPECIES

The complete classification of humans is:

**Kingdom:** *Animalia*

**Phylum:** *Chordata*

**Subphylum:** *Vertebrata*

**Class:** *Mammalia*

**Order:** *Primates*

**Family:** *Hominidae*

**Genus:** *Homo*

**Species:** *Sapiens*

| | The Kingdoms |
|---|---|
| Moneran | Includes bacteria, blue green algae, and primitive pathogens. Considered the most primitive kingdom, it represents prokaryotic (as opposed to eukaryotic) life forms—that is, the cells of Moneran organisms do not have distinct nuclei. |
| Protista | The simplest eukaryotes (cells have nuclei). Includes protozoa, unicellular and multicellular algae, and slime molds. Ancestor organisms to plants, animals, and fungi; most can move around by means of flagella. |
| Fungi | Includes mushrooms, bread molds, and yeasts. Fungi lack the ability to photosynthesize, so they are called decomposers, breaking down and feeding on dead protoplasm. |
| Plantae | Have the ability to photosynthesize, so they are called producers. There are two major phyla, Bryophyta, or mosses, and Tracheophyta, which have vascular systems and include most of the plants you know. |
| Animalia | Produce energy by consuming other organisms, so they are called consumers. Can be either vertebrates, phylum Chordata, or invertebrates such as mollusks, arthropods, sponges, coelenterates, worms, etc. |

## Assignment of Scientific Names

All organisms are assigned a scientific name consisting of the genus and species names of that organism. Thus, a human is a *Homo sapiens*, and the common housecat is *Felis domestica*.

One of the primary groupings of all living organisms separates **prokaryotes** from **eukaryotic** organisms. The prokaryotes include bacteria and another type of organism called archaebacteria. Like the bacteria, archae have no organelles and have a simple circular DNA genome. Archae were relatively unknown until recently, and tend to inhabit harsh environments like hot springs that might resemble the early Earth. Archae are distinct from bacteria in many ways, such as the composition of their membrane lipids, and in some ways appear to be related more closely to eukaryotes than prokaryotes. For this reason, more recent classification schemes break all living things into three **domains**, groups at a higher level than kingdom: bacteria, archaebacteria, and eukaryotes.

### Bacteria

The ubiquitous bacteria are single-celled, lack true nuclei, lack a cytoskeleton, and contain double-stranded circular chromosomal DNA that is not enclosed by a nuclear membrane. These creatures nourish themselves heterotrophically—either saprophytically or parasitically—or autotrophically, depending upon the species. Bacteria are classified by their morphological appearance: cocci (round), bacilli (rods), and spirilla (spiral). Some forms are duplexes (diplococci), clusters (staphylococci), or chains (streptococci).

### The Protist Kingdom

The simplest eukaryotic organisms are the **protists**. Protists probably represent the evolution between prokaryotes and the rest of the eukaryotic kingdoms, including fungi, plants, and animals. Most, but not all, protists are unicellular eukaryotes. One way to define the protists is that the group includes organisms that are eukaryotes but are not plants, animals, or fungi. Protists include heterotrophs like **amoebas** and **paramecia**, photosynthetic autotrophs like **euglenas** and **algae**, and fungi-like organisms like **slime molds**. Some protists are mobile through the use of flagella, cilia, or amoeboid motion. Protists use sexual reproduction in some cases and asexual reproduction in others.

One of the best-known protists are the **amoebas**. Amoebas are large, single-celled organisms that do not have a specific body shape. They move and change their shape through changes in their cytoskeleton and streaming of cytoplasm within the cell into extensions called pseudopods.

**Algae** are an important group of photosynthetic protists that are mostly unicellular. Algae include diatoms, single-celled organisms with intricate silica shells; dinoflagellates with flagella; and brown algae. Algae include large multicellular forms like giant kelp that might be grouped with the protists since they are an algae, but are also grouped with plants by others. It is likely that the plants evolved from one group of algae, the green algae.

### Fungi Kingdom

**Fungi** are heterotrophs that absorb nutrients from their environment. Fungi are often saprophytic, feeding off of dead material, which is their nutrition source; because of this, along with bacteria, they are fundamental components of balanced ecosystems. Without fungi and bacteria, there would be an abundance of decaying material that would hinder ecosystems. Absorptive nutrition involves the secretion of enzymes that digest material in an extracellular environment, followed by cells absorbing the digested material. One of the distinguishing features of fungi is their cell wall made of chitin, unlike the cellulose found in plants. Fungi often form long, slender filaments called hyphae. Mushrooms, molds, and yeasts are all examples of fungi.

**Plant Kingdom**

Plants are multicellular eukaryotes that produce energy in their chloroplasts through photosynthesis, using the energy of the sun to drive the production of glucose. A cell wall of cellulose is a common feature of all plants. Vascular plants have a life cycle featuring alternation of generations between haploid gametophytes and diploid sporophytes. The sporophyte is a diploid form that produces haploid spores, which grow into a complete haploid form, the gametophyte. The gametophyte, in turn, is a haploid form that produces haploid gametes that unite through fertilization during sexual reproduction. The resulting diploid zygote grows into a mature sporophyte once again. Plants are distinct from animals in several ways. First, plants are usually nonmotile, while most animals move. Plants are autotrophic, while animals are heterotrophic. With its ability to branch out extensively, the plant structure is adapted for maximum exposure to light, air, and soil; animals, on the other hand, have adapted to compact structures to ensure minimum surface exposure and maximum motility. Animals have much more centralization in their physiology, while plants often exhibit delocalized control of processes and growth.

The evolution of plants has included an ongoing increase in their ability to conquer land due to modifications that allow them to resist gravity and tolerate drier conditions. The first plants probably evolved from green algae in or near shallow water.

The evolution of vascular systems was a major adaptation in plants. The first vascular plants, tracheophytes, that did not produce seeds included ferns and horsetails—plants with cells called tracheids that form tubes that enable the movement of fluid in the plant tissue called xylem. This vascular system also helps to provide rigid stems that plants need to live on land. These plants colonized land about 400 million years ago, making it possible for animals like arthropods to colonize land soon after.

The evolution of the seed was the next major event in plant evolution, found first in gymnosperms and later in flowering plants, known as angiosperms. The seed is a young sporophyte that becomes dormant early in development. The embryo is usually well protected in the seed and able to survive unfavorable conditions by remaining dormant until conditions become more favorable again. Once those conditions arise, the embryo begins to grow again, sprouting. In some cases seeds can remain viable for many years, waiting for the right conditions for the sporophyte to grow. This increases the ability of plants to deal with the variable conditions found on land.

Following the evolution of the seed, the next big innovation in plant evolution was the flower. Angiosperms represent the flowering plants and are today the predominant plant group in many ecosystems.

## The Animal Kingdom

Animals are fairly easy to recognize, as they are all multicellular heterotrophs. The evolution of animals has included many evolutionary modifications to body plans that aid in fundamental necessities such as getting food, avoiding predators, and reproducing. Members of the animal kingdom have evolved increasingly complex nervous systems that enable complex behaviors in response to the environment. Over time, animals have tended to become larger in size, and more complex, with greater specialization of tissues. Different groups of animals have evolved different body shapes, reflecting their different lifestyles. The body of an animal with **radial symmetry** is organized in a circular shape radiating outward. The echinoderms, such as sea stars and cnidarians like jellyfish, are examples of animals with radial symmetry. Another common body plan is **bilateral symmetry**, in which the body has a left side and a right side that are mirror images of each other.

The human body is a good example of bilateral symmetry. If a plane is drawn vertically through the body, it splits the body into left and right sides that look the same. The front of the body, where the head is located, is the anterior, and the rear of the animal is the posterior. The back of the animal, where the backbone is located in vertebrates, is the dorsal side (like the dorsal fin), and the front of the animal is the ventral side.

## Phylum Chordata

At some stage of their embryologic development, chordates have a stiff, solid dorsal rod called the **notochord,** and paired gill slits. Chordata have hollow dorsal nerve cords, tails extending beyond the anus (at some point in their development), and ventral hearts. These adaptations may not sound impressive but they paved the way for the evolution of vertebrates, a major subphylum of chordates. The chordates probably originated from animals like tunicates, commonly called sea squirts. Adult tunicates are sessile filter feeders that do not resemble vertebrates at all. Tunicate larvae, however, are free-swimming, resemble tadpoles, and have both a notochord and a dorsal nerve cord. Vertebrates are a subphylum of the chordates that includes fish, amphibians, reptiles, birds, and mammals. In vertebrates the notochord is present during embryogenesis but is replaced during development by a bony, segmented vertebral column that protects the dorsal spinal cord and provides anchorage for muscles. Vertebrates have bony or cartilaginous endoskeletons, chambered hearts for circulation, and increasingly complex nervous systems. The vertebrate internal organs are contained in a coelomic body cavity.

The first vertebrates were probably filter-feeding organisms that evolved into swimming, jawless fishes that were still filter feeders. Jawless fish such as lampreys still exist. The evolution of fish with jaws led to the development of the cartilaginous and bony fishes that are dominant today. The jaw allows fish to adopt new life styles other than filter feeding, grabbing food with their jaws. The majority of fish use gills for respiration. The water from which fish extract the oxygen they need to survive moves over their gills through paired gill slits. Cartilaginous fish (class Chondrichthyes) like sharks and rays have an endoskeleton that is made entirely of cartilage rather than hard, calcified bone. Bony fishes (class Osteichthyes) have swim bladders to regulate their buoyancy in water.

Two adaptations were important to set the stage for vertebrates to colonize land. One was the presence of air sacs that allowed some fish in shallow water to absorb oxygen from air for brief periods. The other adaptation was a structural change in fins; fin lobes allowed some degree of movement on land. Fish with these features evolved into **amphibians** about 350 million years ago.

Most amphibians, such as frogs and salamanders, still live in close association with water and have only simple lungs or gills. Their intake of oxygen is supplemented by the ability to absorb it through the skin. Another reason that amphibians are mostly associated with water is that amphibian eggs lack hard shells and dry out on land. Amphibian larvae often live in water and then metamorphose into an adult form that lives primarily on land.

**Reptiles**, on the other hand, have evolved to produce hard-shelled eggs that do not dry out on land. The eggshell protects the developing embryo but still allows a gas exchange with the environment. The heart and lungs of reptiles also evolved to be more effective, particularly for the climates and environments in which they live. Their thick, dry skin allows them greater metabolic activity than amphibians and the ability to survive on land.

The development of wings, feathers, and light bones that allowed for flight distinguished **birds** from their reptilian relatives—dinosaurs. Birds also have four-chambered hearts and uniquely adapted lungs to supply the intense metabolic needs of flight. Birds produce hard-shelled eggs and usually provide a great deal of parental care during embryonic development and the maturation that takes place after hatching.

**Mammals** are the major class of vertebrates. Mammals have hair, sweat glands, mammary glands, and four-chambered hearts. The fossil record indicates that mammals evolved 200 million years ago and coexisted with dinosaurs up until they became extinct 65 million years ago. When mammals no longer had to compete with dinosaurs for dominance, they diversified and occupied many environmental niches, becoming the dominant terrestrial vertebrate present in many ecosystems. Mammals have highly effective regulation systems to control their body temperature, and most mammals provide extensive care for their young. One small group of mammals, the Monotremes (for example, the duck-billed platypus), lays eggs. The embryos of most other mammals undergo internal gestation and are then birthed. **Marsupial** mammals give birth after a short time and complete development of young in an external pouch. **Placental** mammals gestate their young to a more mature state, providing nutrition to the embryo with the exchange of material in the placenta. Marsupial mammals were once widespread across the globe, but were replaced in most cases by placental mammals. As Australia is isolated, it was a haven for marsupial mammals, and continues to be in the present day.

Among mammals, the primates have opposable thumbs and stereoscopic vision for depth perception, adaptations that evolved to support their existence in their preferred environment: trees. Adaptations displayed by primates are traits that have been important factors in the evolution of humans. Many primates also have complex social structures.

Ancestors of humans include **australopithecines**. Fossils indicate these ancestors were able to walk upright on two legs. Fossil remains of hominids such as *Homo habilus*, which lived 2–3 million years ago, show that this human ancestor had a cerebral cortex that had greatly increased in size. *Homo habilus* probably used tools, setting the stage for modern humans, *Homo sapiens*.

Now that you have reviewed the basics of biology, you can review strategies for this part of the test. After reviewing the strategies, and completing the questions at the end of this chapter, you are ready to study the Physical Sciences—chemistry and physics.

# STRATEGIES FOR LIFE SCIENCE TESTING

It's important to know that the science portions of the nursing school entrance exams contain knowledge-based questions. What that means is you can't always reason your way to the correct answer—most likely, you will either know the answer or you will not.

Don't panic! That doesn't mean that there are no strategies to use on test day. It just means the strategies for this part of the test are slightly different from those for other sections. Here are Kaplan's favorite strategies for knowledge-based test questions.

- Mnemonic devices.
- Review of terms and concepts commonly confused for each other.
- Building blocks.
- Quiz yourself.
- General test-taking strategies.

Keep reading to find out how each one of these works for the Life Science section of the test.

## Mnemonic Devices

A mnemonic device is a way to remember something. You may remember the mnemonic tool PEMDAS (Please Excuse My Dear Aunt Sally) that was presented in Chapter Six, Mathematics Review. This phrase could help you remember the order of operations: Parentheses, Exponents, Multiplication, Division, Addition, Subtraction. This same approach can be applied to concepts that might be presented in the Life Science section of the test. Try to come up with mnemonic tools for lists of terms or concepts that are difficult to remember on their own. In the following section we present several examples of how this method could help you tackle science.

### Concept: What hormones are secreted by the anterior pituitary?

The anterior pituitary gland secretes several hormones, including: **F**SH, **L**H, **A**CTH, **T**SH, **P**rolactin, **G**rowth.

Take the first letter of each hormone; write it out in a list: F-L-A-T-P-G. Sound that combination of letters out. Doesn't it sound like "flat pig"? There is your device. Simply add an "I" to your device to help you remember how to sound it out.

**Mnemonic device: FLAT PIG**

### Concept: The correct order of taxonomic classifications.

The order is: **K**ingdom, **P**hylum, **S**ubphylum, **C**lass, **O**rder, **F**amily, **G**enus, **S**pecies.

Again, make a list of the first letters of each group. You are left with K-P-S-C-O-F-G-S. Unlike the last example, when this combination of letters is sounded out, it doesn't mean anything. The easiest thing to do is to build a sentence around the letters you need to remember.

**Mnemonic device:** King Phillip Swiftly Came Over For Good Sushi.

This sentence may act as a tool to help you remember the correct order of classification. If this sentence is hard for you to remember because you do not have mental associations with the words we chose, try building your own sentence.

## Terms That Are Commonly Confused for Each Other

After long hours of study, you might not even care what the difference between mitosis and meiosis is. However, you would care if that were something you were facing on test day. Here are a few biology terms that are commonly misidentified and confused for one another.

### Don't Mix These Up on Test Day

- **Stomata** are pores in the surface of a leaf through which carbon dioxide enters and oxygen exits the plant.
- **Stroma** is the dense fluid within the chloroplast in which carbon dioxide is converted into sugars.

- **mRNA**, or messenger RNA, carries messages that encode proteins.
- **tRNA**, or transfer RNA, carries amino acids to make proteins.
- **rRNA**, or ribosomal RNA, is a structural component of ribosomes.

- **Transcription** involves DNA being read, and that information being transcribed or transferred to RNA.
- **Translation** is when RNA is read, leading to the process of protein synthesis.

- **Prokaryotes** have no nucleus and no membrane-bound organelles, but do have ribosomes and cell walls made up of peptidoglycans.
- **Eukaryotes** have a nucleus, membrane-bound organelles, and ribosomes. Examples include protists, fungi, plants, and animals. Fungi and plant eukaryotic cells have cell walls made of cellulose.

- **Spermatogenesis** is characterized by several things, including:
  - *The production of four mature sperm; each sperm has an X or Y chromosome and does not donate mitochondria to the embryo.*
  - *The process is continuous.*
  - *Fresh sperm are created daily.*

- **Oogenesis** is characterized by the following:
  - *The process produces one egg and two to three polar bodies.*
  - *Only ova with X chromosomes are produced.*
  - *The process is discontinuous.*
  - *The process produces ova that donate mitochondria to embryos.*
  - *A limited supply of ova is produced early in life and the development of ova is arrested later in life.*

- The **right ventricle** pumps blood to the lungs in the pulmonary artery.
- The **left ventricle** pumps blood through the aorta to the rest of the body.

- **Atria** receive blood from veins.
- **Ventricles** pump blood out of arteries.

- **Arteries** have the following characteristics and functions:
  - *Thick-walled.*
  - *Oxygenated.*
  - *Conduct blood at high pressures.*
  - *Have a pulse.*
  - *Have no valves to prevent backflow.*

- **Veins** have the following characteristics and functions:
  - *Thin-walled.*
  - *Deoxygenated.*
  - *Conduct blood at low pressures.*
  - *Have no pulse.*
  - *Have valves to prevent backflow.*

- The **sympathetic nervous system** has the following characteristics and functions:
  - *Associated with the fight-or-flight response.*
  - *Increases the heart rate.*
  - *Increases the breathing rate.*
  - *Lowers the digestive rate.*
  - *Causes pupil dilation.*

- The **parasympathetic nervous system** has the following characteristics and functions:
  - *Is associated with the rest-and-digest response.*
  - *Lowers the heart rate.*
  - *Does not affect the breathing rate.*
  - *Increases the digestive rate.*
  - *Does not cause pupil dilation.*

- **Cones** are photoreceptors that respond to high-intensity illumination and color.
- **Rods** respond to low-intensity illumination (they are important in night vision), but do not detect color well.

- **Smooth muscle** is involuntary muscle present in the arteries, gastrointestinal tract, and elsewhere.
- **Skeletal muscles** are voluntary muscles that cause body movement.
- **Cardiac muscle** is the tissue that makes up the heart.

- **Mitosis** has the following characteristics and functions:
  - *Produces diploid cells from diploid cells.*
  - *Occurs in all dividing cells.*
  - *Does not involve the pairing up of homologous chromosomes.*
  - *Does not involve crossing over (recombination).*

- **Meiosis** has the following characteristics and functions:
  - *Produces haploid cells from diploid cells.*
  - *Occurs only in sex cells (gametocytes).*
  - *Involves the pairing up of homologous chromosomes at the metaphase plate, forming tetrads.*
  - *Involves crossing over.*

- **Incomplete dominance** is when two traits are blended together; both are partially expressed, and neither dominates.
- **Codominance** is when both traits are fully expressed and neither dominates.

- **Homologous** structures share a common ancestry.
- **Analogous** structures are not inherited from a common ancestor, but perform similar functions.

## REVIEW QUESTIONS

The following questions are not meant to mimic actual test questions. Instead, these questions will help you review the concepts and terms covered in this chapter.

1.  List five biological molecules.

    _____

    _____

    _____

    _____

    _____

2.  Which of the following is NOT a biochemical reaction that makes ATP?

    (A)  Krebs cycle

    (B)  Glycolysis

    (C)  Transcription

    (D)  Electron transport

3.  Fill in the blank. In plants, photosynthesis occurs in the _____, an organelle that is specific to plants.

4.  Which of the following is NOT a part of the Central Dogma?

    (A)  RNA is produced when DNA is read during a process called transcription.

    (B)  DNA contains the genes that are responsible for the physical traits (phenotype) observed in all living organisms.

    (C)  RNA serves as the key used to decode and transmit the genetic information, as well as synthesize proteins according to the encoded information. This process of protein synthesis is called translation.

    (D)  The structure of DNA was elucidated by Watson and Crick in 1953 and it became clear how DNA could play a role as the source of genetic material.

    (E)  DNA is replicated from existing DNA to produce new genomes.

5.  Name the four types of nucleotides that make up DNA.

    _____

    _____

    _____

    _____

6.  Match each type of RNA with its description.

    ____  mRNA

    ____  rRNA

    ____  RNA

    (A)  Plays a role in protein synthesis.

    (B)  Part of the structure of ribosomes and is involved in translation (protein synthesis).

    (C)  Encodes gene messages that are to be decoded during protein synthesis to form proteins.

7.  True or False? Humans are composed of prokaryotic cells.

8.  Explain what purpose the organelle mitochondria serves.

    _____

    _____

9.  Fill in the blank. _____ is the simple diffusion of water from a region of lower solute concentration to a region of higher solute concentration.

10. Which of the following is NOT one of the four stages of mitosis?

    (A) Cytokinesis
    (B) Prophase
    (C) Metaphase
    (D) Anaphase
    (E) Telophase

11. True or False? Vertebrates have closed circulatory systems.

12. Name at least three of the air passages involved in respiration.

    _____

    _____

    _____

13. What system enables organisms to receive and respond to stimuli from their external and internal environments?

    _____

14. Name the three different muscle types vertebrates possess.

    _____

    _____

    _____

15. Which of the following is NOT one of the three basic principles of genetics developed by Gregor Mendel?

    (A) Dominance
    (B) Phenotype
    (C) Segregation
    (D) Independent assortment

16. Write out the Law of Segregation.

    _____

    _____

17. True or False? The populations within a community interact with each other in a variety of ways, including predation, competition, or symbiosis.

18. Fill in the blank. A _____ is a group of organisms that is able to successfully interbreed with each other and not with other organisms.

19. Write the taxonomic classifications in order, from least specific to most specific.

    _____

    _____

    _____

    _____

    _____

    _____

    _____

20. List at least two characteristics of mammals.

    _____

    _____

THE ANSWERS APPEAR ON THE FOLLOWING PAGE.

# REVIEW ANSWERS

1. Carbohydrates
   Lipids
   Proteins
   Enzymes
   Nucleic acids

2. (C) Transcription is not a biochemical reaction that makes ATP. Transcription occurs when DNA is read in order to produce RNA.

3. Photosynthesis occurs in the chloroplast, an organelle that is specific to plants.

4. Although (D) is true, it is not a part of the Central Dogma.

5. Adenine (A)
   Guanine (G)
   Thymine (T)
   Cytosine (C)

6. (C) = mRNA encodes gene messages that are to be decoded in protein synthesis to form proteins.
   (B) rRNA is a part of the structure of ribosomes and is involved in translation (protein synthesis).
   (A) tRNA also play a role in protein synthesis.

7. False. Humans are composed of eukaryotic cells.

8. Mitochondria are sites of aerobic respiration within the cell and are important suppliers of energy.

9. Osmosis is the simple diffusion of water from a region of lower solute concentration to a region of higher solute concentration.

10. (A) Cytokinesis is not one of the four stages of mitosis. During cytokinesis, the cytoplasm and all the organelles of the cell are divided as the plasma membrane pinches inward and seals off to complete the separation of the two newly formed daughter cells from each other.

11. True.

12. Answers may vary. The air passages involved in respiration consist of the nose, pharynx, larynx, trachea, bronchi, bronchioles, and the alveoli.

13. The nervous system enables organisms to receive and respond to stimuli from their external and internal environments.

14. Vertebrates possess three different types of muscle tissues: smooth, skeletal, and cardiac.

15. (B) A phenotype is the appearance and physical expression of genes in an organism.

16. The Law of Segregation states that if there are two alleles in an individual that determine a trait, these two alleles will separate during gamete formation and act independently.

17. True. The populations within a community interact with each other in a variety of ways, including predation (the consumption of one organism by another, usually resulting in the death of the organism that is eaten); competition (a competitive relationship between populations in a community existing when different populations in the same location use a limited resource.); and symbiosis (symbionts live together in an intimate, often permanent, association that may or may not be beneficial to them).

18. A species is a group of organisms that is able to successfully interbreed with each other and not with other organisms.

19. Kingdom
    Phylum
    Subphylum
    Class
    Order
    Family
    Genus
    Species

20. Mammals have hair, sweat glands, mammary glands, and four-chambered hearts.

# Chapter Eight: **Physical Science Review**

In the last chapter, you reviewed all the basics about Life Science, or biology. In this chapter, you will learn about the two major subjects of Physical Science: chemistry and physics. This chapter has a separate lesson for both of those divisions, followed by strategies to help you on the test, as well as a review of topics covered in this chapter. Before you get started, here's some information you may find helpful for tackling chemistry and physics.

## MATH FOR SCIENCE

Before starting the following lessons, let's review some of the basic mathematical concepts often used in both chemistry and physics: exponents, the metric system and SI units, scientific notation, and powers of ten.

If you believe your math skills in these areas are strong, and you are confident you do not need to review any further, jump ahead to the chemistry lesson.

### Exponents

For any nonzero number $a$ and any integer $n$:

Exponent of zero: $a^0 = 1$

Exponent of one: $a^1 = a$

Negative exponent: $a^{-n} = \dfrac{1}{a^n}$

If $a, b, x, y,$ and $z$ are all integers:

Product of powers: $(a^x)(a^y) = a^{x+y}$

Power of powers: $(a^x)^y = a^{xy}$

Quotient of powers: $\dfrac{a^x}{a^y} = a^{x-y}$

Power of a product: $(ab)^x = a^x b^x$

Power of a monomial: $(a^x b^y)^z = a^{xz} b^{yz}$

The $n^{\text{th}}$ root of powers: $\sqrt[y]{a^x} = a^{x/y}$

KAPLAN

## Powers of Ten

When $a = 10$, the rules listed on the previous page can also be used. For example:

$$10^0 = 1$$

$$10^1 = 10$$

$$10^2 = 100$$

$$10^3 = 1,000, \text{ and so on. Also:}$$

$$10^{-1} = \frac{1}{10}$$

$$10^{-2} = \frac{1}{100}$$

$$10^{-3} = \frac{1}{1,000}, \text{ and so on.}$$

## Scientific Notation

Very large and very small numbers are often used in both chemistry and physics. Scientific notation is a convention for expressing numbers that simplifies the calculation of equations and standardizes their results. To express a number in scientific notation, convert it into a number between 1 and 10 (the **mantissa** or **coefficient**) multiplied by the number 10; raised to the appropriate **exponent** (a number raised to a power).

For example, with scientific notation, the number 7,000,000,000 would be expressed as: $7 \times 10^9$. In this example, the number 7 is the mantissa, and the number 10 is raised to an exponent of 9. Scientific notation can also be used for numbers smaller than one; for example, the number 0.042 would be expressed as $4.2 \times 10^{-2}$.

## The Metric System and Systeme Internationale (SI) Units

The metric system involves measurement organized in multiples and submultiples related by powers of 10. The system is structured to measure six base units: length, mass, temperature, time, electric current, and substance. The metric system includes other units, but they are all tied to the core six units.

SI Base Units of the Metric System

| Base Quantity | Base Unit | Symbol |
|---|---|---|
| Length | meter | m |
| Mass | kilogram | kg |
| Time | second | s |
| Temperature | Kelvin | K |
| Amount of Substance | mole | mol |
| Electric Current | ampere | A |

The metric system employs a system whereby powers of ten are assigned specific names or prefixes. These prefixes are placed before a unit to indicate the power of 10 that is the fraction or multiplier of that unit. A short list of these prefixes is listed below.

Common Metric Prefixes

| Prefix | Symbol | Power of Ten | Example |
|---|---|---|---|
| nano | n | $10^{-9}$ | nanosecond (ns) |
| micro | μ | $10^{-6}$ | microfarad (μF) |
| milli | m | $10^{-3}$ | milligram (mg) |
| centi | c | $10^{-2}$ | centimeter (cm) |
| kilo | k | $10^{3}$ | kilogram (kg) |
| mega | M | $10^{6}$ | megawatt (MW) |

Now that you have the basics down, let's get started.

# CHEMISTRY LESSON

## Atomic Structure

The atom is the basic building block of matter, representing the smallest unit of a chemical element. In 1911, Ernest Rutherford provided experimental evidence that an atom has a dense, positively charged nucleus that accounts for only a small portion of the volume of the atom. The nucleus, which is the core of the atom, is formed by two subatomic particles, called protons and neutrons. A third form of subatomic particle known as electrons exist outside the nucleus in characteristic regions of space called orbitals. All atoms of an element show similar chemical properties and cannot be further broken down by chemical means.

### Subatomic Particles

#### Protons

Protons carry a single positive charge and have a mass of approximately one atomic mass unit (abbreviated as amu, see table below). The atomic number Z of an element is equal to the number of protons found in an atom of that element. All atoms of a given element have the same atomic number; in other words, the number of protons an atom has defines the element. The atomic number of an element can be found in the periodic table (see the section about the periodic table that is found later in the lesson) as an integer above the symbol for the element.

#### Neutrons

Neutrons carry no charge and have a mass only slightly heavier than that of protons. The total number of neutrons and protons in an atom, known as the mass number, determines its mass.

#### Electrons

Electrons carry a charge equal in magnitude but opposite in charge to that of protons. An electron has a very small mass, approximately $\frac{1}{1,837}$ the mass of a proton or neutron, which is negligible for most purposes. The electrons farthest from the nucleus are known as valence electrons. The further the valence electrons are from the nucleus, the weaker the attractive force of the positively charged nucleus and the more likely the valence electrons are to be influenced by other atoms. Generally, valence electrons and their activity determine the reactivity of an atom. In a neutral atom, the number of electrons is equal to the number of protons. A positive or negative charge on an atom is due to a loss or gain of electrons; the result is called an ion. A positively charged ion (one that has lost electrons) is known as a cation; a negatively charged ion (one that has gained electrons) is known as an anion.

| Subatomic Particle | Relative Mass | Charge | Location |
|---|---|---|---|
| Proton | 1 | 1 | Nucleus |
| Neutron | 1 | 0 | Nucleus |
| Electron | 0 | −1 | Electron orbitals |

### Atomic Weight and Isotopes

To report the mass of something, a number is generally presented with a unit of measurement, such as pounds (lbs), kilograms (kg), grams (g), etc. Because the mass of an atom is so small, these units are not very convenient, and new ways have been devised to describe how much an atom weighs. A unit that can be used to report the mass of an atom is the atomic mass unit (amu). One amu is approximately the same as $1.66 \times 10^{-24}$ g. How is this particular value chosen? The answer is that it is chosen so that a carbon-12 atom, with 6 protons and 6 neutrons, will have a mass of 12 amu. In other words, the amu is defined as one-twelfth the mass of the carbon-12 atom. It does not convert nicely to grams because the mass of a carbon-12 atom in grams is not a round number. In addition, since the mass of an electron is negligible, the mass of the carbon-12 atom is considered to come from protons and neutrons.

Since the mass of a proton is about the same as that of a neutron, and there are six of each in the carbon-12 atom, protons and neutrons are considered to have a mass of $\frac{1}{12} \times 12$ amu $= 1$ amu each.

While it is necessary to have a way of describing the weight of an individual atom, in real life one generally works with a huge number of them at a time. Atomic weight is the mass, in grams, of one mole (mol) of atoms. Just like a pair corresponds to two, and a dozen corresponds to twelve, a mole corresponds to about $6.022 \times 10^{23}$. The atomic weight of an element, expressed in terms of g/mol, therefore, is the mass in grams of $6.022 \times 10^{23}$ atoms of that element. The product of the equation (presented using scientific notation) that corresponds to a mole is known as **Avogadro's number**. Why is this particular value not something like $1 \times 10^{24}$, for example? Once again, the answer lies in the carbon-12 atom. A mole of carbon-12 atoms weighs exactly 12 g. In other words, a mole is defined as the number of atoms in 12 g of carbon-12. If an element were made of a mole of atoms heavier than carbon-12 (such as oxygen), it would have an atomic weight greater than 12 g/mol. If, on the other hand, an element were composed of a mole of atoms lighter than carbon-12 (such as helium), it would have an atomic weight less than 12 g/mol.

The atomic weight of an element is also found in the periodic table—it is the number that appears below an element's symbol. Notice, however, that these numbers are not whole numbers, which is odd considering that a proton and a neutron each have a mass of 1 amu and an atom can only have a whole number of these. Furthermore, even carbon, the element with which we have set the standards, does not have an exact mass of 12. This is due to the presence of isotopes. For a given element, the various nuclei with different numbers of neutrons are called isotopes of that element. The masses listed in the periodic table are weighted averages that account for the relative abundance of various isotopes. The word weighted is important: It is not simply the average of the masses of individual isotopes, it also takes into account how frequently one encounters a particular form of isotope in a sample of an element. There are, for example, three isotopes of hydrogen, with zero, one, and two neutrons respectively. Together with the one proton that makes it hydrogen in the first place, the mass numbers for these isotopes are 1, 2, and 3. The atomic weight of hydrogen, however, is not simply 2 (the average of 1, 2 and 3) but about 1.008, that is, much closer to 1. This is because the isotope with no neutrons is so much more abundant that we count it much more heavily in calculating the average.

## Nuclear Chemistry

Now that you understand atomic structure, it's time to review nuclear chemistry.

### The Nucleus

At the center of an atom lies its nucleus, consisting of one or more nucleons (protons or neutrons) held together with considerably more energy than what is needed to hold electrons in orbit around the nucleus. The radius of a nucleus is about 100,000 times smaller than the radius of an atom. Before we go on, let's review some concepts we've just read about.

### Atomic Number Z

An element's atomic number is defined by the number of protons in its nucleus; the name atomic number Z is used to represent this number. The letter Z represents an integer that is equal to the number of protons in a nucleus. The number of protons is what defines an element: An atom, ion, or nucleus is identified as carbon, for example, only if it has six protons. Each element has a unique number of protons. The letter Z is used as a presubscript to the chemical symbol in isotopic notation; that is, it appears as a subscript before the chemical symbol. The chemical symbols and the atomic numbers of all the elements are given in the periodic table. You will find more information about the periodic table later in the lesson.

### Mass Number A

When calculating mass number, **A** is an integer equal to the total number of nucleons (neutrons and protons) in a nucleus. Let **N** represent the number of neutrons in a nucleus. The equation relating **A**, **N**, and **Z** is simply:

$$A = N + Z$$

### Isotopes

Different nuclei of the same element will by definition all have the same number of protons. The number of neutrons, however, can be different. Nuclei of the same element can therefore have different mass numbers. For a nucleus of a given element with a particular number of protons (atomic number Z), the various nuclei with different numbers of neutrons are called isotopes of that element.

For example, the three isotopes of hydrogen are:

$^{1}_{1}$H: A single proton; the nucleus of ordinary hydrogen.

$^{2}_{1}$H: A proton and a neutron together; the nucleus of one type of heavy hydrogen called deuterium.

$^{3}_{1}$H: A proton and two neutrons together; the nucleus of a heavier type of heavy hydrogen called tritium.

Note that despite the existence of names like deuterium and tritium, they are all considered hydrogen because they have the same number of protons (one). The example shown here is a little bit of an anomaly because in general isotopes do not have specific names of their own.

### Atomic Mass And Atomic Mass Unit

Atomic mass is most commonly measured in atomic mass units (abbreviated amu). By definition, 1 amu is exactly one-twelfth the mass of the neutral carbon-12 atom. In terms of more familiar mass units:

$1 \text{ amu} = 1.66 \times 10^{-27}$

$\text{kg} = 1.66 \times 10^{-24} \text{ g}$

### Atomic Weight

Elements have different masses because of isotopes. Atomic weight refers to a weighted average of the masses of an element. The average is weighted according to the natural abundances of the various isotopic species of an element. The atomic weight can be measured in amu.

## Nuclear Reactions

Nuclear reactions such as fusion, fission, and radioactive decay involve either combining or splitting the nuclei of atoms. Since the binding energy per nucleon is greatest for intermediate-sized atoms, when small atoms combine or large atoms split a great amount of energy is released.

### Fusion

Fusion occurs when small nuclei combine into a larger nucleus. As an example, many stars—including the sun—power themselves by fusing four hydrogen nuclei to make one helium nucleus. Through this method, the sun produces $4 \times 10^{26}$ joules (J) every second. Here on Earth, researchers are trying to find ways to use fusion as an alternative energy source.

### Fission

Fission is a process in which a large nucleus splits into smaller nuclei. Spontaneous fission rarely occurs. However, by the absorption of a low-energy neutron, fission can be induced in certain nuclei. Of special interest are those fission reactions that release more neutrons, since these other neutrons will cause other atoms to undergo fission. This, in turn, releases more neutrons, creating a chain reaction. Such induced fission reactions power commercial electricity-generating nuclear plants.

Nuclear decay will be covered later in the lesson.

# Periodic Table of the Elements

Group

| Period | 1 IA 1A | 2 | | | | | | | | | | | | 13 | 14 | 15 | 16 | 17 | 18 vIIIA 8A |
|---|---|---|---|---|---|---|---|---|---|---|---|---|---|---|---|---|---|---|---|
| 1 | 1 **H** 1.008 | IIA 2A | | | | | | | | | | | | 13 IIIA 3A | 14 IVA 4A | 15 VA 5A | 16 VIA 6A | 17 VIIA 7A | 2 **He** 4.003 |
| 2 | 3 **Li** 6.941 | 4 **Be** 9.012 | | | | | | | | | | | | 5 **B** 10.81 | 6 **C** 12.01 | 7 **N** 14.01 | 8 **O** 16.00 | 9 **F** 19.00 | 10 **Ne** 20.18 |
| 3 | 11 **Na** 22.99 | 12 **Mg** 24.31 | 3 IIIB 3B | 4 IVB 4B | 5 VB 5B | 6 VIB 6B | 7 VIIB 7B | 8 ------- | 9 VIII -- | 10 ----- | 11 IB 1B | 12 IIB 2B | | 13 **Al** 26.98 | 14 **Si** 28.09 | 15 **P** 30.97 | 16 **S** 32.07 | 17 **Cl** 35.45 | 18 **Ar** 39.95 |
| 4 | 19 **K** 39.10 | 20 **Ca** 40.08 | 21 **Sc** 44.96 | 22 **Ti** 47.88 | 23 **V** 50.94 | 24 **Cr** 52.00 | 25 **Mn** 54.94 | 26 **Fe** 55.85 | 27 **Co** 58.47 | 28 **Ni** 58.69 | 29 **Cu** 63.55 | 30 **Zn** 65.39 | 31 **Ga** 69.72 | 32 **Ge** 72.59 | 33 **As** 74.92 | 34 **Se** 78.96 | 35 **Br** 79.90 | 36 **Kr** 83.80 |
| 5 | 37 **Rb** 85.47 | 38 **Sr** 87.62 | 39 **Y** 88.91 | 40 **Zr** 91.22 | 41 **Nb** 92.91 | 42 **Mo** 95.94 | 43 **Tc** (98) | 44 **Ru** 101.1 | 45 **Rh** 102.9 | 46 **Pd** 106.4 | 47 **Ag** 107.9 | 48 **Cd** 112.4 | 49 **In** 114.8 | 50 **Sn** 118.7 | 51 **Sb** 121.8 | 52 **Te** 127.6 | 53 **I** 126.9 | 54 **Xe** 131.3 |
| 6 | 55 **Cs** 132.9 | 56 **Ba** 137.3 | 57 **La*** 138.9 | 72 **Hf** 178.5 | 73 **Ta** 180.9 | 74 **W** 183.9 | 75 **Re** 186.2 | 76 **Os** 190.2 | 77 **Ir** 190.2 | 78 **Pt** 195.1 | 79 **Au** 197.0 | 80 **Hg** 200.5 | 81 **Tl** 204.4 | 82 **Pb** 207.2 | 83 **Bi** 209.0 | 84 **Po** (210) | 85 **At** (210) | 86 **Rn** (222) |
| 7 | 87 **Fr** (223) | 88 **Ra** (226) | 89 **Ac~** (227) | 104 **Rf** (257) | 105 **Db** (260) | 106 **Sg** (263) | 107 **Bh** (262) | 108 **Hs** (265) | 109 **Mt** (266) | 110 --- 0 | 111 --- 0 | 112 --- 0 | | 114 --- 0 | | 116 --- 0 | | | 118 --- 0 |

| Lanthanide Series* | 58 **Ce** 140.1 | 59 **Pr** 140.9 | 60 **Nd** 144.2 | 61 **Pm** (147) | 62 **Sm** 150.4 | 63 **Eu** 152.0 | 64 **Gd** 157.3 | 65 **Tb** 158.9 | 66 **Dy** 162.5 | 67 **Ho** 164.9 | 68 **Er** 167.3 | 69 **Tm** 168.9 | 70 **Yb** 173.0 | 71 **Lu** 175.0 |
|---|---|---|---|---|---|---|---|---|---|---|---|---|---|---|
| Actinide Series~ | 90 **Th** 232.0 | 91 **Pa** (231) | 92 **U** (238) | 93 **Np** (237) | 94 **Pu** (242) | 95 **Am** (243) | 96 **Cm** (247) | 97 **Bk** (247) | 98 **Cf** (249) | 99 **Es** (254) | 100 **Fm** (253) | 101 **Md** (256) | 102 **No** (254) | 103 **Lr** (257) |

The periodic table has been mentioned earlier in this lesson. Now it's time to find out more about it. The periodic table arranges elements in increasing atomic numbers. Its spatial layout is such that a lot of information about an element's properties can be deduced simply by examining its position. The vertical columns are called **groups**, while the horizontal rows are called **periods**. There are seven periods, representing the principal quantum numbers $n = 1$ to $n = 7$, and each period is filled more or less sequentially. The period an element is in tells us the highest shell that is occupied, or the highest principal quantum number. Elements in the same group (same column) have the same electronic configuration in their valence, or outermost shell. For example, both magnesium (Mg) and calcium (Ca) are in the second column; they both have two electrons in the outermost s subshell, the only difference being that the principal quantum number is different for Ca ($n = 4$) than for Mg ($n = 3$). Because these outermost electrons, or valence electrons, are involved in chemical bonding, they determine the chemical reactivity and properties of the element. In short, elements in the same group will tend to have similar levels of chemical reactiveness.

## Valence Electrons and the Periodic Table

The valence electrons of an atom are those electrons in its outer energy shell. The visual layout of the periodic table is convenient for determining the electron configuration of an atom (especially the valence electron configuration).

## Periodic Trends of the Elements

The properties of elements exhibit certain trends, which can be explained in terms of the element's position in the periodic table or its electron configuration. In general, elements seek to gain or lose valence electrons so as to achieve the stable octet formation possessed by the inert or noble gases of Group VIII (last column of the periodic table). Two other important general trends exist. First, as one goes from left to right across a period, it becomes clear that the number of electrons for each element increases one at a time; the electrons of the outermost shell experience an increasing amount of nuclear attraction, becoming closer and more tightly bound to the nucleus. Second, scanning a given column for a group element from top to bottom shows that with each element the outermost electrons become less tightly bound to the nucleus. This is because the number of filled principal energy levels (which shield the outermost electrons from attraction by the nucleus) increases downward within each group. These trends help explain elemental properties such as atomic radius, ionization potential, electron affinity, and electronegativity.

## Atomic Radius

The atomic radius is an indication of the size of an atom. In general, with each element in a period the atomic radius decreases across a period (from left to right on the table). Within each group, the atomic radius increases (from top to bottom on the table). The atoms with the largest atomic radii are found in the last period (bottom line) of Group I (furthest to the left).

As one moves from left to right across a period, the number of electrons in the outer shell increases one at a time. Electrons in the same shell cannot shield one another from the attractive pull of protons very efficiently. As the number of protons increases, a greater positive charge is produced and the effective nuclear charge increases steadily across a period. This means the valence electrons feel an increasingly strong attraction towards the nucleus, which causes the atomic radius to decrease.

As one moves down a group of the periodic table, the number of electrons and filled electron shells will increase, but the number of valence electrons will remain the same. Thus, the outermost electrons in a given group will feel the same amount of effective nuclear charge, but electrons will be found further from the nucleus as the number of filled energy shells increases. Thus, the atomic radius increases. As such, the atomic radius increases.

## Ionization Energy

The **ionization energy** (IE), or **ionization potential**, is the energy required to completely remove an electron from an atom or ion. Removing an electron from an atom always requires an input of energy, since it is attracted to the positively charged nucleus. The closer and more tightly bound an electron is to the nucleus, the more difficult it is to remove, and the higher its level of ionization energy. Ionization energies grow successively. The **first ionization energy** is the energy required to remove one valence electron from a parent atom; the **second ionization energy** is the energy needed to remove a second valence electron from an ion with a +1 charge to form an ion with a +2 charge, and so on.

Ionization energy increases from left to right across a period as the atomic radius decreases. Moving down a group, ionization energy decreases as the atomic radius increases. Group I elements have low ionization energies because the loss of an electron results in the formation of a stable octet.

## Electron Affinity

Electron affinity is the energy released when an electron is added to a gaseous atom. It represents the ease with which an atom can accept an electron. The stronger the attractive pull of the nucleus for electrons, the greater the electron affinity will be. A positive electron affinity value represents energy release when an electron is added to an atom.

A crude way of describing the difference between ionization energy and electron affinity is that the former tells us how attached the atom is to the electrons it already has, while the latter tells us how the atom feels about gaining another electron.

## Electronegativity

Electronegativity is a measure of the attraction an atom has for electrons in a chemical bond. The greater the electronegativity of an atom, the greater its attraction for bonding electrons. This concept is related to ionization energy and electron affinity: Elements with low ionization energies and low electron affinities will have low levels of electronegativity because their nuclei do not attract electrons strongly, while elements with high ionization energies and high electron affinities will have higher levels of electronegativity because of the strong pull the nucleus has on electrons. Therefore, electronegativity increases from left to right across periods. In any group, electronegativity decreases as the atomic number increases, as a result of the increased distance between the valence electrons and the nucleus—that is, greater atomic radius.

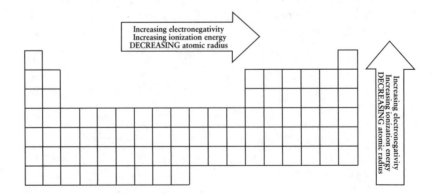

## Categories of Elements

The elements of the periodic table may be classified into three categories: metals, located on the left side and the middle of the periodic table; nonmetals, located on the right side of the table; and metalloids (semimetals), found along a diagonal line between the other two.

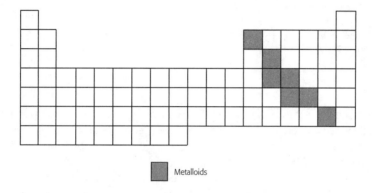

Metalloids

## Metals

Metals are shiny solids at room temperature (except for mercury, which is a liquid) and generally have high melting points and densities. Metals have the characteristic ability to be deformed without breaking. Metal's ability to be hammered into shapes is called **malleability;** its ability to be drawn into wires is called **ductility**. Many of the characteristic properties of metals, such as large atomic radius, low ionization energy, and low electronegativity, are due to the fact that the few electrons in the valence shell of a metal atom can easily be removed. Because valence electrons can move freely, metals are good conductors of heat and electricity. Group IA and IIA represent the most reactive metals. The transition elements are metals that have partially filled **d orbitals**.

## Nonmetals

Nonmetals are generally brittle in a solid state and show little or no metallic luster. They have high ionization energies and electronegativities, and are usually poor conductors of both heat and electricity. Most nonmetals share the ability to gain electrons easily (i.e., they tend to form negative ions), but otherwise they display a wide range of chemical behaviors and reactiveness. Nonmetals are located on the upper right side of the periodic table; they are separated from the metals by a line cutting diagonally through the region of the periodic table containing elements with partially filled **p orbitals**.

## Metalloids

In the periodic table, the metalloids, or semimetals, are found along the line between the metals and nonmetals. The properties of metalloids vary considerably; their densities, boiling points, and melting points fluctuate widely. Their ionization energies and electronegativities lie between those of metals and nonmetals; therefore, these elements possess characteristics of both those classes. For example, silicon has a metallic luster, yet it is brittle and not an efficient conductor. The reactivity of metalloids is dependent upon the element with which they are reacting. For example, boron (B) behaves as a nonmetal when reacting with sodium (Na) and as a metal when reacting with fluorine (F). The elements classified as metalloids are boron, silicon (Si), germanium (Ge), arsenic (As), antimony (Sb), polonium (Po) and tellurium (Te).

## The Chemistry of Groups

Elements in the same group have the same number of valence electrons, and hence tend to have very similar chemical properties.

### Alkali Metals

The alkali metals are the elements of Group IA. They possess most of the physical properties common to metals, yet their densities are lower than those of other metals. The alkali metals have only one loosely bound electron in their outermost shell, giving them the largest atomic radii of all the elements in their respective periods. Their metallic properties and high levels of reactivity are determined by the fact that they have low ionization energies; thus, they easily lose their valence electron to form univalent **cations** (cations with a +1 charge). Alkali metals have low levels of electronegativity and react very readily with nonmetals, especially halogens.

### Alkaline Earth Metals

The alkaline earth metals are the elements of Group IIA. They also possess many characteristically metallic properties. Like the alkali metals, these properties are dependent upon the ease with which they lose electrons. The alkaline earth metals have two electrons in their outer shell and thus have smaller atomic radii than the alkali metals. Alkaline earths have low electronegativities and low electron affinities.

### Halogens

The halogens, Group VIIA (second to last column of the periodic table), are highly reactive nonmetals. They have seven valence electrons, one short of the favored octet configuration. Halogens are highly variable in their physical properties. For instance, at room temperature, the halogens range from gaseous ($F_2$ and $Cl_2$) to liquid ($Br_2$) to solid ($I_2$). Their chemical properties are more uniform: The electronegativities of halogens are very high, and they are particularly reactive with alkali metals and alkaline earth metals that *want* to donate electrons to the halogens to form stable ionic crystals.

### Noble Gases

The noble gases, also called inert gases, are found in Group VIII. They are fairly nonreactive because they have a complete valence shell, which is an energetically favored arrangement. As a result, they have high ionization energies. They possess low boiling points and are all gases at room temperature.

### Transition Elements

The transition elements are those that are found between the alkaline earth metals (the last six columns of the periodic table). The numbering of the groups can get rather confusing because of the existence of two conventions, but you needn't be too concerned with this. These elements are metals known as transition metals. They are very hard and have both high melting and boiling points. As one moves across a period, the five **d orbitals** become progressively more filled. The **d electrons** are held only loosely by the nucleus and are relatively mobile, contributing to the malleability and high electrical conductivity of these elements. Chemically, transition elements have low ionization energies and may exist in a variety of positively charged forms or oxidation states.

## Chemical Bonding

The atoms of many elements can combine to form molecules. The atoms in most molecules are held together by strong attractive forces called chemical bonds. These bonds are formed via the interaction of the valence electrons of combining atoms. The chemical and physical properties of the resulting molecules are often very different from those of their constituent elements. In addition to the very strong forces within a molecule, there are weaker intermolecular forces between molecules. These intermolecular forces, although weaker than the intramolecular chemical bonds, are of considerable importance for understanding the physical properties of many substances.

Processes that involve the breaking and forming of chemical bonds are generally considered chemical processes, while those that only involve interactions between molecules are generally considered physical processes.

In the formation of chemical bonds, many molecules contain atoms bonded according to the octet rule, which states that an atom tends to bond with other atoms until it has eight electrons in its outermost shell. These chemical bonds form a stable electron configuration similar to that of noble gas elements. Exceptions to this rule are as follows: hydrogen, which can have only two valence electrons (the configuration of He); lithium and beryllium, which bond to attain two and four valence electrons, respectively; boron, which bonds to attain six; and elements beyond the second row, such as phosphorus and sulfur, which can expand their octets to include more than eight electrons by incorporating **d** orbitals.

When classifying chemical bonds, it is helpful to introduce two distinct types: **ionic bonds** and **covalent bonds**. During ionic bonding, one or more electrons from an atom with a lower level of ionization energy are transferred to an atom with great electron affinity; the resulting ions are held together by electrostatic forces. During covalent bonding, an electron pair is shared between two atoms. In many cases, the bond is partially covalent and partially ionic; such bonds are called polar covalent bonds.

### Ionic Bonds and Compounds

When two atoms with large differences in electronegativity react, the atom that is less electronegative completely transfers its electrons to the atom that is more electronegative. The elements with higher degrees of electronegativity remove electrons from less electronegative elements. The atom that loses electrons becomes a positively charged ion, or **cation**, and the atom that gains electrons becomes a negatively charged ion, or **anion**. In general, the elements of Groups I and II (low electronegativities) bond ionically to elements of Group VII (high electronegativities).

Ionic compounds have characteristic physical properties. They have high melting and boiling points due to the strong electrostatic forces between ions. They can conduct electricity in liquid and aqueous states, though not in solid states. Ionic solids form crystal lattices consisting of infinite arrays of positive and negative ions. In this arrangement, the attractive forces between ions of opposite charge are maximized, while the repulsive forces between ions of like charge are minimized.

### Covalent Bonds

When two or more atoms with similar electronegativities interact, they often achieve a noble gas electron configuration by sharing electrons in what is known as a covalent bond. However, noble gas configuration is not always attained; there are exceptions to this rule. The binding force between two atoms results from the attraction that each electron of the shared pair has for the two positive nuclei. A covalent bond can be characterized by two features: bond length and bond energy. Bond length is the average distance between the two nuclei of atoms involved in forming the bond; bond energy is the energy required to separate two bonded atoms. As bond length decreases, bond strength increases.

### Types Of Covalent Bonding

The nature of a covalent bond depends on the relative electronegativities of the atoms sharing the electron pairs. Whether or not covalent bonds are considered polar or nonpolar depends on the difference in electronegativities between the atoms. Polar covalent bonding occurs between atoms with small differences in electronegativity. Nonpolar covalent bonding occurs between atoms that have the same electronegativities. This occurs between all of the diatomic elements, such as oxygen, nitrogen, etc.

## Chemical Reactions

In the last section, we discussed how atoms combine and are held together by bonds that can be either ionic or covalent. When atoms combine, that process may result in the loss of some individual properties, while new characteristics may be gained. Water, for example, is formed from two hydrogen atoms and an oxygen atom, but it does not really behave like the elements hydrogen or oxygen.

A compound is a pure substance that is composed of two or more elements in fixed proportion. Compounds can be broken down chemically to produce their constituent elements or other compounds. All elements, except for some of the noble gases, can form new compounds by reacting with other elements or compounds. These new compounds can also react with elements or compounds to form yet more compounds.

### Molecules

A molecule is a combination of two or more atoms held together by covalent bonds. It is the smallest unit of a compound that displays the properties of that compound. Molecules may contain two atoms of the same element, as in $N_2$ and $O_2$, or may be comprised of two or more different atoms, as in $CO_2$ and $SOC_{l2}$.

Earlier, we discussed the concept of atomic weight. Like atoms, molecules can also be characterized by their weight. Molecular weight is simply the sum of the weights of the atoms that make up a molecule.

### Types of Chemical Reactions

There are many ways in which elements and compounds can react to form other compounds; memorizing every reaction would be impossible, as well as unnecessary. However, nearly every inorganic reaction can be classified into at least one of four general categories.

### Combination Reactions

Combination reactions are those in which two or more reactants form one product. The formation of sulfur dioxide by burning sulfur in air is an example of a combination reaction.

$$S\ (s) + O_2(g) \xrightarrow{\Delta} SO_2\ (g)$$

The letters in parentheses designate the phase of the species: **s** for solid, **g** for gas, **l** for liquid, and **aq** for aqueous solution. The sign $\xrightarrow{\Delta}$ represents the addition of heat.

### Decomposition Reactions

A decomposition reaction is defined as one in which a compound breaks down into two or more substances, usually as a result of heating. An example of a decomposition reaction is the breakdown of mercury (II) oxide. Typically, energy is released in these types of reactions, known as exothermic reactions. Energy is released in these types of reactions typically; they are exothermic.

$$2HgO(s) \xrightarrow{\Delta} 2Hg(l) + O_2(g)$$

### Single Displacement Reactions

Single displacement reactions occur when an atom (or ion) of one compound is replaced by an atom of another element. For example, zinc metal will displace copper ions in a copper sulfate solution to form zinc sulfate.

$$Zn\ (s) + CuSO4(aq) \xrightarrow{\Delta} Cu\ (s) + ZnSO4\ (aq)$$

### Double Displacement Reactions

In double displacement reactions, also called metathesis reactions, elements from two different compounds displace each other to form two new compounds. For example, when solutions of calcium chloride and silver nitrate are combined, insoluble silver chloride forms in a solution of calcium nitrate.

$$CaCl2\ (aq) + 2\ AgNO3\ (aq) \xrightarrow{\Delta} Ca(NO3)2\ (aq) + 2\ AgCl\ (s)$$

Neutralization reactions are a specific type of double displacement that occurs when an acid reacts with a base to produce a solution of a salt and water. For example, hydrochloric acid and sodium hydroxide react to form sodium chloride and water.

$$HCl\ (aq) + NaOH\ (aq) \xrightarrow{\Delta} NaCl\ (aq) + H_2O\ (l)$$

## Balanced Equations

Chemical equations express how much and what type of reactants must be used to obtain a given quantity of product. According to the law of conservation of mass, the mass of the reactants must be equal to the mass of the products. More specifically, chemical equations must be balanced so that the product contains the same number of atoms as the reactants.

## Phases of Matter

Matter exists in several phases, each with its own characteristics.

### The Gas Phase

Among the different phases of matter, the gaseous phase is the simplest to understand and model, since all gases, to a first approximation, display similar behavior and follow similar laws, regardless of their identity. The atoms or molecules in a gaseous sample move rapidly and are far apart. In addition, intermolecular forces between gas particles tend to be weak; this results in certain characteristic physical properties, such as the ability to expand in order to fill any volume and to take on the shape of a container. Furthermore, gases are easily, though not infinitely, compressible.

### Descriptive Chemistry of Some Common Gases

There are certain miscellaneous facts about the properties of some common gases you should be aware of. These properties are exploited in qualitative tests designed to detect their presence.

- **Oxygen:** Molecular oxygen, $O_2$, is a reactant in combustion reactions. If a glowing splint is lowered into a test tube containing oxygen, it will reignite.
- **Hydrogen:** When ignited in air, $H_2$, burns with a blue flame.
- **Nitrogen:** $N_2$, the largest component of air (a little less than 80% by volume) is relatively inert.
- **Carbon dioxide:** $CO_2$ produces a moderately acidic solution when dissolved in water because of the reaction:

$$CO_2\ (g) + H_2O\ (l) \xrightarrow{\Delta} H_2CO_3\ (aq)$$

When carbon dioxide is passed through limewater, $Ca(OH)_2$, the solution turns cloudy from the formation of insoluble calcium carbonate:

$$CO_2 + Ca(OH)_2 \xrightarrow{\Delta} CaCO_3 + H_2O$$

The precipitation of calcium carbonate, however, does not go on indefinitely. As just mentioned, water containing $CO_2$ is slightly acidic, and this causes calcium carbonate to dissolve:

$$CaCO_3 \ (s) + H_2O(l) + CO_2 \ (g) \xrightarrow{\Delta} Ca_2 + (aq) + 2HCO_3 \xrightarrow{\Delta} (aq)$$

### Kinetic Molecular Theory of Gases

All gases show similar physical characteristics and behavior. A theoretical model to explain why gases behave the way they do was developed during the second half of the nineteenth century. The combined efforts of Ludwig Boltzmann, James Clerk Maxwell, and others led to the **kinetic molecular theory of gases**, which gives us an understanding of the behavior of gases on a microscopic, molecular level. Like the gas laws, this theory was developed in reference to ideal gases, although it can be applied with reasonable accuracy to real gases as well. The assumptions of the kinetic molecular theory of gases are as follows:

1. Gases are made up of particles whose volumes are negligible compared to the container volume.

2. Gas atoms or molecules exhibit no intermolecular attractions or repulsions.

3. Gas particles are in continuous, random motion, undergoing collisions with other particles and with the container walls.

4. Collisions between any two gas particles are elastic, meaning that no energy is dissipated or, equivalently, no kinetic energy is conserved.

5. The average kinetic energy of gas particles is proportional to the absolute temperature of the gas and is the same for all gases at a given temperature.

### Condensed Phase and Phase Changes

When the attractive forces between molecules overcome the random thermal kinetic energy that keeps molecules apart during the gas phase, molecules cluster together, unable to move about freely and then enter the liquid or solid phase. Because of their smaller volume relative to gases, liquids and solids are often referred to as the condensed phases.

## General Properties of Liquids

In a liquid, atoms or molecules are held close together with little space between them. As a result, liquids, unlike gases, have definite volumes and cannot be expanded or compressed easily. However, molecules can still move around and are in a state of relative disorder. Consequently, a liquid can change shape to fit its container, and its molecules are able to diffuse and evaporate.

One of the most important properties of liquids is their ability to mix, both with each other and other phases, forming **solutions**. The degree to which two liquids can mix is called their **miscibility**. Oil and water are almost completely immiscible because of their difference in polarity. When oil and water are mixed, they normally form separate layers, with oil on top because it is less dense. Under extreme conditions, such as violent shaking, two immiscible liquids can form a fairly homogeneous mixture called an emulsion. Although they look like solutions, emulsions are actually mixtures of discrete particles too small to be seen distinctly.

## General Properties of Solids

In a solid, the attractive forces between atoms, ions, or molecules are strong enough to hold them together rigidly; thus, the particles' only motion is vibration about fixed positions, and the kinetic energy of solids is predominantly vibrational energy. As a result, solids have definite shapes and volumes.

## Phase Equilibria and Phase Changes

The different phases of matter interchange upon the absorption or release of energy, and more than one of them may exist in equilibrium under certain conditions. **Dynamic equilibrium** is a condition that permits two opposing processes to occur in a manner that the outcome's net change is zero. In the next sections we will discuss some other types of equilibrium.

### Gas-Liquid Equilibrium

The temperature of a liquid is related to the average kinetic energy of the liquid molecules; however, the kinetic energy of the individual molecules will vary (just as there is a distribution of molecular speeds in a gas). A few molecules near the surface of the liquid may have enough energy to leave the liquid phase and escape into the gaseous phase. This process is known as **evaporation** (or **vaporization**). Each time liquid loses a high-energy particle, the average kinetic energy of the remaining molecules decreases, which means that the temperature of the liquid decreases. Evaporation is thus a cooling process. Given enough kinetic energy, the liquid will completely evaporate.

If a cover is placed on a beaker of liquid, the escaping molecules are trapped above the solution. These molecules exert a countering pressure, which forces some of the gas back into the liquid phase; this process is called **condensation**.

Atmospheric pressure acts on a liquid in a similar fashion as a solid lid. As evaporation and condensation proceed, a state of equilibrium is reached in which the rates of the two processes become equal; that is, the liquid and vapor are in dynamic equilibrium. The pressure the gas exerts when the two phases are at equilibrium is called the **vapor pressure**. Vapor pressure increases as temperature increases because more molecules will have sufficient kinetic energy to escape into the gas phase. The temperature at which the vapor pressure of the liquid equals the external (most often atmospheric) pressure is called the boiling point. In general, then, the temperature at which a liquid boils is dependent on the pressure surrounding it. We know water boils at 100°C because at this temperature its vapor pressure (or the pressure exerted by the gas phase $H_2O$ molecules) is equal to one atmosphere. At places of high elevation, the surrounding pressure is lower than 1 standard atmostpheric pressure (atm), so water boils at a lower temperature. By controlling the ambient pressure, we can change the temperature at which water boils. This is the principle behind pressure cookers. By maintaining high pressure, water can reach a temperature higher than 100°C before it vaporizes, thus making it more effective at heating things.

### Liquid-Solid Equilibrium

The liquid and solid phases can also coexist in equilibrium. Even though the atoms or molecules of a solid are confined to definite locations, each atom or molecule can undergo motions about some equilibrium position. These motions (vibrations) increase when energy (most commonly in the form of heat) is supplied. If atoms or molecules in the solid phase absorb enough energy in this fashion, the solid's three-dimensional structure breaks down and the liquid phase begins. The transition from solid to liquid is called **fusion** or **melting**. The reverse process, from liquid to solid, is called **solidification**, **crystallization**, or **freezing**. The temperature at which these processes occur is called the **melting point** or **freezing point**, depending on the direction of the transition.

Whereas pure crystals have very distinct, sharp melting points, amorphous solids such as glass tend to melt over a larger range of temperatures, due to their less-ordered molecular distribution.

### Gas-Solid Equilibrium

A third type of phase equilibrium exists between gasses and solids. When a solid goes directly into the gas phase, the process is called **sublimation**. Dry ice (solid $CO_2$) sublimes under atmospheric pressure; the absence of a liquid phase makes it a convenient refrigerant. The reverse transition, from a gaseous to solid phase, is called **deposition**.

## Solution Chemistry

Solutions are homogeneous mixtures of substances that combine to form a single phase, generally the liquid phase. Many important chemical reactions, both in the laboratory and in nature, take place in solution (including almost all reactions in living organisms). A solution consists of a **solute** dissolved in a **solvent**. The solvent is the component of the solution whose phase remains the same after mixing. For example, a solid cube of sugar dissolved in water yields a liquid mixture of water and sugar. In this example, water is the solvent and sugar the solute.

If the two substances are already in the same phase, the solvent is generally taken to be the component present in greater quantity. Solute molecules move about freely in solvent and can interact with other molecules or ions; consequently, chemical reactions occur easily in solution.

### Solution Terminology

There are several key ideas and terms relating to solutions you should be familiar with.

**Solvation:** The interaction between solute and solvent molecules is known as solvation or **dissolution**; when water is the solvent, it is also known as **hydration** and the resulting solution is known as an **aqueous solution**.

**Solubility:** The solubility of a substance is the maximum amount of that substance that can be dissolved in a particular solvent at a particular temperature.

**Percent Composition by Mass:** The percent composition by mass of a solution is the mass of the solute divided by the mass of the solution (solute plus solvent), multiplied by 100.

**Dilution:** A solution is diluted when solvent is added to a solution of high concentration to produce a solution of lower concentration.

### Acids and Bases

Many important reactions in chemical and biological systems involve two classes of compounds—acids and bases. The presence of acids and bases can often be easily detected because they lead to color changes in certain compounds called indicators, which may be in solution or on paper. A particular common indicator is litmus paper, which turns red in acidic solution and blue in basic solution. A more extensive discussion of the chemical properties of acids and bases is outlined below.

### Definitions of Acids and Bases

The first definitions of acids and bases were formulated by Svante Arrhenius toward the end of the nineteenth century. Arrhenius defined an acid as a species that produces H+ (protons) in an aqueous solution, and a base as a species that produces OH– (hydroxide ions) in an aqueous solution.

A more general definition of acids and bases was proposed independently by Johannes Brønsted and Thomas Lowry in 1923. A Brønsted-Lowry acid is a species that donates protons, while a Brønsted-Lowry base is a species that accepts protons. At approximately the same time as Brønsted and Lowry, Gilbert Lewis also proposed definitions for acids and bases. Lewis defined an acid as an electron-pair acceptor, and a base as an electron-pair donor. Lewis's are the most inclusive definitions, however; we will focus our attention on Brønsted-Lowry acids and bases.

### Properties of Acids and Bases

The behavior of acids and bases in solution is governed by equilibrium considerations. It's important to know that pH (proton concentration) and pOH (hydrogen ion concentration) are not totally independent of each other: Knowing the value of one allows us to calculate the other.

For example, in pure water ($H_2O$), pH and pOH would be equal, both having a value of 7. A solution with equal concentrations of H+ and OH– is neutral. A pH below 7 indicates a relative excess of H+ ions, and therefore an acidic solution; a pH above 7 indicates a relative excess of OH– ions, and therefore a basic solution.

## Radioactive Decay

Radioactive decay is a naturally occurring and spontaneous. It is characterized by the decay of certain nuclei and the emission of specific particles. It could be classified as a certain type of fission. The **reactant** in radioactive decay is known as the **parent isotope** while the product is the daughter isotope.

### Alpha Decay

Alpha decay is the emission of an alpha ($\alpha$) particle, which is a $^4$He nucleus that consists of two protons and two neutrons. The alpha particle is very massive (compared to a beta particle, see below) and doubly charged. Alpha particles interact with matter very easily; hence they do not penetrate shielding (such as lead sheets) very far.

### Beta Decay

Beta decay is the emission of a beta particle (β). Despite the similarity between electrons and beta particles, it is important to realize that these particles are not electrons that would normally be found around the nucleus in a neutral atom. Rather, they are products of decay emitted by the nucleus. This is particularly true when a neutron in the nucleus decays into a proton and an electron. Since an electron is singly charged, and about 1,836 times lighter than a proton, the beta radiation from radioactive decay is more penetrating than alpha radiation.

### Gamma Decay

Gamma decay is the emission of gamma rays (γ), which are high-energy photons. They carry no charge and simply lower the energy of the emitting (parent) nucleus without changing the mass number or the atomic number. In other words, the daughter's **A** is the same as the parent's, and the daughter's **Z** is the same as the parent's.

### Radioactive Decay Half-Life ($t_{1/2}$)

In a collection of a great many identical radioactive isotopes, the half-life of a sample is the time it takes for half of the sample to decay. For example: If the half-life of a certain isotope is four years, what fraction of a sample of that isotope will remain after 12 years?

Solution: If four years is one half-life, then 12 years is three half-lives. During the first half-life—the first four years—half of the sample will have decayed. During the second half-life (years five to eight), another half will decay, leaving one-fourth of the original. During the third and final period (years nine to 12), half of the remaining fourth will decay, leaving one-eighth of the original sample.

The fact that different radioactive species have different characteristic half-lives is what enables scientists to determine the age of organic materials. The long-lived radioactive carbon Isotope $^{14}C$, for example, is generated from nuclear reactions induced by high-energy cosmic rays from outer space. There is always a certain fraction of this isotope in the carbon found on Earth. Living things, like trees and animals, are constantly exchanging carbon with the environment, and thus will have the same ratio of carbon-14 to carbon-12 within them as is present in the atmosphere. Once they die, however, they stop incorporating carbon from the environment, and start to lose carbon-14 because of its radioactivity. The longer the species has been dead, the less carbon-14 it will still have. For example, if a sample is taken from an item or the body and the ratio of $^{14}C$ to $^{12}C$ is half of that present in the atmosphere, we would conclude that the species existed about one half-life of $^{14}C$ ago.

## Organic Chemistry

Organic chemistry is the study of compounds containing the element carbon. This covers a wide range of compounds, including proteins, alcohols, steroids, sugars, and compounds found in petroleum, just to name a few. The reason we can study them as facets of one subject is because of the unifying bonding properties of carbon.

## Hydrocarbons

Hydrocarbons are compounds that contain only carbon and hydrogen atoms. Depending on the kinds of bonds found between carbon atoms (only single bonds can exist between carbon and hydrogen), hydrocarbons can be classified into one of four classes: alkanes, alkenes, alkynes, and aromatics.

### Alkanes, Alkenes, and Alkynes

Alkanes are hydrocarbons that contain only single bonds. They are all named by attaching the suffix *-ane* to a prefix that indicates the number of carbon atoms. These prefixes will be used again in the naming of other hydrocarbons and it is therefore worth knowing at least a few.

| # of C Atoms | Prefix | Name of Alkane | Molecular Formula |
|:---:|:---:|:---:|:---:|
| 1 | *meth-* | methane | $CH_4$ |
| 2 | *eth-* | ethane | $C_2H_6$ |
| 3 | *prop-* | propane | $C_3H_8$ |
| 4 | *but-* | butane | $C_4H_{10}$ |
| 5 | *pent-* | pentane | $C_5H_{12}$ |
| 6 | *hex-* | hexane | $C_6H_{14}$ |

Alkenes are hydrocarbons involving carbon-carbon double bonds. They are named using the same scheme as alkanes, except that their suffix is *-ene*.

Alkynes are hydrocarbons involving carbon-carbon triple bonds. They follow the same naming scheme as alkanes and alkenes, but use the suffix *-yne*.

### Aromatics

Certain unsaturated cyclic hydrocarbons are known as aromatics. We need not concern ourselves with exactly what makes a compound aromatic, but all such compounds have a cyclic, planar structure in common and possess a higher degree of stability than expected.

### Oxygen-Containing Compounds

Organic compounds that include oxygen in addition to carbon and hydrogen include alcohols, ethers, carbohydrates, and carbonyl compounds such as aldehydes, ketones, esters, and carboxylic acids.

### Nitrogen-Containing Compounds

Nitrogen-containing compounds are another large class of organic compounds. The most important nitrogen-containing functional group is the amine group, $-NH_2$, which is found in amino acids, the basic building blocks of proteins.

Now that you have reviewed the basics of chemistry, you can start to review the basics of physics.

# PHYSICS LESSON

## Kinematics

*Kinematics* is the branch of mechanics dealing with motion. It is the study of how things move: *how far* things move, *how fast* they move, how fast they move, and *how long* it takes them to move.

## Distance and Displacement

While **distance** is the total amount of space moved, without a particular direction, displacement is very different. **Displacement** is a vector quantity that describes a change in position, and it has both direction and magnitude.

## Speed and Velocity

**Average speed** is scalar. To calculate the average speed of an object, take the total distance covered, and divide it by the total time it took to cover the distance:

$$\text{Average Speed} = \frac{\text{Total Distance}}{\text{Total Time}}$$

$$V = \frac{D}{T}$$

In the equation above, *V* stands for speed, *D* is for distance, and *T* is time.

**Average velocity** is the ratio of the displacement vector over the change in time and is a vector quantity. **Acceleration** (a) is the rate of change of an object's velocity. To calculate acceleration, divide an object's **velocity** (v) or **change in velocity** (v) by the change in **time** (t). The equation is as follows.

$$\text{Acceleration} = \frac{\text{Change in Velocity}}{\text{Change in Time}}$$

## Newtonian Mechanics

**Dynamics** is the study of what causes motion; that is, the **forces** that lead to motion, such as pulling or pushing. Dynamics is often referred to as Newtonian mechanics or Newton's laws of motion, after Isaac Newton, who published his groundbreaking three laws of motion in 1687.

Force is a vector quantity. Forces are observed as the push or pull on an object. Forces can either be exerted between bodies in contact (such as the force a person exerts to push a box across the floor), or between bodies not in contact (such as the force of gravity holding the Earth in its orbit). The unit for force, in SI, is the Newton (N).

### Newton's First Law of Motion

A body either at rest or in motion with constant velocity will remain that way unless a **net force** acts upon it. This law is often known as the law of inertia.

### Newton's Second Law of Motion

A net force applied to a body of a mass will result in that body undergoing acceleration in the same direction as the net force. The magnitude of the body's acceleration is directly proportional to the magnitude of the net force and inversely proportional to the body's mass. This can be expressed as:

$$F_{net} = \Sigma F = m\mathbf{a}$$

### Newton's Third Law of Motion

If body (A) exerts a force (F) on body (B), then body (B) exerts a force (-F), that is equal in magnitude and opposite in direction, back on (A). In Newtown's own words, "to every action there is always an opposed but equal reaction." The concept can be expressed as:

$$F_B = -F_A$$

### Gravity

**Gravity** is an attractive force felt by all forms of matter. The magnitude of the **gravitational force** (F) is given as:

$$F = \frac{Gm^1 m^2}{r^2}$$

In this approach, (G) is the gravitational constant ($6.67 \times 10^{-11}$ N $\cdot$ m$^2$/kg$^2$), m$^1$ and m$^2$ are the masses of the two objects, and (r) is the distance between their centers.

### Friction

Whenever two objects are in contact, their surfaces rub together creating a friction force. **Static friction** ($f_s$) is the force that must be overcome to set an object in motion. For example, to make a book that is at rest start to slide across a table, a force greater than the maximum static force is required. However, once the book starts to slide, the friction force is not as strong. This new friction force is called **kinetic friction**.

## Work And Energy

There are many words in physics that may be used quite differently outside the context of a physics course—work and energy are two such words.

## Work

Essentially, you can think of work as responsible for changing the energy of an object. Work is defined as the scalar product of force (F) and displacement (s):

$$W = Fs$$

Work is expressed in **joules** (J) as it is the product of force and displacement; it has units of Newton-meters, or **joules** (J). A joule is a unit of work or energy equal to the work done by a force of one Newton acting through a distance of one meter. The work done by applying a force of one newton through a displacement of one meter. Work can be written out in the following equation:

$$W = Fd \cos \theta$$

In this approach, $\theta$ is the angle between the applied force and the displacement.

## Energy

A body in motion possesses energy. This energy of motion is called **kinetic energy**. A body can also possess **potential energy**, which depends on a body's position rather than motion. An example of potential energy is the gravitational potential energy an object has when it is raised to a particular height. Objects on Earth have greater potential energy the further they are from the surface.

## Conservation of Energy

When the work done by nonconservative forces is equal to zero or there are no nonconservative forces (such as an object falling without air resistance), the total amount of energy, also known as the total mechanical energy, remains constant. In such a situation, there in a conservation of energy.

## Power

The amount of work required to perform an operation is less important than the amount of time required to do the work. **Power** is the rate at which work is done and the equation to calculate it is:

$$P = \frac{\text{Work}}{\text{Time}}$$

## Waves

Waves contain individual particles that move back and forth with simple harmonic motion. In **transverse waves** the particles oscillate perpendicular to the direction of the wave motion. String elements move at right angles to the direction of travel of a wave. In the case of **longitudinal waves**, particles oscillate along the direction of the wave motion.

**Traveling waves** are best described by example: If a string that is fixed at one end is moved from side to side, a wave travels down the string. When the wave reaches a fixed boundary, it is reflected and inverted. If the free end of the string is continuously moved from side to side, two waves are created—the original wave moving down the string, and a reflected wave moving the other way. These waves interfere with each other.

If a string is fixed on both ends, and waves are created, certain wave frequencies can result in a waveform remaining in a stationary position—known as **standing waves**.

### Sound Waves

Sound is transmitted by the movement of particles along the direction of motion of a sound wave. As such, sound is a longitudinal wave. More generally, sound is a mechanical disturbance that is dependent upon a medium for travel. It can be transmitted through solids, liquids, and gases; it cannot be transmitted through vacuum. The speed of sound in a medium is determined by the spacing of particles. The smaller the spacing between particles, the faster sound will travel in that medium. For this reason, sound travels faster in a solid than in a liquid, and faster in a liquid that in a gas.

For sound to be produced, there must me a longitudinal movement of air molecules—produced by the vibration of a solid object that sets adjacent molecules into motion, or by means of an acoustic vibration in an enclosed space. Sound produced by string and percussion instruments such as the guitar, violin, and piano, comes from solid objects. Using these instruments as an example, a string or several strings are set into motion and vibrate at their normal mode frequencies. Since the strings are very thin, they are ineffective in transmitting their vibration to the surrounding air. A solid body is employed to provide a better coupling to the air. In the case of a guitar, the vibration is transmitted through the bridge to the body of the instrument, which vibrates at the same frequency as the string.

Sound created by acoustic vibration includes sound from instruments such as organ pipes, the flute, and the recorder. There are no moving parts—sound is produced by a vibrating motion of air within the instrument. In the case of an organ pipe, pitch is determined by the length of the pipe. However, instruments such as the recorder and the flute are able to generate more than one pitch by the opening and closing of holes. The sound of the human voice is created by air passing between vocal cords. Pitch is controlled by varying tension of the cords.

## Electric Charge

**Charge** may be either positive or negative. A positive charge and a negative charge attract one another; positive repels positive; and negative repels negative. These fundamental concepts are the foundation of Coulomb's law, which is essential to understanding all electrical phenomena. The SI unit of charge is the **Coulomb** (C).

## Current, Voltage, and Resistance

The flow of a charge is called an **electric current**. There are two types of basic currents: **direct** and **alternating**. The charge of a direct current flows in one direction only; the flow of an alternating current changes periodically. When two points at different electric potentials are connected by a conductor (such as a metal wire), charge flows between the two points. In a conductor, only negatively charged electrons are free to move. These acts as charge carriers and move from low to high potentials. The direction of the current is taken as the direction in which positive charge would flow, from high to low. Thus the direction of current is opposite to the direction of electron flow.

Resistance is the opposition within a conductor to the flow of an electric current. The opposition takes the form of an energy loss or drop in potential. **Ohm's law** states the voltage drop across a resistor is proportional to the current it carries. Current is unchanged as it passes through a resistor. This is because no charge is lost inside a resistor. The SI derived unit of electrical resistance is the **Ohm** ($\Omega$).

Although the topic of electricity may not seem directly related to nursing, you should have a general understanding of it.

Now that you have completed your review of basic chemistry and physics, you're ready to learn some strategies for test day.

## PHYSICAL SCIENCE STRATEGIES

If you read the strategies we present in Chapter Seven, Life Sciences, you know the science portions of the nursing school entrance exams contain knowledge-based questions. You also know that doesn't mean that there are no strategies to use on test day. It just means they have slightly different approach because they have to deal with a test of knowledge. Here are our favorite strategies for knowledge-based test questions.

- Intense review of terms or concepts commonly confused for each other.
- Quizzing yourself.
- General test-taking strategies.

Here is how each one of these works for Physical Science.

### Terms Commonly Confused for Each Other

After long hours of study, you might not even care what the difference between an ionic bond and a covalent bond is. However, you would care if that were something you were facing on test day. Here are a few of the terms and concepts in chemistry and physics that are commonly confused or mistaken for each other. Familiarize yourself with them in preparation for the test.

#### Don't Mix These Up on Test Day

- **Atomic number**: number of protons
- **Mass number**: number of protons and neutrons

- **Ionic bond:** transfer of electron(s)
- **Covalent bond:** sharing of electron(s)

- **Solute**: substance being dissolved (often solid)
- **Solvent**: substance doing the dissolving (often liquid)
- **Solution**: solvent and a dissolved solute

- **Arrhenius** defined an acid as a species that produces H+ in an aqueous solution, and a base as a species that produces OH– in aqueous solution.
- A **Brønsted-Lawry** acid is a species that donates protons, while a **Brønsted-Lawry base** is a species that accepts protons.
- A **Lewis acid** is an electronpair acceptor, and a **Lewis base** is an electron-pair donor.

- **Mass** is the measure of the amount of substance in an object, and is measured in kilograms.
- **Weight** is the gravitational force pulling down on an object, and is measured in Newtons (N).

- **Heat** is the kinetic energy of molecules transferred from a warmer substance to a cooler one.
- **Temperature** is a measure of the average kinetic energy of the molecules in a substance.

- The **atomic number Z** is the number of protons.
- The **mass number A** is the number of protons and neutrons.

- **Fusion** is the combining of small nuclei into larger ones, releasing energy.
- **Fission** is the splitting of a large nucleus into smaller ones, with the release of neutrons and energy.

## General Test-Taking Strategies

At this stage, you might want to go back to Chapter One and review some tips that are likely to help on any type of question. These include answering easier questions first, making an educated guess, and using the process of elimination to find the right answer.

For the Physical Science questions, your very best option is going to be to study hard and prepare yourself for test day. Don't forget to use the Learning Resources in the back of the book to help you. If you're ready to start reviewing, try to answer as many of the review questions from this chapter as you can.

# REVIEW QUESTIONS

Because you are being tested on your knowledge, you are going to need consistent review of things you are studying. Make flashcards, create lists, or write notes on what you have studied. You can ask friends or family to quiz you to make sure that you have mastered the concepts and really know the material. By reviewing your study materials and completing the following review questions, you are on your way to test day success.

The following questions are not meant to mimic actual test questions. Instead, these questions will help you review the concepts and terms covered in this chapter.

1.  List the three types of subatomic particles.

    _____

    _____

    _____

2.  True or False? The periodic table arranges elements in decreasing atomic numbers.

3.  The elements of the periodic table may be classified into three categories; list them below.

    _____

    _____

    _____

4.  Define the chemical term **compound**.

    _____

    _____

5.  Which of the following is NOT a gas law?

    The assumptions of the kinetic molecular theory of gases are as follows:

    (A) Gases are made up of particles whose volumes are negligible compared to the container volume.

    (B) Gas atoms or molecules exhibit no intermolecular attractions or repulsions.

    (C) Gas particles are in continuous, random motion, undergoing collisions with other particles and with the container walls.

    (D) Because gases can take on the shape of a container, they are infinitely compressible.

    (E) Collisions between any two gas particles are elastic, meaning that no energy is dissipated or, equivalently, that kinetic energy is conserved.

    (F) The average kinetic energy of gas particles is proportional to the absolute temperature of the gas, and is the same for all gases at a given temperature.

6.  Fill in the blank. The transition from liquid to solid is called _____.

7.  Define half-life.

    _____

    _____

8.  True or false? Kinematics is the study of why things move.

9. Give the equation for acceleration.

   _____

   _____

10. Put Newton's Three Laws of Motion in order.

    _____ Law of action and reaction

    _____ Law of inertia

    _____ Force equals mass times acceleration

11. True or False? The law of conservation of energy states that when work is done on a system, the energy of that system changes from one form to another, but the total amount of energy remains the same.

12. Match the type of wave with its description.

    _____ Transverse wave

    _____ Longitudinal wave

    (A) A wave that vibrates in a direction that is perpendicular to the direction of motion of the wave.

    (B) A wave that vibrates in a direction that is parallel to the direction of motion of the wave.

13. Check all that apply to a sound wave.

    _____ It is a longitudinal wave.

    _____ It is a mechanical wave.

    _____ It is a transverse wave.

    _____ It does not need a medium to travel through.

14. True or False?

    Heat is the kinetic energy of molecules transferred from a cooler substance to a warmer one.

15. Write the law of charges.

    _____

    _____

THE ANSWERS APPEAR ON THE FOLLOWING PAGE.

## REVIEWS ANSWERS

1.  A.  Protons
    B.  Neutrons
    C.  Electrons

2.  False. The periodic table arranges the elements in **increasing** atomic numbers.

3.  A.  Metals
    B.  Nonmetals
    C.  Metalloids

4.  A compound is a pure substance that is composed of two or more elements in a fixed proportion.

5.  Option (D) is not a gas law.

6.  Possible answers include: solidification, crystallization, or freezing.

7.  The half-life of a sample is the time it takes for half of the sample to decay.

8.  False. Kinematics is the study of how things move. The study of why things move is called dynamism.

9.  $\text{Acceleration} = \dfrac{\text{Change in Velocity}}{\text{Change in Time}}$.

10. (C)  Law of action and reaction.
    (A)  Law of inertia.
    (B)  Force equals mass times acceleration.

11. True.

12. (A)  Transverse Wave
    (B)  Longitudinal Wave

13. The correct selections are:
    It is a longitudinal wave.
    It is a mechanical wave.

14. False.
    Heat is the kinetic energy of molecules transferred from a warmer substance to a cooler one.

15. The law of charges states that like charges repel each other and unlike charges attract each other.

# Practice Tests and Explanations

This is the first full-length practice test in this book. There is an answer sheet on the following page. At the end of the test, you will find an answer key as well as detailed answer explanations. Use these explanations to understand what questions you missed and why. By scoring your test and reading through the answer explanations, you should be able to further diagnose your strengths and weaknesses as you prepare for test day.

# Nursing School Entrance Exams
## Practice Test One
## Answer Sheet

### Reading Comprehension

| | | | | |
|---|---|---|---|---|
| 1. Ⓐ Ⓑ Ⓒ Ⓓ | 10. Ⓐ Ⓑ Ⓒ Ⓓ | 19. Ⓐ Ⓑ Ⓒ Ⓓ | 28. Ⓐ Ⓑ Ⓒ Ⓓ | 37. Ⓐ Ⓑ Ⓒ Ⓓ |
| 2. Ⓐ Ⓑ Ⓒ Ⓓ | 11. Ⓐ Ⓑ Ⓒ Ⓓ | 20. Ⓐ Ⓑ Ⓒ Ⓓ | 29. Ⓐ Ⓑ Ⓒ Ⓓ | 38. Ⓐ Ⓑ Ⓒ Ⓓ |
| 3. Ⓐ Ⓑ Ⓒ Ⓓ | 12. Ⓐ Ⓑ Ⓒ Ⓓ | 21. Ⓐ Ⓑ Ⓒ Ⓓ | 30. Ⓐ Ⓑ Ⓒ Ⓓ | 39. Ⓐ Ⓑ Ⓒ Ⓓ |
| 4. Ⓐ Ⓑ Ⓒ Ⓓ | 13. Ⓐ Ⓑ Ⓒ Ⓓ | 22. Ⓐ Ⓑ Ⓒ Ⓓ | 31. Ⓐ Ⓑ Ⓒ Ⓓ | 40. Ⓐ Ⓑ Ⓒ Ⓓ |
| 5. Ⓐ Ⓑ Ⓒ Ⓓ | 14. Ⓐ Ⓑ Ⓒ Ⓓ | 23. Ⓐ Ⓑ Ⓒ Ⓓ | 32. Ⓐ Ⓑ Ⓒ Ⓓ | 41. Ⓐ Ⓑ Ⓒ Ⓓ |
| 6. Ⓐ Ⓑ Ⓒ Ⓓ | 15. Ⓐ Ⓑ Ⓒ Ⓓ | 24. Ⓐ Ⓑ Ⓒ Ⓓ | 33. Ⓐ Ⓑ Ⓒ Ⓓ | 42. Ⓐ Ⓑ Ⓒ Ⓓ |
| 7. Ⓐ Ⓑ Ⓒ Ⓓ | 16. Ⓐ Ⓑ Ⓒ Ⓓ | 25. Ⓐ Ⓑ Ⓒ Ⓓ | 34. Ⓐ Ⓑ Ⓒ Ⓓ | 43. Ⓐ Ⓑ Ⓒ Ⓓ |
| 8. Ⓐ Ⓑ Ⓒ Ⓓ | 17. Ⓐ Ⓑ Ⓒ Ⓓ | 26. Ⓐ Ⓑ Ⓒ Ⓓ | 35. Ⓐ Ⓑ Ⓒ Ⓓ | 44. Ⓐ Ⓑ Ⓒ Ⓓ |
| 9. Ⓐ Ⓑ Ⓒ Ⓓ | 18. Ⓐ Ⓑ Ⓒ Ⓓ | 27. Ⓐ Ⓑ Ⓒ Ⓓ | 36. Ⓐ Ⓑ Ⓒ Ⓓ | 45. Ⓐ Ⓑ Ⓒ Ⓓ |

### Vocabulary and Spelling

| | | | | |
|---|---|---|---|---|
| 1. Ⓐ Ⓑ Ⓒ Ⓓ | 14. Ⓐ Ⓑ Ⓒ Ⓓ | 27. Ⓐ Ⓑ Ⓒ Ⓓ | 40. Ⓐ Ⓑ Ⓒ Ⓓ | 53. Ⓐ Ⓑ Ⓒ Ⓓ |
| 2. Ⓐ Ⓑ Ⓒ Ⓓ | 15. Ⓐ Ⓑ Ⓒ Ⓓ | 28. Ⓐ Ⓑ Ⓒ Ⓓ | 41. Ⓐ Ⓑ Ⓒ Ⓓ | 54. Ⓐ Ⓑ Ⓒ Ⓓ |
| 3. Ⓐ Ⓑ Ⓒ Ⓓ | 16. Ⓐ Ⓑ Ⓒ Ⓓ | 29. Ⓐ Ⓑ Ⓒ Ⓓ | 42. Ⓐ Ⓑ Ⓒ Ⓓ | 55. Ⓐ Ⓑ Ⓒ Ⓓ |
| 4. Ⓐ Ⓑ Ⓒ Ⓓ | 17. Ⓐ Ⓑ Ⓒ Ⓓ | 30. Ⓐ Ⓑ Ⓒ Ⓓ | 43. Ⓐ Ⓑ Ⓒ Ⓓ | 56. Ⓐ Ⓑ Ⓒ Ⓓ |
| 5. Ⓐ Ⓑ Ⓒ Ⓓ | 18. Ⓐ Ⓑ Ⓒ Ⓓ | 31. Ⓐ Ⓑ Ⓒ Ⓓ | 44. Ⓐ Ⓑ Ⓒ Ⓓ | 57. Ⓐ Ⓑ Ⓒ Ⓓ |
| 6. Ⓐ Ⓑ Ⓒ Ⓓ | 19. Ⓐ Ⓑ Ⓒ Ⓓ | 32. Ⓐ Ⓑ Ⓒ Ⓓ | 45. Ⓐ Ⓑ Ⓒ Ⓓ | 58. Ⓐ Ⓑ Ⓒ Ⓓ |
| 7. Ⓐ Ⓑ Ⓒ Ⓓ | 20. Ⓐ Ⓑ Ⓒ Ⓓ | 33. Ⓐ Ⓑ Ⓒ Ⓓ | 46. Ⓐ Ⓑ Ⓒ Ⓓ | 59. Ⓐ Ⓑ Ⓒ Ⓓ |
| 8. Ⓐ Ⓑ Ⓒ Ⓓ | 21. Ⓐ Ⓑ Ⓒ Ⓓ | 34. Ⓐ Ⓑ Ⓒ Ⓓ | 47. Ⓐ Ⓑ Ⓒ Ⓓ | 60. Ⓐ Ⓑ Ⓒ Ⓓ |
| 9. Ⓐ Ⓑ Ⓒ Ⓓ | 22. Ⓐ Ⓑ Ⓒ Ⓓ | 35. Ⓐ Ⓑ Ⓒ Ⓓ | 48. Ⓐ Ⓑ Ⓒ Ⓓ | 61. Ⓐ Ⓑ Ⓒ Ⓓ |
| 10. Ⓐ Ⓑ Ⓒ Ⓓ | 23. Ⓐ Ⓑ Ⓒ Ⓓ | 36. Ⓐ Ⓑ Ⓒ Ⓓ | 49. Ⓐ Ⓑ Ⓒ Ⓓ | 62. Ⓐ Ⓑ Ⓒ Ⓓ |
| 11. Ⓐ Ⓑ Ⓒ Ⓓ | 24. Ⓐ Ⓑ Ⓒ Ⓓ | 37. Ⓐ Ⓑ Ⓒ Ⓓ | 50. Ⓐ Ⓑ Ⓒ Ⓓ | 63. Ⓐ Ⓑ Ⓒ Ⓓ |
| 12. Ⓐ Ⓑ Ⓒ Ⓓ | 25. Ⓐ Ⓑ Ⓒ Ⓓ | 38. Ⓐ Ⓑ Ⓒ Ⓓ | 51. Ⓐ Ⓑ Ⓒ Ⓓ | 64. Ⓐ Ⓑ Ⓒ Ⓓ |
| 13. Ⓐ Ⓑ Ⓒ Ⓓ | 26. Ⓐ Ⓑ Ⓒ Ⓓ | 39. Ⓐ Ⓑ Ⓒ Ⓓ | 52. Ⓐ Ⓑ Ⓒ Ⓓ | 65. Ⓐ Ⓑ Ⓒ Ⓓ |

## Mathematics

1. Ⓐ Ⓑ Ⓒ Ⓓ   16. Ⓐ Ⓑ Ⓒ Ⓓ   31. Ⓐ Ⓑ Ⓒ Ⓓ   46. Ⓐ Ⓑ Ⓒ Ⓓ   61. Ⓐ Ⓑ Ⓒ Ⓓ
2. Ⓐ Ⓑ Ⓒ Ⓓ   17. Ⓐ Ⓑ Ⓒ Ⓓ   32. Ⓐ Ⓑ Ⓒ Ⓓ   47. Ⓐ Ⓑ Ⓒ Ⓓ   62. Ⓐ Ⓑ Ⓒ Ⓓ
3. Ⓐ Ⓑ Ⓒ Ⓓ   18. Ⓐ Ⓑ Ⓒ Ⓓ   33. Ⓐ Ⓑ Ⓒ Ⓓ   48. Ⓐ Ⓑ Ⓒ Ⓓ   63. Ⓐ Ⓑ Ⓒ Ⓓ
4. Ⓐ Ⓑ Ⓒ Ⓓ   19. Ⓐ Ⓑ Ⓒ Ⓓ   34. Ⓐ Ⓑ Ⓒ Ⓓ   49. Ⓐ Ⓑ Ⓒ Ⓓ   64. Ⓐ Ⓑ Ⓒ Ⓓ
5. Ⓐ Ⓑ Ⓒ Ⓓ   20. Ⓐ Ⓑ Ⓒ Ⓓ   35. Ⓐ Ⓑ Ⓒ Ⓓ   50 Ⓐ Ⓑ Ⓒ Ⓓ   65. Ⓐ Ⓑ Ⓒ Ⓓ
6. Ⓐ Ⓑ Ⓒ Ⓓ   21. Ⓐ Ⓑ Ⓒ Ⓓ   36. Ⓐ Ⓑ Ⓒ Ⓓ   51. Ⓐ Ⓑ Ⓒ Ⓓ   66. Ⓐ Ⓑ Ⓒ Ⓓ
7. Ⓐ Ⓑ Ⓒ Ⓓ   22. Ⓐ Ⓑ Ⓒ Ⓓ   37. Ⓐ Ⓑ Ⓒ Ⓓ   52. Ⓐ Ⓑ Ⓒ Ⓓ   67. Ⓐ Ⓑ Ⓒ Ⓓ
8. Ⓐ Ⓑ Ⓒ Ⓓ   23. Ⓐ Ⓑ Ⓒ Ⓓ   38. Ⓐ Ⓑ Ⓒ Ⓓ   53. Ⓐ Ⓑ Ⓒ Ⓓ   68. Ⓐ Ⓑ Ⓒ Ⓓ
9. Ⓐ Ⓑ Ⓒ Ⓓ   24. Ⓐ Ⓑ Ⓒ Ⓓ   39. Ⓐ Ⓑ Ⓒ Ⓓ   54. Ⓐ Ⓑ Ⓒ Ⓓ   69. Ⓐ Ⓑ Ⓒ Ⓓ
10. Ⓐ Ⓑ Ⓒ Ⓓ   25. Ⓐ Ⓑ Ⓒ Ⓓ   40. Ⓐ Ⓑ Ⓒ Ⓓ   55. Ⓐ Ⓑ Ⓒ Ⓓ   70. Ⓐ Ⓑ Ⓒ Ⓓ
11. Ⓐ Ⓑ Ⓒ Ⓓ   26. Ⓐ Ⓑ Ⓒ Ⓓ   41. Ⓐ Ⓑ Ⓒ Ⓓ   56. Ⓐ Ⓑ Ⓒ Ⓓ   71. Ⓐ Ⓑ Ⓒ Ⓓ
12. Ⓐ Ⓑ Ⓒ Ⓓ   27. Ⓐ Ⓑ Ⓒ Ⓓ   42. Ⓐ Ⓑ Ⓒ Ⓓ   57. Ⓐ Ⓑ Ⓒ Ⓓ   72. Ⓐ Ⓑ Ⓒ Ⓓ
13. Ⓐ Ⓑ Ⓒ Ⓓ   28. Ⓐ Ⓑ Ⓒ Ⓓ   43. Ⓐ Ⓑ Ⓒ Ⓓ   58. Ⓐ Ⓑ Ⓒ Ⓓ   73. Ⓐ Ⓑ Ⓒ Ⓓ
14. Ⓐ Ⓑ Ⓒ Ⓓ   29. Ⓐ Ⓑ Ⓒ Ⓓ   44. Ⓐ Ⓑ Ⓒ Ⓓ   59. Ⓐ Ⓑ Ⓒ Ⓓ   74. Ⓐ Ⓑ Ⓒ Ⓓ
15. Ⓐ Ⓑ Ⓒ Ⓓ   30. Ⓐ Ⓑ Ⓒ Ⓓ   45. Ⓐ Ⓑ Ⓒ Ⓓ   60. Ⓐ Ⓑ Ⓒ Ⓓ   75. Ⓐ Ⓑ Ⓒ Ⓓ

## Science

1. Ⓐ Ⓑ Ⓒ Ⓓ   14. Ⓐ Ⓑ Ⓒ Ⓓ   27. Ⓐ Ⓑ Ⓒ Ⓓ   40. Ⓐ Ⓑ Ⓒ Ⓓ   53. Ⓐ Ⓑ Ⓒ Ⓓ
2. Ⓐ Ⓑ Ⓒ Ⓓ   15. Ⓐ Ⓑ Ⓒ Ⓓ   28. Ⓐ Ⓑ Ⓒ Ⓓ   41. Ⓐ Ⓑ Ⓒ Ⓓ   54. Ⓐ Ⓑ Ⓒ Ⓓ
3. Ⓐ Ⓑ Ⓒ Ⓓ   16. Ⓐ Ⓑ Ⓒ Ⓓ   29. Ⓐ Ⓑ Ⓒ Ⓓ   42. Ⓐ Ⓑ Ⓒ Ⓓ   55. Ⓐ Ⓑ Ⓒ Ⓓ
4. Ⓐ Ⓑ Ⓒ Ⓓ   17. Ⓐ Ⓑ Ⓒ Ⓓ   30. Ⓐ Ⓑ Ⓒ Ⓓ   43. Ⓐ Ⓑ Ⓒ Ⓓ   56. Ⓐ Ⓑ Ⓒ Ⓓ
5. Ⓐ Ⓑ Ⓒ Ⓓ   18. Ⓐ Ⓑ Ⓒ Ⓓ   31. Ⓐ Ⓑ Ⓒ Ⓓ   44. Ⓐ Ⓑ Ⓒ Ⓓ   57. Ⓐ Ⓑ Ⓒ Ⓓ
6. Ⓐ Ⓑ Ⓒ Ⓓ   19. Ⓐ Ⓑ Ⓒ Ⓓ   32. Ⓐ Ⓑ Ⓒ Ⓓ   45. Ⓐ Ⓑ Ⓒ Ⓓ   58. Ⓐ Ⓑ Ⓒ Ⓓ
7. Ⓐ Ⓑ Ⓒ Ⓓ   20. Ⓐ Ⓑ Ⓒ Ⓓ   33. Ⓐ Ⓑ Ⓒ Ⓓ   46. Ⓐ Ⓑ Ⓒ Ⓓ   59. Ⓐ Ⓑ Ⓒ Ⓓ
8. Ⓐ Ⓑ Ⓒ Ⓓ   21. Ⓐ Ⓑ Ⓒ Ⓓ   34. Ⓐ Ⓑ Ⓒ Ⓓ   47. Ⓐ Ⓑ Ⓒ Ⓓ   60. Ⓐ Ⓑ Ⓒ Ⓓ
9. Ⓐ Ⓑ Ⓒ Ⓓ   22. Ⓐ Ⓑ Ⓒ Ⓓ   35. Ⓐ Ⓑ Ⓒ Ⓓ   48. Ⓐ Ⓑ Ⓒ Ⓓ   61. Ⓐ Ⓑ Ⓒ Ⓓ
10. Ⓐ Ⓑ Ⓒ Ⓓ   23. Ⓐ Ⓑ Ⓒ Ⓓ   36. Ⓐ Ⓑ Ⓒ Ⓓ   49. Ⓐ Ⓑ Ⓒ Ⓓ   62. Ⓐ Ⓑ Ⓒ Ⓓ
11. Ⓐ Ⓑ Ⓒ Ⓓ   24. Ⓐ Ⓑ Ⓒ Ⓓ   37. Ⓐ Ⓑ Ⓒ Ⓓ   50. Ⓐ Ⓑ Ⓒ Ⓓ   63. Ⓐ Ⓑ Ⓒ Ⓓ
12. Ⓐ Ⓑ Ⓒ Ⓓ   25. Ⓐ Ⓑ Ⓒ Ⓓ   38. Ⓐ Ⓑ Ⓒ Ⓓ   51. Ⓐ Ⓑ Ⓒ Ⓓ   64. Ⓐ Ⓑ Ⓒ Ⓓ
13. Ⓐ Ⓑ Ⓒ Ⓓ   26. Ⓐ Ⓑ Ⓒ Ⓓ   39. Ⓐ Ⓑ Ⓒ Ⓓ   52. Ⓐ Ⓑ Ⓒ Ⓓ   65. Ⓐ Ⓑ Ⓒ Ⓓ

# Practice Test One

## READING COMPREHENSION

**Questions 1–4 are based on the following passage.**

City parks were originally created to provide the local populace with a convenient refuge from the crowding and chaos of their surroundings. Until quite recently, these parks served their purpose admirably. Whether city dwellers wanted to sit under a shady tree to think or take a vigorous stroll to get some exercise, they looked forward to visiting these nearby oases. Filled with trees, shrubs, flowers, meadows, and ponds, city parks were a tranquil spot in which to unwind from the daily pressures of urban life. They were places where people met their friends for picnics or sporting events. And they were also places to get some sun and fresh air in the midst of an often dark and dreary environment, with its seemingly endless rows of steel, glass, and concrete buildings.

For more than a century, the importance of these parks to the quality of life in cities has been recognized by urban planners. Yet city parks around the world have been allowed to deteriorate to an alarming extent in recent decades. In many cases, they have become centers of crime; some city parks are now so dangerous that local residents are afraid even to enter them. And the great natural beauty that was once their hallmark has been severely damaged. Trees, shrubs, flowers, and meadows have withered under the impact of intense air pollution and littering, and ponds have been fouled by untreated sewage.

This process of progressive decline, however, is not inevitable. A few changes can turn the situation around. First, special police units, whose only responsibility would be to patrol city parks, should be created to ensure parks remain safe for those who wish to enjoy them. Second, more caretakers should be hired to care for the grounds and, in particular, to collect trash. Beyond the increased staffing requirements, it will also be necessary to insulate city parks from their surroundings. Total isolation is, of course, impossible; but many beneficial measures in that direction could be implemented without too much trouble. Vehicles, for instance, should be banned from city parks to cut down on air pollution. And sewage pipes should be rerouted away from park areas to prevent the contamination of land and water. If urban planners are willing to make these changes, city parks can be restored to their former glory for the benefit of all.

1. The author uses the phrase *convenient refuge* to suggest that parks were:

   (A) Built in order to preserve plant life in cities.
   (B) Designed with the needs of city residents in mind.
   (C) Meant to end the unpleasantness of city life.
   (D) Supposed to help people make new friends.

2. By mentioning crime and pollution, the author primarily emphasizes:

   (A) How rapidly the city parks have deteriorated.
   (B) How city parks can once again be made safe and clean.
   (C) Why people can no longer rest and relax in city parks.
   (D) Why urban planners should not be in charge of city parks.

GO ON TO THE NEXT PAGE

**KAPLAN**

3. In the last paragraph, the author acknowledges which problem in restoring city parks?

   (A) The constant need to collect trash.

   (B) The difficulty in rerouting sewage pipes.

   (C) The congestion caused by banning vehicular traffic.

   (D) The lack of total separation from the surrounding city.

4. The passage focuses primarily on all of the following EXCEPT:

   (A) Criticizing certain aspects of the city.

   (B) Romanticizing city life in a bygone era.

   (C) Exploring the origins of urban decay.

   (D) Pointing out how city life could be improved.

GO ON TO THE NEXT PAGE ⟫

KAPLAN)

**Questions 5–11 are based on the following passage.**

When the first of the two Viking landers touched down on Martian soil on July 20, 1976, and began to send camera images back to Earth, the scientists at the Jet Propulsion Laboratory could not suppress a certain nervous anticipation, like people who hold a ticket to a lottery they have a one-in-a-million chance of winning. The first photographs that arrived, however, did not contain any evidence of life. What revealed itself to them was merely a barren landscape littered with rocks and boulders. The view resembled nothing so much as a flat section of desert—in fact, the winning entry in a contest at J.P.L. for the photograph most accurately predicting what Mars would look like was a snapshot taken in a particularly arid section of the Mojave Desert.

The scientists were soon ready to turn their attention from visible life to microorganisms. The twin Viking landers carried three experiments designed to detect biological activity and one to detect organic compounds, because researchers thought it possible that life had developed on early Mars just as it is thought to have developed on Earth, through the gradual chemical evolution of complex organic molecules. To detect biological activity, Martian soil samples were treated with various nutrients that would produce characteristic by-products if life forms were active in the soil. The results from all three experiments were inconclusive. The fourth experiment heated a soil sample to look for signs of organic material but found none, an unexpected result because at least organic compounds from the steady bombardment of the Martian surface by meteorites were thought to have been present.

The absence of organic materials, some scientists speculated, was the result of intense ultraviolet radiation penetrating the atmosphere of Mars and destroying organic compounds in the soil. Although Mars' atmosphere was at one time rich in carbon dioxide and thus thick enough to protect its surface from the harmful rays of the Sun, the carbon dioxide had gradually left the atmosphere and been converted into rocks. This means that even if life had gotten a start on early Mars, it could not have survived the exposure to ultraviolet radiation when the atmosphere thinned. Mars never developed a protective layer of ozone as Earth did.

Despite the disappointing Viking results, there are those who still keep open the possibility of life on Mars.

They point out that the Viking data cannot be considered the final word on Martian life because the two landers only sampled two limited—and uninteresting—sites. The Viking landing sites were not chosen for what they might tell of the planet's biology. They were chosen primarily because they appeared to be safe for landing a spacecraft. The landing sites were on parts of the Martian plains that appeared relatively featureless from orbital photographs.

The type of Martian terrain that these researchers suggest may be a possible hiding place for active life has an Earthly parallel: The ice-free region of southern Victoria Land, Antarctica, where the temperatures in some dry valleys average below zero. Organisms known as endoliths, a form of blue-green algae that has adapted to this harsh environment, were found living inside certain translucent, porous rocks in these Antarctic valleys. The argument based on this discovery is that if life did exist on early Mars, it is possible that it escaped worsening conditions by similarly seeking refuge in rocks. Skeptics object, however, that Mars in its present state is simply too dry, even compared with Antarctic valleys, to sustain any life whatsoever.

Should Mars eventually prove to be completely barren of life, as some suspect, then this would have a significant impact on the current view of the chemical origin of life. It could be much more difficult to get life started on a planet than scientists thought before the Viking landings.

5.  The major purpose of the passage is to:

   (A) Relate an account of an extraordinary scientific achievement.

   (B) Undermine the prevailing belief that life may exist on Mars.

   (C) Discuss the efforts of scientists to determine whether Martian life exists.

   (D) Show the limitations of the scientific investigation of other planets.

GO ON TO THE NEXT PAGE

6. The reference to "people who hold a ticket to a lottery" serves to:

   (A) Point out the human facet of a scientific enterprise.

   (B) Indicate the expected likelihood of visible Martian life.

   (C) Show that there was doubt as to whether the camera would function.

   (D) Imply that any mission to another planet is a risky venture.

7. The author uses the evidence from the four Viking experiments to establish that:

   (A) Meteorites do not strike the surface of Mars as often as scientists had thought.

   (B) Current theory as to how life developed on Earth is probably flawed.

   (C) There was no experimental confirmation of the theory that life exists on Mars.

   (D) Biological activity has been shown to be absent from the surface of Mars.

8. The third paragraph of the passage provides:

   (A) An analysis of a theory proposed earlier.

   (B) Evidence supporting a statement made earlier.

   (C) A theory about findings presented earlier.

   (D) Criticism of experiments discussed earlier.

9. The author suggests that an important difference between Mars and Earth is that, unlike Earth, Mars:

   (A) Accumulated organic compounds from the steady bombardment of meteorites.

   (B) Possessed at one time an atmosphere rich in carbon dioxide.

   (C) Is in the path of the harmful rays of ultra-violet radiation.

   (D) Could not have sustained any life that developed.

10. The author mentions the Viking landing sites in order to emphasize which point?

    (A) Although evidence of life was not found by the landers, this does not mean that Mars is devoid of life.

    (B) Although the landing sites were uninteresting, they could have harbored Martian life.

    (C) The Viking mission was unsuccessful largely due to poor selection of the landing sites.

    (D) The detection of life on Mars was not a primary objective of the scientists who sent the Viking landers.

11. In the fifth paragraph, the researchers' argument that life may exist in Martian rocks rests on the idea that:

    (A) Organisms may adopt identical survival strategies in comparable environments.

    (B) Life developed in the form of blue-green algae on Mars.

    (C) Life evolved in the same way on two different planets.

    (D) Endoliths are capable of living in the harsh environment of Mars.

GO ON TO THE NEXT PAGE

**Questions 12–13 are based on the following passage.**

Many mammals instinctively raise their fur when they are cold—a reaction produced by tiny muscles just under the skin that surround hair follicles. When the muscles contract, the hairs stand up, creating an increase in air space under the fur. The air space provides more effective insulation for the mammal's body, thus allowing it to retain more heat for longer periods of time. Some animals also raise their fur when they are challenged by predators or even other members of their own species. The raised fur makes the animal appear slightly bigger, and, ideally, more powerful. Interestingly, though devoid of fur, humans still retain this instinct. So, the next time a horror movie gives you "goosebumps," remember that your skin is following a deep-seated mammalian impulse now rendered obsolete.

12. The "increased air space under the fur" mentioned in the passage serves primarily to:

    (A) Combat cold.

    (B) Intimidate other animals.

    (C) Render goosebumps obsolete.

    (D) Cool over-heated predators.

13. Based on the passage, the author would most likely describe "goosebumps" in humans as:

    (A) An unnecessary and unexplained phenomenon.

    (B) A harmful but necessary measure.

    (C) An amusing but dangerous feature.

    (D) A useless but interesting remnant.

**Questions 14–15 are based on the following passage.**

While it is often helpful to think of humans as simply another successful type of mammal, a vital distinction remains. When a pride of lions enjoys a surfeit of food, they are likely to hunt quickly, eat all they can, and then spend the remainder of the day sleeping. When people enjoy such easy living, we see a markedly different pattern—our big brains cause us to be restless, and we engage in play. This takes the form of art, philosophy, science, even government. So the intelligence and curiosity that allowed early humans to develop agriculture, and thus a caloric surplus, also led to the use of that surplus as a foundation for culture.

14. The author most likely cites the behavior of lions in order to:

    (A) Provide an example of an even more successful mammalian species.

    (B) Question the efficiency of the lion's feeding behavior.

    (C) Provide a contrast to the image of humans as industrious and resourceful.

    (D) Help illustrate the distinguishing characteristic of humans that led to the development of culture.

15. The final sentence ("So, the intelligence…for culture") primarily serves to:

    (A) Illustrate the significance of a distinction.

    (B) Counter a likely objection.

    (C) Provide an alternative explanation.

    (D) Suggest future implications of a phenomenon.

GO ON TO THE NEXT PAGE

**KAPLAN**

**Questions 16–26 are based on the following passage.**

The relationship between humans and animals dates back to the misty morning of history. The caves of southern France and northern Spain are full of wonderful depictions of animals. Early African petroglyphs depict recognizable mammals and so does much American Indian art. But long before art, we have evidence of the closeness of humans and animals. The bones of dogs lie next to those of humans in the excavated villages of northern Israel and elsewhere. This unity of death is terribly appropriate. It marks a relationship that is the most ancient of all, one that dates back at least to the Mesolithic Era.* With the dog, the hunter acquired a companion and ally very early on, before agriculture, and long before the horse and the cat. The companion animals were followed by food animals, and then by those that provided enhanced speed and range, and those that worked for us.

How did it all come about? A dog of some kind was almost inevitable. Consider its essence: A social carnivore, hunting larger animals across the broad plains it shared with our ancestors. Because of its pack structure, it is susceptible to domination by, and attachment to, a pack leader—the top dog. Its young are born into the world dependent, must be reared without too much skill, and best of all, they form bonds with those that rear them. Dogs have a set of appeasement behaviors that elicit affective reactions from even the most hardened and unsophisticated humans. Puppies share with human babies the power to transform cynics into cooing softies. Furthermore, the animal has a sense of smell and hearing several times more acute than our own, great advantages to a hunting companion and intrusion detector. The dog's defense behavior makes it an instinctive guard animal.

No wonder the dog was first and remains so close to us. In general, however, something else was probably important in narrowing the list—the candidates had to be camp followers or cohabitants. When humankind ceased to be continually nomadic, when we put down roots and established semi-permanent habitations, hut clusters and finally villages, we created an instant, rich food supply for guilds of opportunistic feeders. Even today, many birds and mammals parasitize our wastes and feed from our stores. They do so because their wild behaviors provide the mechanisms for opportunistic exploitation. A striking example occurred in Britain during the 1940s and 50s. In those days, milk was delivered to a person's doorstep in glass bottles with aluminum-foil caps. Rich cream topped the milk, the paradise before homogenization. A chickadee known as the blue tit learned to puncture the cap and drink the cream. The behavior soon spread among the tits, and soon milk bottles were being raided in the early morning throughout Britain. If the birds had been so specialized that they only fed in deep forest, it never would have happened. But these were forest-edge opportunists, pioneers rather than conservatives. It is from animals of this ilk that we find our allies and our foes.

Returning to the question of how it all came about, my instincts tell me that we first domesticated those individual animals that were orphaned by our hunting ancestors. In my years in the tropics, I have seen many wild animals raised by simple people in their houses. The animals were there, without thought of utility or gain, mainly because the hunter in the family had brought the orphaned baby back for his wife and children. In Panama it was often a beautiful small, spotted cat that bounced friskily out of a peasant's kitchen to play at my feet. The steps from the home-raised wolfling to the domestic dog probably took countless generations. I bet it started with affection and curiosity. Only later did it become useful.

When we consider that there are more than 55 million domestic cats and 50 million dogs in this country, and that they support an industry larger than the total economy of medieval Europe, we must recognize the strength of the ancient bond. Without the "aid" of goats, sheep, pigs, cattle, and horses we would never have reached our present population densities. The parasitic and symbiotic relationships we share with other species made civilization possible. That civilization, in turn, is increasingly causing the extinction of many animals and plant species—an ironic paradox indeed.

*Mesolithic Era: the Middle Stone Age, between 8,000 and 3,000 years B.C.E.

GO ON TO THE NEXT PAGE ⇨

16. The author most likely describes the archaeological discoveries mentioned as "terribly appropriate" because:

    (A) Dogs were always buried next to their owners in the Mesolithic Era.

    (B) Few animals were of religious significance in prehistoric cultures.

    (C) They illustrate the role of dogs on a typical hunting expedition.

    (D) Our relationship with dogs goes back farther than with any other animal.

17. According to the first paragraph, the first animals that humans had a close relationship with were those that:

    (A) Acted as companions.

    (B) Provided a source of food.

    (C) Helped develop agriculture.

    (D) Enabled humans to travel further.

18. According to the author, why was some kind of dog "inevitable" as a companion animal for humans?

    (A) It survived by maintaining its independence.

    (B) It was stronger than other large animals.

    (C) It shared its prey with our ancestors.

    (D) It was suited for human domination.

19. Judging from the passage, the phrase "affective reactions" most probably means:

    (A) Callous decisions

    (B) Rational judgments

    (C) Emotional responses

    (D) Juvenile behavior

20. The author most likely compares puppies with human babies in order to:

    (A) Criticize an uncaring attitude toward animals.

    (B) Point out ways in which animals dominate humans.

    (C) Support the idea that dogs form bonds with their owners.

    (D) Dispel some misconceptions about the innocence of puppies.

21. In the passage, "the list" most likely refers to the:

    (A) Types of birds that scavenge human food supplies.

    (B) Number of animals that developed relationships with humans.

    (C) Group of species that are able to communicate with dogs.

    (D) Variety of attributes that make dogs good hunters.

22. The author most likely discusses the case of the British blue tit in order to:

    (A) Highlight a waste of valuable food supplies.

    (B) Indicate the quality of milk before homogenization.

    (C) Explain how unpredictable animal behavior can be.

    (D) Provide one example of an opportunistic feeder.

23. In the third paragraph, "animals of this ilk" refers to animals that are:

    (A) Good companions

    (B) Forest inhabitants

    (C) Adaptable feeders

    (D) Efficient hunters

GO ON TO THE NEXT PAGE

**KAPLAN**

24. The author most likely describes his experience in the tropics in order to:

    (A) Portray the simple life led by a hunter's family.

    (B) Show how useful animals can be in isolated places.

    (C) Underline the effort involved in training a wild animal.

    (D) Illustrate how the first domesticated animals were created.

25. In the passage, the use of "aid" in quotation marks emphasizes the point that:

    (A) The animals' help was involuntary.

    (B) Population levels are dangerously high.

    (C) The contribution of animals is rarely recognized.

    (D) Many animals benefited from the relationship.

26. Which of the following best describes the "ironic paradox" mentioned in the passage?

    (A) More money is now spent on domestic animals than on animal livestock.

    (B) Pet ownership will become impractical if population density continues to increase.

    (C) The pet care industry in the United States today is larger than the total economy of medieval Europe.

    (D) Human civilization is currently making extinct many of the other life forms that enabled it to grow.

GO ON TO THE NEXT PAGE

KAPLAN

**Questions 27–29 are based on the following passage.**

With an estimated 250 million cases and 2 million resulting deaths per year, malaria is the world's number-one public health problem, especially in tropical and subtropical regions. The struggle with this infection is nothing new—malaria is mentioned in some of the earliest medical records of Western civilization. We know, for example, that the ancient Greek physician Hippocrates identified three types of malarial fevers in the fifth century B.C.E. By the late fifteenth century, malaria had spread to the Americas, likely as the result of European explorers. In fact, epidemics in Central America were recorded in 1493, only a year after Columbus's first voyage there.

27. According to the passage, malaria is:

   (A) A disease with a long history that remains a serious public health problem today.
   (B) A disease that epidemiologists are steadily bringing under control.
   (C) Likely to spread from the tropics to temperate regions.
   (D) Impossible to eradicate from the tropics.

28. Malaria's long history suggests that it has been:

   (A) Especially well documented in the annals of medicine.
   (B) Spread primarily from locations in Europe to other parts of the world.
   (C) Particularly resistant to efforts to eradicate or control the infection.
   (D) A disorder whose symptoms were misunderstood for many centuries.

29. It can be inferred that:

   (A) Hippocrates had malaria.
   (B) Hippocrates lived in the fifth century B.C.E.
   (C) Hippocrates died from malaria.
   (D) Hippocrates named malaria the number-one public health problem.

**Questions 30–31 are based on the following passage.**

One of the hazards of swimming in the ocean is an unexpected encounter with a jellyfish. Contact with the poison in a jellyfish's tentacles can result in sharp, lingering pain, or even death if the person stung is highly allergic. While everyone, including the jellyfish, would like to avoid these encounters, they are not uncommon. This is hardly surprising considering that jellyfish live in every ocean in the world and have done so for more than 650 million years. The animals are likely so widespread because of their extreme adaptability—they are quite hardy and can withstand a wide range of temperatures and conditions in their environment.

30. The author uses the phrase "including the jellyfish" in order to:

   (A) Introduce a small note of humor to an otherwise serious discussion.
   (B) Encourage the reader's sympathy for the jellyfish.
   (C) Ridicule humans' fear of jellyfish.
   (D) Emphasize the danger that jellyfish pose for swimmers.

31. According to the passage, encounters between humans and jellyfish in the ocean are relatively common because jellyfish:

   (A) Are more than 650 million years old.
   (B) Live in all the world's oceans.
   (C) Are extremely robust.
   (D) Have poisonous tentacles.

GO ON TO THE NEXT PAGE ⟩

**KAPLAN)**

**Questions 32–34 are based on the following passage.**

The four Galilean satellites of Jupiter probably experienced early, intense bombardment. Thus, the very ancient surface of Callisto remains scarred by impact craters. The younger, more varied surface of Ganymede reveals distinct light and dark areas, the light areas featuring networks of intersecting grooves and ridges, probably resulting from later iceflows. The impact sites of Europa have been almost completely erased, apparently by water outflowing from the interior and instantly forming vast, low, frozen seas. Satellite photographs of Io, the closest of the four to Jupiter, were revelatory. They showed a landscape dominated by volcanos, many erupting, making Io the most tectonically active object in the solar system. Since a body as small as Io cannot supply the energy for such activity, the accepted explanation has been that, forced into a highly eccentric orbit, Io is engulfed by tides stemming from a titanic contest between the other three Galilean moons and Jupiter.

32. According to the passage, which of the following is probably NOT true of the surface of Io?

   (A) It is characterized by intense tectonic activity.
   (B) Its volcanos have resulted from powerful tides.
   (C) It is younger than the surface of Callisto.
   (D) It is distinguished by many impact craters.

33. It can be inferred that the geologic features found in the light areas of Ganymede were probably formed:

   (A) Subsequent to the features found in the dark areas.
   (B) In an earlier period than those in the dark areas.
   (C) At roughly the same time as the features found in the dark areas.
   (D) Primarily by early bombardment.

34. It can be inferred that the author regards current knowledge about the satellites of Jupiter as:

   (A) Insignificant and disappointing.
   (B) Grossly outdated.
   (C) Complete and satisfactory.
   (D) Persuasive though incomplete.

GO ON TO THE NEXT PAGE

**Questions 35–36 are based on the following passage.**

Ecology—the study of the relationships among organisms, and between organisms and their environment—is a relatively new branch of science. The name itself was coined by a German biologist, Ernst Haeckel, in 1866. Haeckel postulated the living world is a community where each species has a distinctive role to play. One of the major focuses of ecological study today is fieldwork analyzing relationships within an ecosystem, or a collection of communities, such as a tropical rainforest or a coral reef. The results of such studies have provided conservationists and wildlife managers with important new insights, though many questions remain unanswered.

35. Based on the passage, why might many of the basic questions posed by ecology still remain unanswered today?

    (A) Ecology has received little support from funding agencies and from the general public.
    (B) The areas studied by ecologists are remote and inhospitable.
    (C) Ecologists have found it difficult to enlist the cooperation of other scientists.
    (D) Ecology is a relatively young, developing branch of science.

36. Based on the passage, all of the following might be considered an ecosystem *except*:

    (A) A temperate forest
    (B) A coral reef
    (C) An ice crystal
    (D) A tropical rainforest

**Questions 37–38 are based on the following passage.**

A major story in recent years has been the triumph of electronic mail, commonly known as e-mail. Since the early 1990s, e-mail users have multiplied exponentially. Many major corporations have chosen e-mail as their primary channel for all communications, internal and external. Yet, however effective and inexpensive e-mail may be, it is not without flaws. The medium is impersonal, lacking the intimacy of a letter or the immediacy of a phone call. As an interactive medium, e-mail is less than ideal, since messages allow correspondents to politely ignore points they do not wish to address, or indeed not to respond at all.

37. The attitude of the author of the passage could best be described as:

    (A) Uniformly favorable
    (B) Intensely subjective
    (C) Harshly critical
    (D) Objective and mixed

38. The word *immediacy* most nearly means:

    (A) Quickness
    (B) Precision
    (C) Closeness
    (D) Speed

GO ON TO THE NEXT PAGE

**KAPLAN**

**Questions 39–40 are based on the following passage.**

Coral reefs are created over the course of hundreds or even thousands of years. The main architect in coral reef formation is the stony coral, a relative of sea anemones that lives in tropical climates and secretes a skeleton of almost pure calcium carbonate. It is partnered by green algae, tiny unicellular plants that live within the tissues of coral. The two organisms form a mutually beneficial, symbiotic relationship, with the algae consuming carbon dioxide given off by the coral, and the coral thriving on the abundant oxygen produced photosynthetically by the algae. When the coral dies, its skeleton is left, and other organisms grow on top of it. Over the years the mass of the coral skeletons and the associated organisms combine to form the petrified underwater forest that divers find so fascinating.

39. Which of the following best describes what this passage is about?

    (A) The varieties of animal life that live in coral reefs.

    (B) The formation of coral reefs.

    (C) The life and death cycles of coral reefs.

    (D) The physical beauty of coral reefs.

40. The relationship between the coral and the algae is best described as:

    (A) Parasitic

    (B) Competitive

    (C) Predatory

    (D) Cooperative

**Questions 41–43 are based on the following passage.**

Most life is fundamentally dependent on photosynthetic organisms that store radiant energy from the sun. In almost all the world's ecosystems and food chains, photosynthetic organisms such as plants and algae are eaten by other organisms, which are then consumed by others. The existence of organisms that are not dependent on the sun's light has long been established, but until recently they were regarded as anomalies.

Over the last 20 years, however, research in deep sea areas has revealed the existence of entire ecosystems in which the primary producers are chemosynthetic bacteria dependent on energy from within the earth itself. Indeed, growing evidence suggests that these sub-sea ecosystems model the way in which life first came about on this planet.

41. The passage suggests that most life is ultimately dependent on what?

    (A) Photosynthetic algae

    (B) The world's oceans

    (C) Bacterial microorganisms

    (D) Light from the sun

42. Which of the following conclusions about photosynthetic and chemosynthetic organisms is supported by this passage?

    (A) Both perform similar functions in different food chains.

    (B) Both are known to support communities of higher organisms at great ocean depths.

    (C) Sunlight is the basic source of energy for both.

    (D) Chemosynthetic organisms are less nourishing than photosynthetic organisms.

GO ON TO THE NEXT PAGE

**KAPLAN**

43. According to the passage, which of the following is true?

    (A) Plants and algae are photosynthetic organisms.

    (B) Chemosynthetic bacteria do not exist.

    (C) Deep sea research has been extremely limited.

    (D) Science is unable to explain food chains.

**Questions 44–45 are based on the following passage.**

The existence of Halley's Comet has been known since at least 240 B.C.E., and possibly since 1059 B.C.E. Its most famous appearance was in 1066 C.E., when it appeared right before the Battle of Hastings. It was named after the astronomer Edmund Halley, who calculated its orbit. He determined the comets seen in 1530 and 1606 were the same object following a 76-year orbit. Unfortunately, Halley died in 1742, never living to see his prediction come true when the comet returned on Christmas Eve 1758.

44. It can be inferred from the passage that the last sighting of the Halley's Comet recorded before the death of Edmund Halley took place in:

    (A) 1066

    (B) 1530

    (C) 1606

    (D) 1682

45. According to the passage, Edmund Halley:

    (A) Was born in 1066.

    (B) Witnessed the comet three times.

    (C) Calculated the orbit of the comet.

    (D) Was famous for naming comets.

GO ON TO THE NEXT PAGE

**KAPLAN**

# VOCABULARY AND SPELLING

1. *Foolhardy* most nearly means:

   (A) Stubborn
   (B) Vigorous
   (C) Proud
   (D) Reckless

2. *Truncate* most nearly means:

   (A) Widen
   (B) Shorten
   (C) Pack
   (D) Join

3. *Seclude* most nearly means:

   (A) Isolate
   (B) Tempt
   (C) Acquire
   (D) Emit

4. *Acquit* most nearly means:

   (A) Surrender
   (B) Obtain
   (C) Appraise
   (D) Clear

5. *Simulate* most nearly means:

   (A) Agitate
   (B) Review
   (C) Endure
   (D) Replicate

6. *Erroneous* most nearly means:

   (A) Approximate
   (B) Unplanned
   (C) Mistaken
   (D) Sensual

7. *Garbled* most nearly means:

   (A) Rinsed
   (B) Pointed
   (C) Jumbled
   (D) Whispered

8. *Synthetic* most nearly means:

   (A) Expensive
   (B) Unusual
   (C) Artificial
   (D) Unattractive

9. *Creep* most nearly means:

   (A) Squeak
   (B) Move slowly
   (C) Grip tightly
   (D) Retreat

10. *Leverage* most nearly means:

    (A) Influence
    (B) Height
    (C) Mechanism
    (D) Humor

11. *Viscous* most nearly means:

    (A) Treacherous
    (B) Green
    (C) Syrupy
    (D) Wild

12. *Benefactor* most nearly means:

    (A) Critic
    (B) Recipient
    (C) Supporter
    (D) Mediator

GO ON TO THE NEXT PAGE

13. *Prohibition* most nearly means:

    (A) Shyness
    (B) Ban
    (C) Agreement
    (D) Display

14. *Hypocrite* most nearly means:

    (A) Poser
    (B) Scholar
    (C) Follower
    (D) Dictator

15. *Opulent* most nearly means:

    (A) Luxurious
    (B) Overweight
    (C) Transparent
    (D) Smelly

16. *Interminable* is the opposite of:

    (A) Brief
    (B) Constant
    (C) External
    (D) Physical

17. *Traditional* is the opposite of:

    (A) Improvident
    (B) Unconscionable
    (C) Uninhabitable
    (D) Iconoclastic

18. *Abandon* is the opposite of:

    (A) Arrival
    (B) Presence
    (C) Security
    (D) Restraint

19. *Logy* is the opposite of:

    (A) Irrational
    (B) Upset
    (C) Alert
    (D) Patient

20. *Cede* is the opposite of:

    (A) Make sense of
    (B) Fail
    (C) Get ahead of
    (D) Retain

21. *Proscribe* is the opposite of:

    (A) Risk
    (B) Deny
    (C) Support
    (D) Permit

22. *Eschew* is the opposite of:

    (A) Relax
    (B) Restrain
    (C) Indulge in
    (D) Reunite

23. *Collar* is the opposite of:

    (A) Misstate
    (B) Untwist
    (C) Free
    (D) Abscond

24. *Iota* is the opposite of:

    (A) Molecule
    (B) Plethora
    (C) Dispatch
    (D) Scrap

GO ON TO THE NEXT PAGE

25. *Ambulatory* is the opposite of:

    (A) Surefooted

    (B) Fast moving

    (C) Fixed

    (D) Healthy

26. *Leveling* is the opposite of:

    (A) Darkening

    (B) Illuminating

    (C) Expanding

    (D) Canting

27. *Lull* is the opposite of:

    (A) Upset

    (B) Dislike

    (C) Fool

    (D) Mull over

28. *License* is the opposite of:

    (A) Curb

    (B) Tie

    (C) Rule

    (D) Impress

29. *Insidious* is the opposite of:

    (A) Comparable

    (B) Direct

    (C) External

    (D) Moral

30. *Unguent* is the opposite of:

    (A) Irritant

    (B) Depressant

    (C) Solvent

    (D) Penitent

31. Ominous : Disaster ::

    (A) Auspicious : Success

    (B) Dangerous : Alert

    (C) Difficult : Task

    (D) Corrected : Error

32. Coagulate : Clot ::

    (A) Prosecute : Sentence

    (B) Inject : Needle

    (C) Obstruct : Blockade

    (D) Freeze : Ice

33. Care : Fuss ::

    (A) Talk : Whisper

    (B) Assert : Imply

    (C) Object : Quibble

    (D) Demote : Dismiss

34. Novel : Book ::

    (A) Epic : Poem

    (B) House : Library

    (C) Tale : Fable

    (D) Number : Page

35. Hungry : Ravenous ::

    (A) Thirsty : Desirous

    (B) Large : Titanic

    (C) Famous : Eminent

    (D) Dizzy : Disoriented

36. Bouquet : Flower ::

    (A) Humidor : Tobacco

    (B) Mosaic : Tile

    (C) Tapestry : Color

    (D) Pile : Block

GO ON TO THE NEXT PAGE ⇨

37. Paraphrase : Verbatim ::

    (A) Approximation : Precise
    (B) Description : Vivid
    (C) Quotation : Apt
    (D) Interpretation : Valid

38. Impeccable : Flaw ::

    (A) Impeachable : Crime
    (B) Obstreperous : Permission
    (C) Impetuous : Warning
    (D) Absurd : Sense

39. Seismograph : Earthquake ::

    (A) Stethoscope : Health
    (B) Speedometer : Truck
    (C) Telescope : Astronomy
    (D) Thermometer : Temperature

40. Guzzle : Drink ::

    (A) Elucidate : Clarify
    (B) Ingest : Eat
    (C) Boast : Describe
    (D) Stride : Walk

41. Orator : Articulate ::

    (A) Soldier : Merciless
    (B) Celebrity : Talented
    (C) Judge : Unbiased
    (D) Novice : Unfamiliar

42. Intransigent : Flexibility ::

    (A) Transient : Mobility
    (B) Disinterested : Partisanship
    (C) Dissimilar : Variation
    (D) Progressive : Transition

43. Castigate : Wrongdoing ::

    (A) Congratulate : Success
    (B) Amputate : Crime
    (C) Annotate : Consultation
    (D) Deface : Falsehood

44. Maven : Expertise ::

    (A) Monarch : Wisdom
    (B) Athlete : Determination
    (C) Neophyte : Honesty
    (D) Supplicant : Humility

45. Exculpate : Blame ::

    (A) Abash : Shame
    (B) Forswear : Violence
    (C) Decipher : Code
    (D) Forgive : Debt

GO ON TO THE NEXT PAGE

**KAPLAN**

**Choose the word that is misspelled.**

46. (A) Majestic
    (B) Compromise
    (C) Tuant
    (D) Pacify

47. (A) Collective
    (B) Reasonible
    (C) Broadening
    (D) Dangerous

48. (A) Hilarious
    (B) Confusion
    (C) Illuminate
    (D) Gratefull

49. (A) Cautious
    (B) Acidental
    (C) Helpful
    (D) Determination

50. (A) Patient
    (B) Tangible
    (C) Opress
    (D) Disappeared

51. (A) Intelligent
    (B) Certain
    (C) Cosmapolitan
    (D) Breakable

52. (A) Lively
    (B) Comparison
    (C) Controversial
    (D) Sensable

53. (A) Intrecate
    (B) Accident
    (C) Loyalty
    (D) Summarize

54. (A) Interrupt
    (B) Solemn
    (C) Collossal
    (D) Parallel

55. (A) Friendly
    (B) Condem
    (C) Hazardous
    (D) Restaurant

GO ON TO THE NEXT PAGE

**KAPLAN**

**Choose the sentence that contains a misspelled word. If there are no mistakes, choose (D).**

56. (A) Janet was decidedly perplexed by the note she received.

    (B) Of all the things she could have forgotten, her hat was the worst.

    (C) Henry thought it was wierd that they served pumpkin pie at the 4th of July party.

    (D) No mistake.

57. (A) Jensen had diffuculty finding the hotel's swimming pool.

    (B) Claus insured his automobile for more than the car was worth.

    (C) She is a gracious host.

    (D) No mistake.

58. (A) Hanna did not want to embarass her friend at the party.

    (B) Despite her intention to swim, Hillary never made it to the pool.

    (C) The reappearance of the missing key was mysterious.

    (D) No mistake.

59. (A) No one believed that it was possible.

    (B) Her outfit did not mirror the occasion.

    (C) There are several occupational hazards to be aware of.

    (D) No mistake.

60. (A) The possibility of rain is a factor in planning the picnic.

    (B) The train conducter was known for his cautious driving.

    (C) The reception was beautiful.

    (D) No mistake.

61. (A) His attitude was always upbeat.

    (B) Her perspective on the situation was tainted.

    (C) It is impossible to ascertain the situation.

    (D) No mistake.

62. (A) Rosa was unable to contact her relatives.

    (B) Stefanie was persistant in her desire for more information.

    (C) The ultimate outcome of the debate is still undecided.

    (D) No mistake.

63. (A) The librarian made sure that the computers were accessable to all library patrons.

    (B) For the next century, inflation is expected to rise.

    (C) The growth of the company was exponential.

    (D) No mistake.

64. (A) I am unwilling to negotiate.

    (B) She made sure to follow the pattern exactly.

    (C) Having dinner together was an every day occurrence when I was younger.

    (D) No mistake.

65. (A) The art historian was certain the painting had been altared.

    (B) She preferred to study abroad during college.

    (C) She believed the doctor was infallible.

    (D) No mistake.

GO ON TO THE NEXT PAGE

**KAPLAN**

## MATHEMATICS

1. Which of the following demonstrates the commutative property of addition?

   (A) $1 + 3 = 4$

   (B) $1 + 3 = 3 + 1$

   (C) $1 + 3 = x$

   (D) $1 + 3 = 1 - (-3)$

2. What is the value of $a(b - 2) + 3c$ if $a = 2$, $b = 6$ and $c = 4$?

   (A) 20

   (B) 12

   (C) 24

   (D) 32

3. Andrew bought a camera on sale at a 20% discount. It was marked down from its regular price of $120. If there is an 8% sales tax on the sale price, how much did Andrew pay for the camera?

   (A) $24.00

   (B) $103.68

   (C) $127.68

   (D) $105.68

4. When $z$ is divided by 8, the remainder is 5. What is the remainder when $4z$ is divided by 8?

   (A) 1

   (B) 3

   (C) 4

   (D) 5

5. What is the least common multiple of 12 and 8?

   (A) 12

   (B) 24

   (C) 18

   (D) 96

6. What is the value of $x$ in the equation $6x - 7 = y$, if $y = 11$?

   (A) 12

   (B) 8

   (C) 4

   (D) 3

7. Edward has $400 more than Robert. After Edward spends $60 on groceries, he has 3 times more money than Robert. How much money does Robert have?

   (A) 140

   (B) 120

   (C) 90

   (D) 170

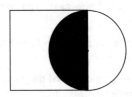

8. A square and a circle are drawn as shown above. The area of the square is 64 in². What is the area of the shaded region?

   (A) $16\pi$ in²

   (B) $8\pi$ in²

   (C) $4\pi$ in²

   (D) $32\pi$ in²

9. John bought a camera on sale that normally costs $160. If the price was reduced 20% during the sale, what was the sale price of the camera?

   (A) $120

   (B) $124

   (C) $128

   (D) $140

GO ON TO THE NEXT PAGE

10. What is the sum of 5 consecutive integers if the middle one is 9?

    (A) 50
    (B) 55
    (C) 45
    (D) 30

11. A dry cleaning store charges $3.50 to clean men's shirts, $4.00 to clean men's pants, and $5.00 to clean men's jackets. If Jose brings 10 items for cleaning and pays a total of $48, what is the average price he has paid per item?

    (A) $3.50
    (B) $2.22
    (C) $5.00
    (D) $4.80

12. Renée's dress shop is suffering from slow business. Renée decides to mark down all her merchandise. The next day, she sells 33 winter coats. That day Renée sold 30% of the winter coats she had in stock. How many winter coats were in stock before the sale?

    (A) 990
    (B) 99
    (C) 110
    (D) 1,110

13. If $x = \sqrt{3}$, $y = 2$, and $z = \frac{1}{2}$, then $x^2 - 5yz + y^2 = ?$

    (A) 1
    (B) 2
    (C) 4
    (D) 7

14. Which of the following is an even multiple of both 2 and 6?

    (A) 435
    (B) 247
    (C) 322
    (D) 426

15. What is 25% of 25% of 72?

    (A) 4
    (B) 4.5
    (C) 5
    (D) 12

16. The price of a stock decreased by 20%. By what percent must the price increase to return to its original value?

    (A) 25%
    (B) 50%
    (C) 20%
    (D) 120%

17. Mrs. Bailer divides the amount of money she has between her 4 children. Mr. Bailer then adds $2 to the amount each one receives so that each child now has a total of $5.25. Which of the following equations shows this relationship?

    (A) $4x + 2 = 5.25$
    (B) $\frac{x}{4} + 2 = 5.25$
    (C) $4x = 5.25 + 2$
    (D) $4(x + 2) = 5.25$

GO ON TO THE NEXT PAGE

**KAPLAN**

18. Which of the following numbers is closest to the product of $52.3 \times 10.4$?

    (A) 5,000
    (B)   500
    (C) 6,000
    (D)    60

19. A subway car passes 3 stations every 10 minutes. At this rate, how many stations will it pass in 1 hour?

    (A) 15
    (B) 18
    (C) 20
    (D) 30

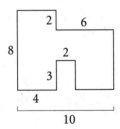

20. What is the area of the polygon above, in square units, if each corner of the polygon is a right angle?

    (A) 40
    (B) 62
    (C) 68
    (D) 74

21. If 40% of $x$ is 8, what is $x$% of 40?

    (A) 80
    (B) 30
    (C) 10
    (D)  8

22. Four people shared a taxi to the airport. The fare was $36.00, and they gave the driver a tip equal to 25% of the fare. If they equally shared the cost of the fare and tip, how much did each person pay?

    (A)  $9.75
    (B) $10.25
    (C) $10.75
    (D) $11.25

23. After spending $\frac{5}{12}$ of his salary, a man has $420 left. What is his salary?

    (A)   175
    (B)   245
    (C)   720
    (D) 1,008

24. If 48 is divided by 0.08, the result is:

    (A) 0.06
    (B) 0.6
    (C)  60
    (D) 600

25. Ms. Smith drove a total of 700 miles on a business trip. If her car averaged 35 miles per gallon of gasoline and gasoline cost $1.25 per gallon, what was the cost in dollars of the gasoline for the trip?

    (A) $20.00
    (B) $24.00
    (C) $25.00
    (D) $40.00

26. If $100 \div x = 10n$, then which of the following is equal to $nx$?

    (A)  10
    (B)  10$x$
    (C) 100
    (D)  10$xn$

GO ON TO THE NEXT PAGE ▷

**KAPLAN**

27. If the number 9,899,399 is increased by 2,082, the result will be:

    (A) 9,901,481

    (B) 9,901,471

    (C) 9,902,481

    (D) 9,902,471

28. If 50% of $x$ is 150, what is 75% of $x$?

    (A) 225

    (B) 250

    (C) 275

    (D) 300

29. Melissa took $5n$ photographs on a trip. If she gives $n$ photographs to each of her 3 friends, how many photographs will she have left?

    (A) $2n$

    (B) $3n$

    (C) $4n - 3$

    (D) $4n + 3$

30. Barry is 4 years older than his brother Cole, who is 4 years older than their sister Darcy. If the sum of their three ages is 60, how old is Barry?

    (A) 16

    (B) 20

    (C) 24

    (D) 28

31. The total fare for 2 adults and 3 children on an excursion boat is $14. If each child's fare is one half of each adult's fare, what is the adult fare?

    (A) $2.00

    (B) $3.00

    (C) $3.50

    (D) $4.00

32. Which of the following is closest in value to the decimal 0.40?

    (A) $\dfrac{1}{3}$

    (B) $\dfrac{4}{7}$

    (C) $\dfrac{3}{8}$

    (D) $\dfrac{1}{2}$

33. What is the value of $(-ab)(a)$ when $a = -2$ and $b = 3$?

    (A) $-12$

    (B) $-6$

    (C) $6$

    (D) $12$

34. A rectangular picture that is 4 inches wide and 6 inches long is enlarged so that it is 10 inches long without changing the width. What is the perimeter, in inches, of the enlarged picture?

    (A) 20

    (B) 24

    (C) 28

    (D) 40

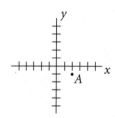

35. What are the coordinates of point $A$ on the graph above?

    (A) $(-1, 2)$

    (B) $(2, -1)$

    (C) $(-2, -1)$

    (D) $(-2, 1)$

GO ON TO THE NEXT PAGE

**KAPLAN**

36. Three lottery winners decide to split a cash prize in the ratio $1 : 2 : 3$. If the cash prize is $12,000, what is the greatest amount earned by one of the three winners?

    (A) $2,000
    (B) $3,000
    (C) $4,000
    (D) $6,000

**Use the table below to answer questions 37 and 38.**

## LUNCHEON SPECIALS

| Meal | Price |
|------|-------|
| Hamburger | $3.00 |
| Chicken | $2.75 |
| Tuna Salad | $2.50 |
| Pasta Salad | $2.25 |
| Pizza | $1.50 |

37. If the table above represents the luncheon prices at a certain cafeteria, what is the average (arithmetic mean) price for a meal at this cafeteria?

    (A) $2.40
    (B) $2.50
    (C) $2.60
    (D) $2.70

38. If three people each ordered a different meal from the table above, which of the following could NOT be the total cost of the meals, excluding tax?

    (A) $7.00
    (B) $6.75
    (C) $6.25
    (D) $6.00

39. Team A had 4 times as many losses as it had ties in a season. If Team A won none of its games, which could be the total number of games it played that season?

    (A) 15
    (B) 18
    (C) 21
    (D) 24

40. If the average of 5 consecutive odd numbers is 11, then the largest number is:

    (A) 17
    (B) 15
    (C) 13
    (D) 11

41. The price of a newspaper rises from 5¢ to 15¢. What is the percent increase in price?

    (A) 75%
    (B) 150%
    (C) 200%
    (D) 300%

42. $0.123 \times 10^4 = ?$

    (A) 12.3
    (B) 123
    (C) 1,234
    (D) 1,230

43. $(3d - 7) - (5 - 2d) = ?$

    (A) $d - 12$
    (B) $5d - 2$
    (C) $5d + 12$
    (D) $5d - 12$

GO ON TO THE NEXT PAGE

**KAPLAN**

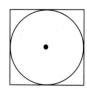

44. If the perimeter of the above square is 36, what is the circumference of the circle?

    (A)  6π
    (B)  9π
    (C)  12π
    (D)  18π

45. Douglas receives a 6% raise. If his old monthly salary was $2,250, what is his monthly salary now?

    (A)  $2,256
    (B)  $2,385
    (C)  $2,400
    (D)  $2,650

46. If $x$ is an integer, which of the following expressions is always even?

    (A)  $2x + 1$
    (B)  $3x + 2$
    (C)  $5x + 3$
    (D)  $6x + 4$

47. For all $a$, $(3a + 4)(3a - 4)$

    (A)  $6a$
    (B)  $3a^2 - 4$
    (C)  $9a^2 - 4$
    (D)  $9a^2 - 16$

48. The average (arithmetic mean) weight of Jake, Ken, and Larry is 60 kilograms. If Jake and Ken both weigh 50 kilograms, how much, in kilograms, does Larry weigh?

    (A)  50
    (B)  60
    (C)  70
    (D)  80

49. A measuring cup contains $1\frac{2}{3}$ cups of water. It needs to be filled to the $3\frac{3}{4}$ cup mark. How much water must be added?

    (A)  A little more than 1 cup.
    (B)  A little less than 2 cups.
    (C)  A little more than 2 cups.
    (D)  A little less than 3 cups.

50. If the average of 7 consecutive even numbers is 24, then the largest number is:

    (A)  26
    (B)  28
    (C)  30
    (D)  34

51. Five less than 3 times a certain number is equal to the original number plus 7. What is the original number?

    (A)  2
    (B)  6
    (C)  11
    (D)  12

52. $[(12 - 11) - (10 - 9)] - [(12 - 11 - 10) - 9] = ?$

    (A)  −20
    (B)  0
    (C)  16
    (D)  18

GO ON TO THE NEXT PAGE

**KAPLAN**

53. If $abc \neq 0$, then $\dfrac{a^2bc + ab^2c + abc^2}{abc} = ?$

    (A) $a + b + c$

    (B) $abc$

    (C) $a^3b^3c^3$

    (D) $a^2 + b^2 + c^2$

54. The cube of 9 is:

    (A)  27

    (B)  81

    (C)  243

    (D) 729

55. The user's manual for a stereo set includes a scale diagram in which 2 scaled inches represent 8 actual inches. If the speakers of the stereo set measure 6 inches in the diagram, how tall are they in reality?

    (A)  1 foot 6 inches

    (B)  1 foot 8 inches

    (C)  1 foot 10 inches

    (D)  2 feet

56. If $s - t = 5$ what is the value of $3s - 3t + 3$?

    (A)  11

    (B)  12

    (C)  15

    (D)  18

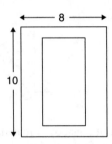

57. What is the area of the frame in the above diagram if the inside picture has a length of 8 and a width of 4?

    (A)  16

    (B)  24

    (C)  48

    (D)  56

58. When $D$ is divided by 15, the result is 6 with a remainder of 2. What is the remainder when $D$ is divided by 6?

    (A)  0

    (B)  2

    (C)  3

    (D)  4

59. A bicycle rider travels 8 miles due north, then 6 miles due east. How many miles is she from her starting point?

    (A)  16

    (B)  12

    (C)  10

    (D)  14

GO ON TO THE NEXT PAGE

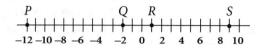

60. What is the distance from the midpoint of $\overline{PQ}$ to the midpoint of $\overline{RS}$?

    (A) 12

    (B) 14

    (C) 16

    (D) 18

61. A tailor has 20 yards of shirt fabric. How many shirts can she complete if each shirt requires $2\frac{2}{3}$ yards of fabric?

    (A) 7

    (B) 8

    (C) 9

    (D) 10

62. $(x-4)(x-4) = ?$

    (A) $x^2 + 8x - 16$

    (B) $x^2 - 8x - 16$

    (C) $x^2 - 8x + 16$

    (D) $x^2 - 16x + 8$

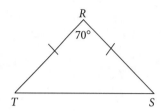

63. In triangle $RST$ above, if $RS = RT$, what is the degree measure of angle $S$?

    (A) 40

    (B) 55

    (C) 70

    (D) Cannot be determined from the information given.

64. Which of the following represents 89,213 written in scientific notation?

    (A) $8.9213 \times 10^2$

    (B) $8.9213 \times 10^3$

    (C) $8.9213 \times 10^4$

    (D) $8.9213 \times 10^5$

65. $\sqrt{100} - \sqrt{64} = ?$

    (A) 2

    (B) 4

    (C) 6

    (D) 8

66. A painter charges $12 an hour while his son charges $6 an hour. If the father and son worked the same amount of time together on a job, how many hours did each of them work if their combined charge for their labor was $108?

    (A) 6

    (B) 9

    (C) 12

    (D) 18

GO ON TO THE NEXT PAGE

**KAPLAN**

67. If $3ab = 6$, what is the value of $a$ in terms of $b$?

(A) $\dfrac{2}{b}$

(B) $\dfrac{2}{b^2}$

(C) $2b$

(D) $2b^2$

68. The ratio of $3\frac{1}{4}$ to $5\frac{1}{4}$ is equivalent to the ratio of:

(A)  3 to 5

(B)  4 to 7

(C)  8 to 13

(D)  13 to 21

69. If $x \neq 0$, then $\dfrac{6x^6}{2x^2} = ?$

(A) $4x^4$

(B) $4x^3$

(C) $3x^4$

(D) $3x^3$

70. If the perimeter of a square is 32 meters, then what is the area of the square, in square meters?

(A) 16

(B) 32

(C) 48

(D) 64

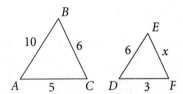

71. If triangle $ABC$ is similar to triangle $DEF$, then $EF = ?$

(A) 6

(B) 3.6

(C) 4.1

(D) 5

72. At garage $A$, it costs \$8.75 to park a car for the first hour and \$1.25 for each additional hour. At garage $B$, it costs \$5.50 to park a car for the first hour and \$2.50 for each additional hour. What is the difference between the cost of parking a car for 5 hours at garage $A$ and parking it for the same length of time at garage $B$?

(A) \$2.25

(B) \$1.75

(C) \$1.50

(D) \$1.25

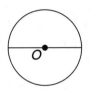

73. Circle $O$ above has a diameter of 6, an area of $b$ square units, and a circumference of $c$ units. What is the value of $b + c$?

(A) $9\pi$

(B) $15\pi$

(C) $18\pi$

(D) $42\pi$

74. If each digit 5 is replaced with the digit 7, how much will 258,546 be increased?

(A) 2,020

(B) 2,200

(C) 20,020

(D) 20,200

75. A 25-ounce solution is 20% alcohol. If 50 ounces of water are added to it, what percent of the new solution is alcohol?

(A) $6\frac{2}{3}\%$

(B) $7\frac{1}{2}\%$

(C) 10%

(D) $13\frac{1}{3}\%$

GO ON TO THE NEXT PAGE ⇨

KAPLAN

## SCIENCE

1. There is a recessive allele for a gene that made people more susceptible than normal to smallpox. Only homozygous recessive people display this trait; heterozygotes are indistinguishable from homozygous dominant people, with normal resistance to smallpox. After the point at which the smallpox virus was eliminated from the Earth, which of the following occurred to the allele frequency for the allele that caused smallpox susceptibility?

   (A) The allele declined in frequency for several generations and then disappeared.

   (B) The allele remained at a constant frequency in the gene pool.

   (C) The allele increased in frequency, since it was no longer selected against.

   (D) The number of homozygous recessive people remained the same, but the number of heterozygous people increased for several generations.

2. A black male mouse (I) is crossed with a black female mouse, and they produce 20 offspring: 15 black and 5 white. A different black male mouse (II) is crossed with the same female, and the offspring from this mating are 30 black mice. Which of the following must be true?

   (A) The female mouse is homozygous.

   (B) Male mouse II is heterozygous.

   (C) Two of the mice are heterozygous.

   (D) All the progeny of mouse II are homozygous.

3. Which of the following is found in all forms of life?

   I.   Genetic material
   II.  Protein
   III. Water

   (A) I only

   (B) II only

   (C) III only

   (D) I, II, and III

4. Water diffuses into and out of cells via:

   (A) Carrier proteins

   (B) Symport systems

   (C) Ion channels

   (D) Osmosis

5. Members of a class are more alike than members of:

   (A) An order

   (B) A phylum

   (C) A genus

   (D) A species

6. Albinos have a genotype of *aa*, while all other members of a population are either *AA* or *Aa*. The offspring of a cross between a heterozygous male and an albino female would be:

   (A) 100% albino

   (B) 100% normal pigmentation

   (C) 50% normal pigmentation, 50% albino

   (D) 25% normal pigmentation, 75% albino

7. In humans, normal sperm must contain:

   I.   An *X* chromosome
   II.  23 chromosomes
   III. A *Y* chromosome

   (A) I only

   (B) II only

   (C) III only

   (D) I and II

8. Stomata in plant leaves close at night to prevent the loss of:

   (A) $O_2$

   (B) $H_2O$

   (C) $CO_2$

   (D) Energy

GO ON TO THE NEXT PAGE

**KAPLAN**

9. Meiosis differs from mitosis in that:

    I. Two cell divisions take place.
    II. DNA replicates during interphase.
    III. Haploid cells are produced from diploid cells.

  (A) I only

  (B) II only

  (C) III only

  (D) I and III only

10. All organisms utilize:

  (A) $CO_2$.

  (B) A triplet genetic code to produce proteins.

  (C) Oxygen.

  (D) ADP as cellular energy.

11. Sexually reproducing species can have a selective advantage over asexually reproducing species because sexual reproduction:

  (A) Is more energy efficient.

  (B) Allows for more genetic diversity.

  (C) Decreases the likelihood of mutations.

  (D) Always decreases an offspring's survival ability.

12. The genes encoding for eukaryotic protein sequences are passed from one generation to the next via:

  (A) Other proteins

  (B) rRNA

  (C) tRNA

  (D) DNA

13. In humans, the site of successful fertilization is most commonly the:

  (A) Ovary

  (B) Fallopian tube

  (C) Uterus

  (D) Cervix

14. Which are correctly related?

  (A) White blood cell: No nucleus

  (B) Smooth muscle cell: Multinuclear

  (C) Smooth muscle: Voluntary action

  (D) Cardiac muscle: Involuntary action

15. To test whether a tall plant (in which the allele that determines tallness is dominant and the allele that determines shortness is recessive) is homozygous or heterozygous, you could:

    I. Cross it with a tall plant that had a short parent.
    II. Cross it with a tall plant that had two tall parents.
    III. Cross it with a short plant.

  (A) I only

  (B) II only

  (C) III only

  (D) I and III only

16. Which of the following associations of brain structure and function is false?

  (A) Hypothalamus: Appetite

  (B) Cerebellum: Motor coordination

  (C) Cerebral cortex: Higher intellectual function

  (D) Medulla: Basic emotional drives

GO ON TO THE NEXT PAGE

17. Which of the following is NOT characteristic of fermentation?

    (A) It is anaerobic.

    (B) It requires glucose.

    (C) It produces energy.

    (D) It requires oxygen.

18. Which order of classificatory divisions is correct?

    (A) Kingdom, subphylum, genus, family.

    (B) Phylum, class, order, genus.

    (C) Species, order, family, phylum.

    (D) Subphylum, kingdom, family, order.

19. Tall is dominant over short in a certain plant. A tall plant was crossed with a short plant, and both tall and short offspring were produced. This demonstrates:

    (A) The law of segregation

    (B) Incomplete dominance

    (C) Linkage

    (D) Mutation

20. Living in a close nutritional relationship with another organism in which one organism benefits while the other is neither harmed nor benefited is best defined as:

    (A) Symbiosis

    (B) Mutualism

    (C) Saprophytism

    (D) Commensalism

21. Ribosomes function in clusters called:

    (A) Histones

    (B) Nucleoli

    (C) Endoplasmic reticulum

    (D) Polysomes

22. The best description of identical twins is that they are:

    (A) Twins of the same sex.

    (B) Twins from a single egg.

    (C) Twins from two eggs that have been fertilized by the same sperm.

    (D) Twins from two eggs fertilized by two separate sperm.

23. The notochord is:

    (A) Present in all adult chordates.

    (B) Present in all echinoderms.

    (C) Present in chordates during embryonic development.

    (D) Always a vestigial organ in chordates.

24. The absorption of oxygen from the atmosphere into the blood takes place in the:

    (A) Pulmonary artery

    (B) Pulmonary vein

    (C) Alveoli

    (D) Trachea

25. Which of the following is a correct association?

    (A) Mitochondria: Transport of materials form the nucleus to the cytoplasm.

    (B) Golgi apparatus: Modification and glycosylation of proteins.

    (C) Endoplasmic reticulum: Selective barrier for the cell.

    (D) Ribosomes: Digestive enzymes most active at acidic pH.

GO ON TO THE NEXT PAGE

**KAPLAN**

26. Enzymes in human cells:

    I. Are proteins.
    II. Typically work best at pH 7.2.
    III. Are changed during a reaction.
    IV. Are found in the nucleus only.

    (A) I only
    (B) II only
    (C) I and II only
    (D) I, II, and III only

27. Which statement about the plasma membrane is false?

    (A) It serves as a selectively permeable barrier to the external environment.
    (B) It serves as a mediator between internal and external environments.
    (C) In eukaryotes, it contains the cytochrome chain of oxidative phosphorylation.
    (D) It contains phospholipids as a structural component.

28. Straight tail ($T$) is dominant over bent tail ($t$) in mice, and long-tailed mice ($L$) are dominant over short-tailed mice ($l$). Which cross must produce all straight, long-tailed mice?

    (A) $TtLl \times TtLl$
    (B) $Ttll \times TTLl$
    (C) $TtLL \times ttLL$
    (D) $TtLl \times TTLL$

29. Red is dominant over white in a certain flower. To test whether a red offspring is homozygous or heterozygous in this flower, one would:

    (A) Cross it with a red plant that had a white parent.
    (C) Cross it with a red plant that had two red parents.
    (C) Cross it with a white plant.
    (D) Two of the above will work.

30. A process that CANNOT take place in haploid cells is:

    (A) Mitosis
    (B) Meiosis
    (C) Cell division
    (D) Growth

31. In humans, brown eyes are dominant over blue eyes. In the cross of $BB \times bb$, what percentage of the offspring will have brown eyes?

    (A) 75%
    (B) 50%
    (C) 0%
    (D) 100%

32. Which of the following is NOT an organelle?

    (A) Nucleus
    (B) Golgi apparatus
    (C) Lysosome
    (D) Chlorophyll

33. The source of oxygen given off in photosynthesis is:

    (A) Water
    (B) Carbon dioxide
    (C) Glucose
    (D) Starch

34. Which of the following associations is correct?

    (A) Mitochondria: Transports materials from the nucleus to the cytoplasm.
    (B) Lysosome: Digestive enzymes for intracellular use.
    (C) Endoplasmic reticulum: Selective barrier for the cell.
    (D) Ribosome: Electron transport chain.

GO ON TO THE NEXT PAGE

KAPLAN

35. Which is NOT a characteristic of proteins?

    (A) They contain genetic information.
    (B) They can act as hormones.
    (C) They can catalyze chemical reactions.
    (D) They act in cell membrane trafficking.

36. Which part of cellular respiration directly produces a pH gradient during the oxidative metabolism of glucose?

    (A) Glycolysis
    (B) Anaerobic respiration
    (C) Krebs cycle
    (D) Electron transport chain

37. All of the following statements underlie the kinetic molecular theory of gases EXCEPT:

    (A) Gas molecules have no intermolecular forces.
    (B) Gas particles are in random motion.
    (C) Gas particles have no volume.
    (D) The average kinetic energy is proportional to the temperature (°C) of the gas.

38. The major portion of an atom's mass consists of:

    (A) Neutrons and protons
    (B) Electrons and protons
    (C) Electrons and neutrons
    (D) Neutrons and positrons

39. What happens when a radioactive element decays?

    (A) The nucleus gives off particles.
    (B) The ribosomes give off particles.
    (C) The mitochondria give off particles.
    (D) The Golgi apparatus gives off particles.

40. Which of the following is the best example of heat transferring from one source to another?

    (A) Making ice cubes.
    (B) Turning on a fan to cool the room.
    (C) Taking a hot bath.
    (D) Putting salt on snow to melt it.

41. Which of the following is the best example of potential energy changing to kinetic energy?

    (A) Pushing a rock off a cliff.
    (B) Sitting in a rocking chair.
    (C) Observing a bird fly.
    (D) Standing on a table.

42. The number of electrons revolving around the nucleus of an atom in an unionized state is equal to the number of positively charged protons within the nucleus. Which of the following elements would be considered an isotope?

    (A) 6 protons + 6 neutrons
    (B) 6 electrons + 6 neutrons
    (C) 7 protons + 6 neutrons
    (D) 7 protons + 6 electrons

GO ON TO THE NEXT PAGE

**KAPLAN**

43. Because the law of conservation of matter tells us that matter can be neither created nor destroyed, all equations must be balanced; that is, the number and kinds of atoms appearing on one side of the equation cannot be destroyed and so must appear in the same number and kind on the other side. In representing the formation of water by the simple addition of hydrogen and oxygen we might select the equation:

    $$H_2 + O_2 \rightarrow H_2O$$

    However, this equation is not balanced, because there are different numbers of atoms on each side of the equation. Balance is achieved by manipulating the coefficients, which indicate how many of each of the molecules is involved in the equation:

    $$2H_2 + O_2 \rightarrow 2H_2O$$

    Now the equation is balanced.

    According to the correctly balanced equation above, how many atoms of hydrogen are present in the reaction?

    (A) One
    (B) Two
    (C) Three
    (D) Four

44. Water at sea level boils at what temperature?

    (A) 100° F
    (B) 180° F
    (C) 212° C
    (D) 373° K

45. Which of the following subatomic particles has the largest mass?

    (A) Proton
    (B) Electron
    (C) Positron
    (D) Neutrino

46. Which one of the following processes includes all others in the list?

    (A) Diffusion
    (B) Osmosis
    (C) Passive transport
    (D) Facilitated transport

47. The Atomic Theory could be used to analyze which of the following?

    (A) Properties of hydrogen.
    (B) The proliferation of bacteria.
    (C) The AIDS epidemic.
    (D) The motion of an object.

48. As you move from left to right across a period (horizontal row) in the periodic table:

    (A) The number of electrons doubles.
    (B) The number of electrons is one more than the previous element.
    (C) The number of electrons stays the same.
    (D) The number of electrons is one less than the previous element.

49. Ionization energy is:

    (A) The energy required to completely remove an electron from an atom or ion.
    (B) The energy created by an ion.
    (C) The same as kinetic energy.
    (D) The attraction between a proton and neutron.

GO ON TO THE NEXT PAGE

50. Which of the following is true about compounds?

    (A) Compounds are pure substances that are composed of two or more elements in a fixed proportion.

    (B) Compounds can be broken down chemically to produce their constituent elements or other compounds.

    (C) Both A and B are correct.

    (D) Neither A nor B is correct.

51. Evaporation can best be described as:

    (A) The process in which molecules may have enough energy to leave the liquid phase and escape into the gaseous phase.

    (B) A heating process.

    (C) Fusion.

    (D) The process in which molecules in the solid phase absorb enough energy to begin the liquid phase.

52. If the half-life of a certain isotope is 5 years, what fraction of a sample of that isotope will remain after 15 years?

    (A) $\frac{1}{5}$

    (B) $\frac{1}{8}$

    (C) $\frac{1}{15}$

    (D) $\frac{1}{20}$

53. Which of the following represents 1 amu?

    (A) $1.66 \times 10^{-24}$ g

    (B) $1.66 \times 10^{-27}$ kg

    (C) Neither A nor B is correct.

    (D) Both A and B are correct.

54. Force exists only:

    (A) In a vacuum

    (B) In pairs

    (C) In two dimensions

    (D) Without movement

55. Speed is different from velocity because:

    (A) Speed is a scalar quantity, and velocity is a vector quantity.

    (B) Velocity involves speed and direction.

    (C) Speed only expresses a magnitude.

    (D) All of the above are correct.

56. Whenever a current passes through a resistance, _____ is generated.

    (A) Voltage

    (B) Capacitance

    (C) Heat

    (D) Light

57. While attempting to push a heavy box across the floor:

    (A) The amount of force required to start the box sliding is more than that required to keep it sliding.

    (B) Pushing on the box without moving it results in no work being done.

    (C) The coefficient of static friction is dependent on the nature of the surface the box is resting on.

    (D) All of the above.

GO ON TO THE NEXT PAGE

**KAPLAN**

58. A larger mass requires _____ force to achieve the same acceleration rate.

   (A) Less
   (B) More
   (C) The same
   (D) None of the above

59. A vehicle travels at a constant speed on the highway. It can be said that:

   (A) Its acceleration rate is zero.
   (B) The net forces acting on the vehicle are zero.
   (C) The force applied by the vehicle's drive wheels is equal and opposite to the forces that act to slow the vehicle.
   (D) All of the above are correct.

60. Vector quantities express:

   (A) Magnitude
   (B) Direction
   (C) Both A and B are correct.
   (D) Neither A nor B is correct.

61. All of the following statements about force are true EXCEPT:

   (A) Force is a scalar quantity.
   (B) Force is a push or pull.
   (C) Greater force results in greater acceleration.
   (D) Smaller masses require less force to achieve the same acceleration.

62. An astronaut has less _____ when in outer space.

   (A) Weight
   (B) Mass
   (C) Velocity
   (D) Speed

63. _____ voltage drops occur at higher resistances.

   (A) Higher
   (B) Lower
   (C) Zero
   (D) None of the above

64. An object at rest:

   (A) Has no forces acting on it.
   (B) Is not subject to the law of gravity.
   (C) Has no net force acting on it.
   (D) Has no mass.

65. A circuit with flowing current in it is considered:

   (A) Open
   (B) Closed
   (C) Short
   (D) Dead

END OF TEST. STOP

THE ANSWER KEY APPEARS ON THE FOLLOWING PAGE.

# Practice Test One: **Answer Key**

| Reading Comprehension | | Vocabulary and Spelling | | Mathematics | | | | Science | | | |
|---|---|---|---|---|---|---|---|---|---|---|---|
| 1. B | 24. D | 1. D | 34. A | 1. B | 26. A | 51. B | | 1. B | 34. B | | |
| 2. C | 25. A | 2. B | 35. B | 2. A | 27. A | 52. D | | 2. C | 35. A | | |
| 3. D | 26. D | 3. A | 36. B | 3. B | 28. A | 53. A | | 3. D | 36. D | | |
| 4. C | 27. A | 4. D | 37. A | 4. C | 29. A | 54. D | | 4. D | 37. D | | |
| 5. C | 28. C | 5. D | 38. D | 5. B | 30. C | 55. D | | 5. B | 38. A | | |
| 6. B | 29. B | 6. C | 39. D | 6. D | 31. D | 56. D | | 6. C | 39. A | | |
| 7. C | 30. A | 7. C | 40. D | 7. D | 32. C | 57. C | | 7. B | 40. C | | |
| 8. C | 31. B | 8. C | 41. C | 8. B | 33. A | 58. B | | 8. B | 41. A | | |
| 9. D | 32. D | 9. B | 42. B | 9. C | 34. C | 59. C | | 9. D | 42. C | | |
| 10. A | 33. A | 10. A | 43. A | 10. C | 35. B | 60. A | | 10. B | 43. D | | |
| 11. A | 34. D | 11. C | 44. D | 11. D | 36. D | 61. A | | 11. B | 44. D | | |
| 12. A | 35. D | 12. C | 45. D | 12. C | 37. A | 62. C | | 12. D | 45. A | | |
| 13. D | 36. C | 13. B | 46. C | 13. B | 38. D | 63. B | | 13. B | 46. A | | |
| 14. D | 37. D | 14. A | 47. B | 14. D | 39. A | 64. C | | 14. D | 47. A | | |
| 15. A | 38. C | 15. A | 48. D | 15. B | 40. B | 65. A | | 15. D | 48. B | | |
| 16. D | 39. B | 16. A | 49. B | 16. A | 41. C | 66. A | | 16. D | 49. A | | |
| 17. A | 40. D | 17. D | 50. C | 17. B | 42. D | 67. A | | 17. D | 50. C | | |
| 18. D | 41. D | 18. D | 51. C | 18. B | 43. D | 68. D | | 18. B | 51. A | | |
| 19. C | 42. A | 19. C | 52. D | 19. B | 44. B | 69. C | | 19. A | 52. B | | |
| 20. C | 43. A | 20. D | 53. A | 20. B | 45. B | 70. D | | 20. D | 53. D | | |
| 21. B | 44. D | 21. D | 54. C | 21. D | 46. D | 71. B | | 21. D | 54. B | | |
| 22. D | 45. C | 22. C | 55. B | 22. D | 47. D | 72. B | | 22. B | 55. D | | |
| 23. C | | 23. C | 56. C | 23. C | 48. D | 73. B | | 23. C | 56. C | | |
| | | 24. B | 57. A | 24. D | 49. C | 74. D | | 24. C | 57. D | | |
| | | 25. C | 58. A | 25. C | 50. C | 75. A | | 25. B | 58. B | | |
| | | 26. D | 59. D | | | | | 26. C | 59. D | | |
| | | 27. A | 60. B | | | | | 27. C | 60. C | | |
| | | 28. A | 61. D | | | | | 28. D | 61. A | | |
| | | 29. B | 62. B | | | | | 29. D | 62. A | | |
| | | 30. A | 63. A | | | | | 30. B | 63. A | | |
| | | 31. A | 64. C | | | | | 31. D | 64. C | | |
| | | 32. D | 65. A | | | | | 32. D | 65. B | | |
| | | 33. C | | | | | | 33. A | | | |

# Answers and Explanations

## Reading Comprehension

**1. B**

The author says parks were created to give people a "refuge" from the city. Scanning quickly through the answer choices, (B) jumps out because it fits the opening statement: Parks were designed with the needs of city residents in mind. (A) and (D) are misleading bits of information from the rest of the first paragraph. As for (C), the author never suggests that parks are supposed to end the unpleasantness of city life. They merely provide a refuge.

**2. C**

To answer this question, you have to understand the context in which crime and pollution are mentioned in the second paragraph. The author describes the deterioration of parks, including the effects of crime and pollution, to show that people can no longer use the parks as they were meant to be used. In other words, why people can no longer rest and relax in the parks, (C).

**3. D**

The last paragraph offers suggestions for reversing the decline of the parks: Adding more police units and caretakers, banning vehicles, and rerouting sewage pipes. It is also necessary, the author says, to "insulate city parks from their surroundings," but the problem here is that "total isolation" is "impossible." This is paraphrased in (D). (A), (B), and (C) twist information from the author's suggestions.

**4. C**

Choice (C) can be eliminated because it's not the primary focus of the passage.

**5. C**

The answer here has to be broad enough to cover the entire passage. Review the topics of the individual paragraphs; scientists get pictures, scientists run experiments, scientists propose theories and make suggestions throughout the passage. Clearly, the author is

*discussing* the (C) efforts of scientists. Though the Viking mission may have been an extraordinary scientific achievement, there's much more than a simple *account* of it here, (A). (B) is incorrect because the passage presents a balanced view on the question of life on Mars. (D) is incorrect because the only time the author discusses *limitations of the scientific investigation* of Mars is in the fourth paragraph.

**6. B**

The word *however* in the sentence right after the cited sentence indicates that what the scientists hardly dared to hope for (and didn't get) was some visible sign of Martian life. So the reference to "people who hold a ticket to the lottery" is there to show how likely it was that the photographs would show Martian life (B).

**7. C**

You know by the end of the second paragraph that the experiments designed to detect biological life were inconclusive, and that no organic materials were found either. (C) is the answer. The other choices may have tempted you, but they all involve making unsupported inferences. Just because there weren't organic materials from meteorites on Mars doesn't mean that (A) *meteorites do not strike the surface of Mars* as often as scientists thought. The author never implies (B), and (D) is too sweeping. These four experiments did not provide sufficient evidence to prove or disprove the existence of life on Mars.

**8. C**

Here you need to understand the role of the third paragraph. Reread it, starting from the end of the second paragraph. The author states that a Viking experiment turned up no trace of organic material on the Martian surface. We are then presented with a theory that UV radiation may have destroyed any organic materials once present in the Martian soil. So the third paragraph provides (C) a *theory* about findings presented earlier. The theory is not *proposed* earlier in the passage, so (A) is incorrect. There's no *evidence supporting a statement made earlier*, so (B) is incorrect. Nor is there *criticism* (D).

**9. D**

The author mentions Earth in the passage at the end of the third paragraph, where he says that Mars "never developed a protective layer of ozone as Earth did." Since it is life that the ozone layer protected on Earth, you can infer that Mars was not able to support life, (D), as Earth was. (A) contradicts information from the passage that says that no organic compounds were found on Mars. (B) is incorrect, because although Mars possessed at one time an atmosphere rich in carbon dioxide, the author never suggests that Earth *didn't*. Mars and Earth are both in the path of the ultraviolet radiation of the Sun, so (C) is incorrect.

**10. A**

Reread the sentences surrounding the reference to Viking landing sites, and look for a paraphrase among the answer choices. Those who still think that there might be life on Mars point out that there were only two Viking landers, that the experimental sites were limited and uninteresting, and that scientists were not concerned about finding life when they chose the landing spots. In other words, they are saying that although evidence of life was not found by the landers, this does not mean that Mars is devoid of life, choice (A). Though (B) is a true statement, this isn't why the author mentions the landing sites. The author never says that the Viking mission was unsuccessful or that the selection of landing sites was poor, so (C) is incorrect. (D) focuses on the intentions and expectations of the scientists. All you know is that they wanted to land the spacecrafts safely, not whether they thought *detection of life was a primary objective* (D).

**11. A**

The argument of the researchers in the fifth paragraph is that, if endoliths could adapt to the harsh conditions of Antarctica by living in rocks, maybe some form of life did the same thing to survive on early Mars. The idea here is that Mars and Antarctica are (A) comparable environments and that life may adapt in the same way, or adopt identical strategies, to survive. All of the incorrect choices are based on distortions of the argument. (B) and (D) are incorrect because the argument never states that *blue-green algae* or *endoliths* have anything to do with Mars; they were found in Antarctica and merely became the subject of speculation for the researchers. (C) is too broad.

**12. A**

When you go back to the referenced line, you find that the increased air space *provides more effective insulation…allowing it to retain more heat*. The question is

specifically asking about the increased air space, not raised fur in general. (A) refers to the air space, whereas (B) is more general. So, (A) is correct.

**13. D**

Ask yourself: What does the author think about goosebumps? Because you're asked about the overall point, you probably don't need to go back to a specific part of the passage. Instead, quickly summarize the author's point. (D) looks very good. (The author must think it's pretty interesting or she wouldn't have written the passage in the first place.) Only (D) fits, so that's your answer.

**14. D**

The author says that there's a difference between humans and other mammals, and uses the lions to illustrate this point. Lions sit around or nap after they eat a lot. People get bored and do stuff. Why is this important? Because this led to the ultimate development of culture. (C) and (D) both seem correct, but only (D) includes the author's larger point about culture.

**15. A**

The general purpose of the passage is to explain something, so look for this direction. (A) and (C) both look feasible. On further consideration, (C) doesn't quite work, since only one thesis is presented—the author is not providing an *alternative* to anything. (A), however, fits well. The author shows a *distinction* between the behavior of people and other mammals, and then shows the *significance* of this distinction (it led to culture). (B) is off base, since the author never indicates there might be an objection to the thesis. (D) is out of the scope of the passage—what will happen in the future is never discussed.

**16. D**

The *archaeological discoveries* mentioned in the question are human and dog bones lying next to each other in ancient burial sites. The reason the author feels it's *terribly appropriate* that these bones are found together comes a few lines later, when he says *it marks a relationship that is the most ancient of all*. (D) paraphrases that idea. You can see from this how important it is to read a few lines before and after the line reference in the question. The author says nothing about burial habits in the Mesolithic Era (A), or the religious significance of animals in prehistoric cultures (B). He does mention hunting (C), but the bone finds are not appropriate because they do not *illustrate the role of dogs in hunting expeditions*. (D) is the only possibility.

### 17.  A

The end of the first paragraph provides the answer. The author says that the dog was the first domesticated animal because it served as a *companion and ally* (A). Only after domesticating animals as companions did humans domesticate *food animals* (B), and then *those that provided enhanced speed and range* (D), followed by those that helped us farm (C). The key thing is to see that all these other types of domesticated animals came after animals were domesticated as companions.

### 18.  D

The quote takes you to the beginning of the second paragraph. The author says that having a dog as a companion animal was *almost inevitable*, and then lists several reasons why. One of these is that the dog *is susceptible to domination by, and attachment to, a pack leader—the top dog*. The implication is that humans formed bonds with dogs because they could dominate them (D). None of the other choices gives characteristics that make sense in answer to the question.

### 19.  C

This is definitely a question you need to return to the passage to answer. Back in the second paragraph, the author lists the characteristics that made dogs *inevitable* companions for humans. In addition to being born dependent and forming bonds with those that rear them, dogs *have a set of appeasement behaviors that elicit affective reactions from even the most hardened* humans. The author goes on to talk about puppies transforming *cynics* into *cooing softies*. Even if you weren't sure what *appeasement behaviors* were, you can see the gist of the author's point here: humans form bonds with dogs largely because dogs are cute and loveable. So would it make sense if *affective reactions* were *callous* (A), or *rational* (B)? No. (D) goes too far. The author isn't saying humans become childish around dogs, but that dogs arouse human emotions. (C) is the best answer.

### 20.  C

The easiest way to understand the point of a comparison is to understand the context. What's the author saying in these lines? He's trying to show why it was inevitable that dogs

became human companions. One reason is that dogs form bonds with their owners (C). That's the only reason he compares puppies with babies—to show how emotional people get about dogs. The author's point has nothing to do with *criticizing an uncaring attitude* (A), so that can't be the point of his comparing puppies and babies. The same is true for the rest of the choices, so (C) is correct.

### 21.  B

Go back to the passage. Notice that the start of the third paragraph actually refers back to the end of the *first* paragraph. The first paragraph ended with the author listing the dog as the first domesticated animal, followed by food animals, work animals, etc. The second paragraph talks about why the dog came first. So when the third paragraph begins with *no wonder the dog was first*, it's referring to the dog's status as the first domesticated animal. Similarly, *the list* refers to other domesticated animals, or *the number of animals that developed relationships with humans* (B). The author hasn't yet mentioned *birds that scavenge human food supplies*, and when he does, he only mentions one, not many *types* (A). The passage never mentions species that are able to communicate with dogs (C), or the variety of attributes that make dogs good hunters (D).

### 22.  D

This question might seem more complicated than it really is. If you were confused by the digression the author made to talk about the blue tit, taking a look at the choices first probably would've saved you time. (A) and (B) are fairly easy to eliminate—they have nothing to do with any of the author's main points. The author mentions *opportunistic feeders*. He goes on saying, "even today, many birds…feed from our stores." So (D) must be right; the blue tit is an example of an opportunistic feeder.

### 23.  C

This is a clear reference question. Go back to the passage to see what kind of animals are being referred to. You have to read above a little to find the answer. The author has just finished describing the blue tit as an example of an opportunistic feeder. He reinforces the idea that the tit is an animal that feeds when and where it can by saying, "If all birds had been so specialized that they only fed in deep forest, it never would have happened." In other words, they are *not* so specialized—they'll eat wherever they find a food source (C). The author isn't talking here about companion animals (A). Forest inhabitants, choice (B), is too broad. (D) is incorrect because the birds are not hunting, they're feeding.

**24. D**

Go back to the passage to see in what context the author discusses his experiences in the tropics. At the beginning of the fourth paragraph, the author says that he thinks that the very first domesticated animals were orphaned as a result of hunting. He then tells how, in the tropics, he saw many instances of wild animals raised in homes of hunters. So his experiences illustrate his theory about how *the first domesticated animals were created* (D). None of the other choices relates to the author's argument here (or anywhere in the passage).

**25. A**

Check out the line *aid* is in to see what's going on. The author says that without domesticated animals—goats, sheep, pigs, cattle, and horses—we never would've achieved civilization. These animals helped or *aided* us—but they didn't have much choice in the matter. We dominated them, and then used them for food or labor. That's why *aid* is in quotes, and (A) is correct. The passage never says *population levels are dangerously high* (B). (C) is a better possibility—but it's not a point the author makes; you're inferring too much if you chose (C). It's not clear that animals benefited at all from domestication (D).

**26. D**

The *ironic paradox* is found in the last four lines of the passage. The author says our living with other species—using them for food and labor—is what made our civilization possible. It is ironic then, that our civilization is presently wiping out many plant and animal species (D). Nowhere does the author say anything about (A) or (B). With (C), the author does talk about the pet care industry in the final paragraph, but not to say its size is *ironic.* His point is just to show how big it is.

**27. A**

Reread the paragraph to acquire an overview, and pay special attention to the opening sentences, which introduce the topic. With (B), we have no idea whether scientists are bringing the disease under control. (C) is not discussed. (D) is too extreme; the author doesn't claim that malaria *cannot* be eradicated.

**28. C**

Note the use of the word *suggests*. Draw a reasonable conclusion from the evidence offered in the passage. (A) is tempting. The author refers to two examples of historically documented incidents of the disease, but that is not the same thing as a *well-documented disease*. We have no way of knowing whether the disease is well documented. With (B), we know only that malaria was spread to the Americas from Europe. (D) is incorrect since there's nothing about misunderstanding the symptoms of the disease. (C) is correct. A long history, significant spread, and 250 million cases annually all support this conclusion.

**29. B**

According to the passage, Hippocrates identified three types of malarial fevers in the fifth century B.C.E. Therefore, he must have lived in the fifth century B.C.E.

**30. A**

Since it's clear that a jellyfish couldn't have any feelings about its encounter with humans, the author is apparently using this image to make the reader smile (A). The author doesn't ask us to feel sympathy for either the jellyfish or humans (B), and doesn't discuss whether or not humans are afraid of jellyfish (C). Although the author does discuss the danger of jellyfish, the quote in question doesn't accomplish that purpose (D).

**31. B**

The third and fourth sentences contain the key to answering this question. It is within this passage that you learn the relatively common encounters are not surprising because jellyfish *live in every ocean in the world* (B). (A), (C), and (D) are all details from the passage, but none of them help to explain why encounters are so common.

**32. D**

In this passage, the big contrast is between moons that have remained unchanged since their "early, intense bombardment," and those whose surfaces have been altered in more recent epochs. Io is mentioned in the last three sentences. These sentences stress recent, indeed ongoing, changes in the satellite's surface. By inference, most impact craters from the long-ago bombardments have probably been obliterated (D). Continuing tectonic activity (A) is mentioned explicitly; tides (B) are mentioned in the final sentence as the probable cause of the tectonic activity, and hence the active volcanos. Inferably Io's surface is younger than the "very ancient" surface of Callisto, (C).

### 33. A

Keep your eye on the big contrast. The bombardments, and the craters that record them, were laid down long ago; thus a surface marked by impact craters (the dark areas of Ganymede) is older than one not so marked (the lighter areas). In addition, it's mentioned that some features of the light areas probably result from later iceflows. Thus, (A) is correct, ruling out (B) and (C). The light areas feature grooves and ridges probably resulting from these iceflows, not from early bombardment (D).

### 34. D

The passage conveys a great deal of information, which the author implicitly accepts, ruling out (A). The word used for the photographs of Io—*revelatory*—is enough by itself to eliminate this choice. The fact that information about Io comes from satellite photographs rules out (B). On the other hand, (C) is out because of the cautious language used throughout: *probably* (twice), *apparently*, and *accepted explanation*. Hence the knowledge is persuasive though incomplete, as specified in (D).

### 35. D

The question refers to questions that remain unanswered today. Look for an answer choice that provides an historical perspective on ecology and its concerns. Watch out for incorrect answer choices that confuse the author's perspective with that of someone else. Nowhere does the passage mention funding agencies or the attitudes of the general public, so (A) is incorrect. And though many of these regions may indeed be remote or inhospitable, there's no direct evidence to suggest that that's why questions remain, so (B) is incorrect as well. Nothing in the passage indicates a lack of cooperation, so (C) is incorrect.

### 36. C

Look for a mention of ecosystem in the passage. Ecosystems are described as "collections of communities," with tropical rainforests and coral reefs given as examples. Remember, the question says *except*, so your answer must be a *non-ecosystem*. Rainforests are ecosystems, so it's reasonable to infer that temperate forests would also fit the definition of a "collection of communities." (A) is out. (B)

and (D) are out because coral reefs and tropical rainforests are mentioned as examples of ecosystems.

### 37. D

Examine the key sentence beginning "Yet, however effective and inexpensive email may be …." In the center of the paragraph, the author balances advantages versus disadvantages. (A) is the opposite of what is written. The author mentions several flaws in the text. (B) is out, too: While the author presents a personal opinion, it is too extreme to say the text is *intensely subjective*. With (C), the author criticizes email as impersonal and mediocre, but he admits that e-mail also has advantages. (D) is the answer: The author is objectively analytical, presenting both pros and cons.

### 38. C

The author says e-mail is impersonal, and lacks the immediacy of a phone call, so immediacy here must have something to do with being personal or intimate. Quickness is a common meaning of immediacy, but it doesn't fit in a sentence about why e-mail is impersonal. So (A) is out. With (B), e-mail may lack *precision*, but this doesn't follow from the word *immediacy*. (D) means pretty much the same thing as (A), and they can't both be right.

### 39. B

This is a main idea question, so either the correct answer will make so much sense you will want to pick it, or you can eliminate incorrect answer choices because they are too broad or too specific, or otherwise don't properly describe the passage. Here the correct answer choice does make a lot of sense. The passage describes how coral reefs are created, so choice (B), the formation of coral reefs, describes the passage well. Choice (A) is out because *varieties* of animal life are nowhere described. (C) is incorrect because "death cycles" of coral reefs are never touched upon. And (D) is far too narrow; there's only the barest reference in the passage to "the physical beauty" of coral reefs.

**40. D**

For this question, you just want to pick the answer choice that best paraphrases the relationship between the coral and algae as described in the passage. The passage states that the "two organisms form a mutually beneficial relationship"; in other words, the relationship is cooperative, choice (D).

**41. D**

Although the wording of this question indicates that this is an inference question, the correct answer choice, (D), can be gleaned directly from the first sentence. If most life is "dependent on organisms that store radiant energy from the sun," it doesn't take much to infer that most life is ultimately dependent on light from the sun. Remember that on inference questions you are looking for the one answer that must be true based on what is stated in the passage.

**42. A**

The first paragraph describes ecosystems that are dependent on photosynthetic organisms, while the second paragraph describes ecosystems that are dependent on chemosynthetic organisms. In both cases, the organisms serve similar functions as primary producers within their different food chains, so choice (A) is correct. Choice (B) is incorrect because only chemosynthetic organisms are described in the passage as supporting higher organisms at great ocean depths. (C) is clearly incorrect because chemosynthetic organisms do not rely on sunlight for their basic source of energy. Choice (D) is never discussed in the passage.

**43. A**

The passage states that "photosynthetic organisms such as plants and algae are eaten by other organisms." This means that plant and algae are photosynthetic.

**44. D**

This is a slightly tricky inference question, because a lot of dates are mentioned in the passage. Nonetheless, the passage states that Halley determined that the comet followed a 76-year orbit. He never lived to see the comet that appeared in 1758, so it follows that the last time the comet appeared before his death took place 76 years earlier, or in 1758 − 76 = 1682, choice (D).

**45. C**

The passage clearly states the comet was named after the astronomer Edmund Halley, who calculated its orbit.

## Vocabulary and Spelling

**1. D**

If you know that *foolhardy* has a negative charge, that alone will probably direct you to the correct answer, *reckless* (D). *Foolhardy* and *reckless* both mean "rash" or "overly bold."

**2. B**

Try to think where you've heard *truncate* before. If that doesn't work, ask yourself whether *truncate* could possibly mean each of the various answer choices. Sometimes, even if you have only the vaguest sense of a word, you will still know what the word cannot mean. *Truncate* does mean *shorten*.

**3. A**

Try to come up with a context clue. Have you ever heard of a "secluded island"? Which of the answer choices best describes such an island? Only (A), *isolate*, makes any sense. *Isolate* and *seclude* both mean "to separate" or "keep away from contact with others."

**4. D**

If you have heard that a defendant was "acquitted of all charges," you should know that means the defendant was *cleared* of all charges, and is now free to go.

**5. D**

Even if you've never heard the word *simulate* before and don't know that it means the same as *replicate*, both of which mean "to reproduce or imitate," you might be able to use word roots and associated words to find the correct answer. *Simulate* has the prefix *sim-*, meaning "same," and *replicate* is very close to *replica*, meaning "copy" or "facsimile."

**6. C**

*Erroneous* means mistaken. You should have had no problem with this question if you realized *erroneous* has the same root as "error," meaning "mistake."

**7. C**

*Garbled* means "jumbled" or "all mixed up", as in a "garbled message," which is one that gets messed up during transfer so that it no longer makes any sense.

**8. C**

*Synthetic* means *artificial*, as in the synthetic fabric polyester.

**9. B**

You can tell from the answer choices that *creep* is being used here as a verb, so if you are unsure of the definition, try to use *creep* as a verb in a sentence. You might come up with something like: "He crept up on me carefully so I wouldn't hear him." As this sentence illustrates, the verb *creep* means "to move slowly or crawl quietly."

**10. A**

*Leverage* means *influence* or power. Try to use the word in a sentence: He used his *leverage* to convince skeptical allies. If you are not sure of the meaning, eliminate answer choices you know don't make any sense.

**11. C**

Have you ever heard the phrase "viscous fluid"? Which of the answer choices could logically describe a fluid? Only (C), *syrupy*, makes any sense. And *viscous* literally means "thick or glutinous"—in other words, *syrupy*.

**12. C**

Word roots alone could have gotten you to the correct answer. *Bene-* means "good," and *factor* means "doer," so *benefactor* means "someone who does good things." Of the answer choices, (C) makes the most sense. Specifically, a *benefactor* is one who gives aid, usually in the form of money.

**13. B**

You may have heard of the Prohibition era, which was a constitutionally enacted ban on alcohol the United States experimented with, unsuccessfully, in the early twentieth century. A small "p" *prohibition* refers to any ban, much like *to prohibit* means "to forbid."

**14. A**

A *hypocrite* is someone who says one thing and does another. Perhaps you knew that, but weren't quite happy with the correct answer choice, (A) *poser*. But a *hypocrite* and a *poser* are both phonies, and none of the other answer choices makes any sense.

**15. A**

*Opulent* means *luxurious*. It helps if you've seen the word used in a phrase before, such as "opulent palace." Otherwise, you should make your best guess.

**16. A**

The prefix *in-* usually means "not," so something that is interminable is not terminable, that is, never ending. The correct answer choice will be a word that means "short-lived." *Brief* means "short-lived." This is the correct answer.

**17. D**

Something traditional is well established, such as a custom. The correct answer choice will be a word that means "not well established." *Iconoclastic* means "against tradition," that is, tending to overthrow any kind of established ideals, beliefs, or custom. This is the correct answer. If you needed to guess, remember that the prefixes *im-*, *un-*, and *an-* mean "not." You could use this to eliminate answer choices.

**18. D**

The verb *abandon* means to desert or forsake, to leave behind. However, the answer choices tell you that here, it is being used as a noun; that is, it refers to a complete surrender of inhibitions. The correct answer choice will be a word that means "restraint." Choice (D) is exactly what you are looking for.

**19. C**

*Logy* means *lethargic* or *lacking in energy or vitality*. It usually refers to a combination of mental and physical slowness. The correct answer choice will be a word that means "wakeful" and "fresh." *Alert* works here.

**20. D**

To *cede* is to yield, give up, or transfer title to someone else—one country cedes land to another, for instance. If you don't give something up, you hang onto it, so a synonym for "keep" will be the correct answer. *Retain* is the answer choice you are looking for.

**21. D**

To *proscribe* is to forbid or to prohibit as harmful. It shouldn't be confused with *prescribe*, which means "to set down as a rule," such as when you order someone to take medicine. The correct answer choice will be a word that means "allow." Choice (D) fits well here.

**22. C**

*Eschew* has nothing to do with chewing. To eschew something is to shun, abstain from, or avoid it. The correct answer choice will be a word that means "embrace" or "indulge in." Choice (C) works perfectly.

**23. C**

Aside from what you might wear around your neck, to *collar* is to grab or seize. You may have heard the phrase *police collared the criminal*, meaning that they caught the criminal. The correct answer choice will be a word that means "let go." Choice (C) is the closest match

**24. B**

An *iota* is a tiny amount or a minuscule portion. The correct answer choice will be a word that means "a lot." A *plethora* is a great amount. This is the correct answer.

**25. C**

To be *ambulatory* is to be able to move. The correct answer choice will be a word that means "unable to move." *Fixed* means "immobile" or "stationary." This is the correct answer.

**26. D**

*Leveling* is the act of making something level or flat. The correct answer choice will be a word that means "to make uneven." *Canting* is setting something at an angle; that is, stopping it from being level. (D) is the correct answer.

**27. A**

To *lull* is to soothe. You may have thought of the word *lullaby*, a song that is meant to soothe a child to sleep. The correct answer choice will be a word that means "to cause distress." *Upset* is the correct answer.

**28. A**

In this question, *license* is a verb. It must be, because choice (D), *impress*, can't be a noun, so all the choices in this question must be verbs. As a verb, license means "to allow." The correct answer choice will be a synonym for "prohibit." To *curb* is to restrain.

**29. B**

*Insidious* describes something that spreads harmfully in a subtle or stealthy manner. The correct answer choice will be a synonym for "overt" or "direct." *Direct* is correct.

**30. A**

An *unguent* is an ointment used to soothe or heal. The correct answer choice will be a synonym for something that irritates or aggravates. *Irritant* is the correct answer.

**31. A**

Something *ominous* predicts or foreshadows disaster. Does something *auspicious* foreshadow *success*? Yes. In fact, something *auspicious* is considered a good omen, just as something *ominous* is considered a bad omen.

**32. D**

When a liquid, like blood, *coagulates,* it forms a *clot.* When a liquid *freezes,* it forms *ice.* You may have been tempted by choice (C). People can *obstruct* something by forming a *blockade,* but those words don't refer to changes that a liquid undergoes. When you find a choice like this, don't try to force it to work—it's just a tempting incorrect answer. Let it go, and stick with the one that works best.

**33. C**

By definition, to *fuss* is to pay excessive attention to small details, or to *care* excessively. Likewise, to *quibble* is to raise minor objections, or to *object* excessively.

**34. A**

A *novel* is a type of *book.* That's an easy bridge. In (A), is an *epic* a type of *poem?* Yes, an epic is a long narrative poem, so (A) is right.

**35. B**

*Ravenous* means extremely *hungry*—the second word is an extreme version of the first word. (B) is perfect—*titanic* is an amplification of *large*. *Titanic* means gigantic, so (B) is the answer.

**36. B**

A *bouquet* is an arrangement of *flowers*, so the first word will be an arrangement of the second word. A *mosaic* is made of *tiles*, just as a bouquet is made up of flowers. That's a good match. The correct answer is (B).

**37. A**

*Paraphrase* means restatement of a text using different words. *Verbatim* means word for word or exact. A paraphrase is not verbatim—the words are near opposites. The only choices opposite in meaning are *approximation* and *precise*, in (A). An approximation is an estimate, while something that's precise is exact, so an approximation is not precise. (A) is correct.

**38. D**

Something *impeccable* is perfect, it doesn't have a *flaw*. *Absurd* means without sense, so this is the correct answer.

**39. D**

A *seismograph* is an instrument used to measure an earthquake, so we need another instrument used to measure something. In (D), a *thermometer* measures *temperature*, so (D) is the best answer.

**40. D**

To *guzzle* is to *drink* very quickly, taking big gulps, so the relationship is one of speed or degree. In (D), to *stride* is to *walk* quickly, taking big steps, so (D) is the best answer.

**41. C**

An *orator* is a public speaker and *articulate* means able to express oneself well. You can form the bridge, "A successful orator is one who is articulate." With that in mind, (C) is good—a good *judge* has to be *unbiased*. It's safe to say that a biased judge is a bad judge in the same way that an inarticulate orator is a bad orator. (C) is correct.

**42. B**

*Intransigent* means unyielding—the opposite of *flexible*. Our bridge is "a person who is intransigent is lacking in flexibility." The only pair that looks good is (B), *disinterested* and

partisanship. One who's disinterested is unbiased—he doesn't have an interest in either side of a dispute. *Partisan* means partial to a particular party or cause. That's the opposite of disinterested. So partisanship, the quality of being biased, is lacking in a person who could be described as disinterested.

**43. A**

*Castigate* means *criticize*. Knowing that, we can build the bridge: people castigate others for their wrongdoings. Try this bridge on the choices. People *congratulate* each other for their *successes*.

**44. D**

By definition, a *maven*, or expert, has expertise. Likewise, a *supplicant*, or humble beggar, by definition has *humility*, making choice (D) the right answer.

**45. D**

By definition, to *exculpate* is to clear from blame. If you weren't sure of the meaning of exculpate, you could try breaking the word apart: *ex-* means remove or undo, *culpa-*, as in *culprit*, means guilt or blame. Likewise, *forgive* (secondary meaning: to grant relief from payment) is to clear from *debt*. (D) is correct.

**46. C**

The correct spelling is *taunt*.

**47. B**

The correct spelling is *reasonable*.

**48. D**

The correct spelling is *grateful*.

**49. B**

The correct spelling is *accidental*.

**50. C**

The correct spelling is *oppress*.

**51. C**

The correct spelling is *cosmopolitan*.

**52. D**

The correct spelling is *sensible.*

**53. A**

The correct spelling is *intricate.*

**54. C**

The correct spelling is *colossal.*

**55. B**

The correct spelling is *condemn.*

**56. C**

The correct spelling is *weird.*

**57. A**

The correct spelling is *difficulty.*

**58. A**

The correct spelling is *embarrass.*

**59. D**

No mistake.

**60. B**

The correct spelling is *conductor.*

**61. D**

No mistake.

**62. B**

The correct spelling is *persistent.*

**63. A**

The correct spelling is *accessible.*

**64. C**

The correct spelling is *everyday.*

**65. A**

The correct spelling is *altered.*

## Mathematics

**1. B**

The commutative property of addition states that when adding two or more terms, the sum is the same, no matter the order in which the terms are added.

**2. A**

Plug in $a = 2$, $b = 6$, and $c = 4$

$$a(b - 2) + 3c =$$
$$2(6 - 2) + 3(4) =$$
$$2(4) + 3\,(4) =$$
$$8 + 12 = 20$$

**3. B**

This problem has several steps. First, find out what the sale price of the camera was. It was discounted 20% from $120.

$$x = 0.20 \times \$120 = \$24$$

Next, subtract the discount from the total amount to find out the sale price.

$$\$120 - \$24 = \$96$$

(You could also arrive at the sale price by using the formula part = percent × whole.) Since the camera was discounted 20%, Andrew really paid 80% of the whole.

$$x = 0.80 \times \$120 = \$96$$

Now, multiply the sale price by the tax of 0.08 to find out how much tax Andrew paid.

$$\$96 \times 0.08 = \$7.68$$

Finally, add the tax to the sale price to find the total Andrew paid for his purchase.

$$\$96 + \$7.68 = \$103.68$$

**4. C**

Let $z = 13$ because when $x$ is divided by 8 the remainder is 5, and plug in $4z = 4(13) = 52$, which leaves a remainder of 4 when divided by 8.

**5. B**

The least common multiple of two integers is the product of their prime factors, each raised to the highest power with which it appears. The prime factorization of 12 is $2 \times 2 \times 3$, while the prime of factorization of 8 is $2 \times 2 \times 2$. So their LCM is $2 \times 2 \times 2 \times 3 = 24$. You could also find their LCM by checking out the multiples of the larger integer (12) until you find one that is also a multiple of the smaller.

### 6.  D

We are told that $y = 11$, so first we'll replace the $y$ in the equation with 11, and then we can solve for $x$.

$$6x - 7 = y$$

$$6x - 7 = 11$$

Now, we can add 7 to both sides:

$$6x - 7 + 7 = 11 + 7$$

$$6x = 18$$

Next, we divide both sides by 6:

$$\frac{6x}{6} = \frac{18}{3}$$

$$x = 3$$

### 7.  D

Translate the words into math and solve for the unknown. Let $x =$ the unknown amount of money Robert has.

"Edward has 400 more than Robert": $x + 400$

After he spends $60 on groceries": $x + 400 - 60$

"He has 3 times more than Robert": $x + 400 - 60 = 3x$

Now that you've set up an equation, solve for $x$.

$$x + 400 - 60 = 3x$$

$$x + 340 = 3x$$

$$340 = 2x$$

$$170 = x$$

### 8.  B

The shaded region represents half the area of the circle. Find the length of the radius to determine this area. Notice that the diameter of the circle is equal to a side of the square. Since the area of the square is 64 in², it has a side length of 8 in. So, the diameter of the circle is 8, and its radius is 4. The area of a circle is $\pi r^2$, where $r$ is the radius, so the area of this circle is $\pi(4)^2 = 16\pi$ in². This isn't the answer though; the shaded region is only half the circle, so its area is $8\pi$ in².

### 9.  C

This question asks you to determine the sale price of a camera that normally sells at $160 and is discounted 20%. To solve, determine what 20% of $160 equals. Rewrite 20% as a decimal. 20% = 0.20. So 20% of $160 = 0.20 × $160 = $32. The sale price of the camera would be $160 − $32 = $128, choice (C).

### 10.  C

This is a simple addition problem. If the middle integer is 9, place them in order. You would have:

$7 + 8 + 9 + 10 + 11 = 45$.

### 11.  D

$$\text{Average} = \frac{\text{total sum}}{\text{number of items}}$$

Let $x$ equal the unknown average.

$$x = \frac{48}{10} = \$4.80$$

Notice that the information about how much is charged per item is extraneous. You don't need it to solve the problem.

### 12.  C

Let $x =$ the unknown number of coats in stock before the sale. Use the formula part = percent × whole.

33 winter coats $= 0.30x$

$$\frac{33}{0.30} = 110$$

### 13.  B

Remember, $5yz$ means $5 \times y \times z$. First, we will replace $x$, $y$, and $z$ with the values given. Then, we will carry out the indicated operations using the PEMDAS order of operations—Parentheses, Exponents, Multiplication and Division, Addition and Subtraction.

$$x^2 - 5yz + y^2 = (\sqrt{3})^2 - 5 \times 2 \times \frac{1}{2} + 2^2$$

$$= 3 - 5 \times 2 \times \frac{1}{2} + 4$$

$$= 3 - 5 + 4$$

$$= -2 + 4$$

$$= 2$$

**KAPLAN**

## 14. D

If a number is a multiple of both 2 and 6, it must satisfy the divisibility rules of both: Its last digit must be even, its digits must add up to a multiple of 3. Only choice (D) fits both requirements: $4 + 2 + 6 = 12$. You could have quickly eliminated choice (A) and (B), which are not even numbers.

## 15. B

"25% of 25%" means $(0.25)(0.25)$, so $(0.25)(0.25)(72) = 4.5$

## 16. A

The key here is that while the value of the stock increases and decreases by the same amount, it doesn't increase and decrease by the same percent since the "whole" is different once the stock has lost value. If it seems confusing, this is a good question to pick numbers for. Let's pick $100 for the price of the stock. If the price decreases by 20%, the price is now $80. For the price to return to its original value of $100, it must be increased by $20. What percent of 80 equals $20?

$x\%(80) = 20$

$x\% = \dfrac{20}{80}$

$x\% = \dfrac{1}{4}$ is equal to 25%.

## 17. B

Translate this question using the verbal clues provided. Let the amount of money Mrs. Bailer has $= x$. Mrs. Bailer divides the amount of money she has between her 4 children: $\dfrac{x}{4}$ Mr. Bailer then adds $2 to the amount each one receives: $\dfrac{x}{4} + 2$ so that each child now has a total of 5.25:

$\dfrac{x}{4} + 2 = 5.25$

## 18. B

This is a rounding off question. You can round off 52.3 to 50 and 10.4 to 10; $50 \times 10 = 500$.

## 19. B

Since there are 60 minutes in an hour, the subway will pass $\dfrac{60}{10}$ or 6 times as many stations in 1 hour as it passes in 10 minutes. In 10 minutes it passes 3 stations, so in 60 minutes it must pass $6 \times 3$ or 18 stations.

## 20. B

Think of the figure as a rectangle with two rectangular bites taken out of it. Sketch in lines to make one large rectangle as shown below.

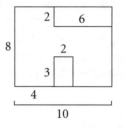

The area of a rectangle is length times width. If we call the length of the large rectangle 10, then its width is 8, so its area is $10 \times 8 = 80$ square units. The rectangle missing from the top right corner has dimensions of 6 and 2, so its area is $6 \times 2 = 12$ square units. The rectangle missing from the bottom has dimensions of 2 and 3, so its area is $2 \times 3 = 6$ square units. To find the area of the polygon, subtract the areas of the two missing shapes from the area of the large rectangle: $80 - (12 + 6) = 80 - 18 = 62$ square units, choice (B).

## 21. D

This problem is not difficult if you remember that $a\%$ of $b = b\%$ of $a$. In this case, $x\%$ of $b$ (the number 40) $= b$ (the number 40)% of $x = 8$.

## 22. D

The total cost of the taxi ride equals $36 + (25\%$ of $36)$, or $36 + \left(\dfrac{1}{4} \times \$36\right) = \$36 + \$9 = \$45$. If four people split the cost equally, then each person paid $\dfrac{\$45}{4}$ or $11.25 each.

## 23. C

You can save valuable time by estimating on this one. Pay special attention to how much you have left and how much you've already spent. If a man spent $\dfrac{5}{12}$ of his salary and was left with $420, that means that he had $\dfrac{7}{12}$ left, and if the man's salary is $x$ dollars, then $\dfrac{7}{12}x = 420$. That means that $420 is a little more than half of his salary. So his salary would be a little less than $2(\$420) = \$840$. Choice (C), $720 is a little less than $840. So (C) works perfectly, and it's the correct answer here.

**24. D**

A question like this one tests your ability to play with decimals. 48 divided by 0.08 is the same as $\frac{4,800}{8} = 600$. (D) is correct. When dividing by a decimal, be sure to move the decimal place the same number of spaces for both numbers.

**25. C**

If Ms. Smith's car averages 35 miles per gallon, she can go 35 miles on 1 gallon. To go 700 miles she will need $\frac{700}{35}$, or 20 gallons of gasoline. The price of gasoline was $1.25 per gallon, so she spent $20 \times \$1.25$, or $25, for her trip.

**26. A**

If $100 \div x = 10n$, that can be rewritten as $\frac{100}{x} = 10n$. Cross-multiply and you get $100 = 10nx$. $nx = \frac{100}{10} = 10$. (A) is correct.

**27. A**

Be careful with your number-crunching here. $9,899,399 + 2,082 = 9,901,481$, choice (A).

**28. A**

The most important thing to keep in mind is that you're solving for 75% of $x$ and not for $x$. First, we are told that 50% of $x$ is 150. That means that half of $x$ is 150, and that $x$ is 300. So 75% of $x = 0.75 \times 300 = 225$. (A) is correct.

**29. A**

If Melissa has $5n$ photographs, and she gives $n$ photographs to each of three friends, she would have given away $3n$ photographs. $5n - 3n = 2n$. (A) is correct.

**30. C**

Use the answer choices to help find the solution. When backsolving you want to start with one of the middle numbers. Start with (C), 24, for Barry's age. If Barry is 24, then his brother Cole is 20, and his sister is 16. Thus, the sum of their ages is $24 + 20 + 16 = 60$, which is the sum we want. Choice (C) is correct.

**31. D**

This is a question where backsolving (working with your answer choices) can save you a lot of time. Let's start with choice (B) and see if it works. If (B) is correct, an adult's ticket would cost $3.00, and a child's ticket would cost $1.50. The total fare we are looking for was for two adults and three children. If an adult's fare were $3.00, that total fare would be $2(\$3.00) + 3(\$1.50) = \$6.00 + \$4.50 = \$10.50$. That's too low since the question states that the total fare is $14.00. Now see what happens if an adult fare were more expensive. If (D) were correct, an adult's ticket would cost $4.00 and a child's ticket would cost $2.00. The total fare would equal $2(\$4.00) + 3(\$2.00) = \$8.00 + \$6.00 = \$14.00$. That's the total fare we're looking for, so (D) is correct.

**32. C**

Some answer choices you should be able to eliminate straight off the bat. $\frac{4}{7}$ is greater than $\frac{1}{2}$, so that's incorrect, as is, for that matter, $\frac{1}{2}$. So you're left with $\frac{1}{3}$, which is about 0.333, and $\frac{3}{8}$, which is 0.375. Choice (C) is closest.

**33. A**

Plug in the values for $a$ and $b$ and remember your order of operations when working through your calculations. When $a = -2$ and $b = 3$, $(-ab)(a) = [-(-2) \times 3](-2) = (2 \times 3)(-2) = (6) \times (-2) = -12$, choice (A).

**34. C**

The original rectangle was 4 inches by 6 inches. It was lengthened to 10 inches with the width remaining at 4 inches. The perimeter of a rectangle can be found by adding twice the length to twice the width (or by adding up each of the four sides). So the perimeter would be $4 + 10 + 4 + 10 = 28$, choice (C).

**35. B**

When giving coordinates, give the $x$-coordinate first, and then the $y$-coordinate second. Point $A$ lies at 2 on the $x$-axis and $-1$ on the $y$-axis. Therefore, $(2, -1)$ is correct.

**36. D**

The textbook approach is to come up with the ratio total by adding together the ratio parts: $1 + 2 + 3 = 6$, so the ratio for the biggest winner is $3 : 6 = \frac{1}{2}$ the entire prize of $12,000, so he or she would earn $\left(\frac{1}{2}\right)$$12,000 = $6,000.

**37. A**

To find the average price for a meal, use the formula:

$$\text{Average} = \frac{\text{sum of terms}}{\text{number of terms}}$$

$$= \frac{$3.00 + $2.75 + $2.50 + $2.25 + $1.50}{5}$$

$$= \frac{$12.00}{5} = $2.40.$$

**38. D**

The three lowest-priced meals—pizza at $1.50, pasta salad at $2.25, and tuna salad at $2.50—add up to $6.25. So it is not possible that a combination of three different meals could cost less than $6.25. Since choice (D), $6.00, is less than this, it could not be the total cost of three different meals.

**39. A**

Let the number of ties Team A had equal $x$. It lost 4 times as many games as it tied, or $4x$ games. It had no wins, so the total number of games played by Team A is $x + 4x = 5x$. The number of games played must be a multiple of 5; the only choice that is a multiple of 5 is (A), 15.

**40. B**

One trick for dealing with consecutive numbers is to realize that the middle number in a group of consecutive numbers is equal to the average of the numbers. So of the five consecutive odd numbers, the middle or third number is 11, the fourth number is 13, and the fifth or final number is 15.

**41. C**

This question can be a bit tricky, but not if you know that percent increase $= \frac{\text{change}}{\text{original number}} \times 100\%$, so in this case, the percent increase equals $\frac{10}{5} \times 100\%$, or 200%.

**42. D**

$10^4 = 10,000$. So $0.123 \times 10^4 = 0.123 \times 10,000 = 1,230$, choice (D).

**43. D**

Eliminate the parentheses by distributing the minus operation over the second set of parentheses: $(3d - 7) - (5 - 2d) = 3d - 7 - 5 - (-2d) = 3d - 7 - 5 + 2d$. Now combine like terms and perform the additions and subtractions: $3d + 2d - 7 - 5 = 5d - 12$.

**44. B**

If the perimeter of the square is 36, then each of the four sides equals 9. The side of the square is the same length as the diameter of the circle, so if the diameter of the circle is 9, the circumference is $9\pi$.

**45. B**

First find 6% of $2,250. You could multiply $2,250 by 0.06, or you could look at it like this. 10% of $2,250 is $225, and 1% of $2,250 is $22.50. So 6% of $2,250 is $22.50 $\times$ 6 = $135. So Douglas's new monthly salary is $2,250 + $135 = $2,385, choice (B).

**46. D**

You could either apply the rules of odds and evens, or you could pick even and odd numbers for $x$ to see which answer choice always works. For instance if $x$ is an odd integer, such as 1, then (A) and (B) add up to odd numbers, so they are incorrect. Now if you pick an even number for $x$ such as 2, then (C) is incorrect because $5x + 3 = 5(2) + 3 = 13$, which is also odd. But choice (D) works in both cases. This only makes sense according to the rules of odds and evens, because $6x$ will always be even, since 6 is even and an even number times any number is even. So $6x + 4$ must be even because an even number plus an even number is always even.

**47. D**

Apply FOIL:

$(3a + 4)(3a - 4) =$
$(3a)(3a) + (3a)(-4) + (3a)(4) + (4)(-4) =$
$9a^2 - 12a + 12a - 16 =$
$9a^2 - 16$

**48. D**

Average $= \dfrac{\text{sum of the terms}}{\text{number of terms}}$, so if the average weight of the three men is 60 kg, the sum of their weights is $60 \times 3 = 180$ kg. Then if Jake and Ken both weigh 50 kg, Larry must weigh $180 - (50 \times 2) = 80$ kilograms.

**49. C**

The question asks for "how much," but looking at the answer choices you'll note that you are not being asked for an exact amount. This is an estimation question. You need to compare the relative values of the two amounts. If the amount were simply 1 cup and 3 cups, it would clearly be 2 cups. But now you have to determine the relationship between $\dfrac{2}{3}$ and $\dfrac{3}{4}$. $\dfrac{3}{4}$ is just a little more than $\dfrac{2}{3}$. Thus, when you go from $1\dfrac{2}{3}$ cups to $3\dfrac{3}{4}$ cups, you are adding slightly more than 2 cups.

**50. C**

The average of 7 consecutive even numbers is 24. That means that 24 must be in the middle of the set of numbers. So the set must be {18, 20, 22, 24, 26, 28, 30}. The largest number is 30, choice (C).

**51. B**

Translate the English into math bit by bit. "Five less than 3 times a certain number" becomes "$3x - 5$"; "is equal to the original number plus 7" becomes "$= x + 7$." So altogether you have $3x - 5 = x + 7$.

Now solve for $x$:

$$3x - 5 = x + 7$$
$$3x - x = 7 + 5$$
$$2x = 12$$
$$x = 6$$

**52. D**

Follow PEMDAS:

$$[(12 - 11) - (10 - 9)] - [(12 - 11 - 10) - 9]$$
$$= [1 - 1] - [-9 - 9]$$
$$= 0 - (-18)$$
$$= 18$$

**53. A**

$$\frac{a^2bc + ab^2c + abc^2}{abc} =$$
$$\frac{a \times abc}{abc} + \frac{b \times abc}{abc} + \frac{c \times abc}{abc} =$$
$$a + b + c$$

**54. D**

The cube of a number is that number multiplied by itself three times. So the cube of 9 would be $9 \times 9 \times 9 = 729$, choice (D).

**55. D**

The best way to solve this one is to set up a proportion, solve it, and then convert the units: $\dfrac{2}{8} = \dfrac{6}{n}$, so $2n = 6 \times 8$, and $n = \dfrac{48}{2} = 24$ inches, which is equal to 2 feet, choice (D).

**56. D**

If $s - t = 5$, and you multiply both sides by 3, you get $3s - 3t = 15$. Thus $3s - 3t + 3 = 15 + 3 = 18$.

**57. C**

The area of the frame is the area of the larger rectangle minus the area of the smaller rectangle, or $(8 \times 10) - (4 \times 8) = 80 - 32 = 48$.

**58. B**

On remainder questions like this one, pick simple numbers and solve. When $D$ is divided by 15, the result is 6 with a remainder of 2. That means that $D = 6(15) + 2$ or 92. When 92 is divided by 6, the remainder is 2. (B) is correct.

**59. C**

This is a geometry word problem. If you draw the path with the directions provided, you'll see a right triangle. The question is asking you how many miles the rider is from her starting point, or the hypotenuse of the triangle. Use the formula $\text{leg}^2 + \text{leg}^2 = \text{hypotenuse}^2$. The legs are 8 and 6, so $8^2 + 6^2 = 64 + 36 = 100 = (\text{hypotenuse})^2$. $\sqrt{100} = 10$. The rider is 10 miles from her starting point.

**60. A**

To find the midpoint of a segment on the number line you can add the endpoints and the divide the sum by 2. So the midpoint of $PQ$ is $\dfrac{(-12) + (-2)}{2} = \dfrac{-14}{2} = -7$. The midpoint of $RS$ is $\dfrac{1 + 9}{2} = \dfrac{10}{2} = 5$. Thus the distance between the two points is the positive difference between their coordinates, or $5 - (-7) = 12$.

**61. A**

This question is really asking you how many times $2\frac{2}{3}$ goes into 20, or what is $20 \div 2\frac{2}{3}$. To divide, first you'll want to turn the mixed fraction into a regular fraction. $2\frac{2}{3} = \frac{8}{3}$. Dividing by a fraction is the same a multiplying by its inverse, so $20 \div 2\frac{2}{3} = 20 \times \frac{3}{8} = \frac{60}{8} = \frac{15}{2} = 7\frac{1}{2}$. Since you can't make half a shirt, the tailor can make a total of 7 shirts with this amount of fabric.

**62. C**

This is a classic product of two binomials. Remember to FOIL.

$(x - 4)(x - 4)$
$= (x)(x) + (x)(-4) + (-4)(x) + (-4)(-4)$
$= x^2 - 4x - 4x + 16$
$= x^2 - 8x + 16$.

Choice (C) is correct.

**63. B**

Since $RS$ and $RT$ are equal, the angles opposite them must be equal. Therefore, angle $T$ = angle $S$. Since the degree measures of the three interior angles of a triangle sum to 180, $70 +$ angle measure $S +$ angle measure $T = 180$, and angle measure $S +$ angle measure $T = 110$. Since the two angles, $S$ and $T$, are equal, each must have angle measures half of 110, or 55.

**64. C**

Scientific notation is correctly represented as a number between 1 and 10 multiplied by a power of 10. To figure out what that power of 10 is, you have to carefully count out the number of decimal places you must move the decimal point of your original number until you reach a number between 1 and 10. To go from 89,213 to 8.9213 you must move the decimal point four places to the left, so that means you must multiply the number by 10 to the exponent 4. In other words, $89,213 = 8.9213 \times 10^4$.

**65. A**

Know your perfect squares. $\sqrt{100} = 10$ and $\sqrt{64} = 8$. So $\sqrt{100} - \sqrt{64} = 10 - 8$, choice (A).

**66. A**

When the painter and his son work together, they charge the sum of their hourly rates, $12 + $6, or $18 per hour. Their bill equals the product of this combined rate and the number of hours they worked. Therefore $108 must equal $18 per hour times the number of hours they worked. We need to divide $108 by $18 per hour to find the number of hours. $108 \div $18 = 6$.

**67. A**

If you're looking for $a$ in terms of $b$, try to isolate the $a$ on one side of the equation.

$$3ab = 6$$
$$ab = 2$$
$$a = \frac{2}{b}$$

(A) is correct.

**68. D**

We are asked which of five ratios is equivalent to the ratio of $3\frac{1}{4}$ to $5\frac{1}{4}$. Since the ratios in the answer choices are expressed in whole numbers, turn this ratio into whole numbers: $3\frac{1}{4} \div 5\frac{1}{4} = \frac{13}{4} \div \frac{21}{4} = \frac{13}{4} \times \frac{4}{21}$ or $13 \div 21$.

**69. C**

$$\frac{6x^6}{2x^2} = \frac{6}{2}\left(\frac{x^6}{x^2}\right) = 3x^4, \text{ choice (C)}.$$

**70. D**

The perimeter of a square is $4s$ where $s$ is the length of a side. If a square has a perimeter of 32, then it has a side length of 8. The area of the square is $s^2 = 8^2 = 64$, choice (D).

**71. B**

Since the triangles are similar, set up a proportion to solve for the unknown side.

$$\frac{10}{6} = \frac{6}{x}$$
$$10x = 36$$
$$x = \frac{36}{10} = 3.6$$

**72. B**

We need to compute the cost of parking a car for 5 hours at each garage. Since the two garages have a split-rate system of charging, the cost for the first hour is different from the cost of each remaining hour.

The first hour at garage $A$ costs $8.75

The next 4 hours cost $4 \times \$1.25 = \$5.00$

The total cost for parking at garage $A = \$8.75 + 5.00 = \$13.75$

The first hour at garage $B$ costs $5.50

The next 4 hours cost $4 \times \$2.50 = \$10.00$

The total cost for parking at garage $B = \$5.50 + \$10.00 = \$15.50$

So the difference in cost $= \$15.50 - \$13.75 = \$1.75$, (B).

**73. B**

Given a diameter of 6, the radius must equal $\frac{1}{2}$ of 6, or 3. Next, the circumference $= \pi r = 2\pi(3) = 6\pi$. The area $= \pi r^2 = \pi(3^2) = 9\pi$. Summing these two we get: $9\pi + 6\pi = 15\pi$.

**74. D**

If you change each digit 5 into a 7 in the number 258,546, the new number would be 278,746. The difference between these two numbers would be $278,746 - 258,546 = 20,200$. Choice (D) is correct.

**75. A**

You're asked what percent of the new solution is alcohol. The *part* is the number of ounces of alcohol; the *whole* is the total number of ounces of the new solution. There were 25 ounces originally. Then 50 ounces were added, so there are 75 ounces of new solution. How many ounces are alcohol?

20% of the original 25-ounce solution was alcohol. 20% is $\frac{1}{5}$, so $\frac{1}{5}$ of 25, or 5 ounces are alcohol. Now you can find the percent of alcohol in the new solution:

$$\% \text{ alcohol} = \frac{\text{alcohol}}{\text{total solution}} \times 100\%$$
$$= \frac{5}{75} \times 100\%$$
$$= \frac{20}{3}\% = 6\frac{2}{3}\%$$

## Science

**1. B**

When an allele is harmful, as this one would be, it will be selected against. In this case, the allele is recessive and is only expressed in the homozygous recessive people, with heterozygotes as carriers. The homozygous recessive people will be selected against, and the allele frequency in the population will decrease slowly over time as long as the selection pressure is maintained. Once the selection pressure is removed by the absence of the virus, the allele frequencies will remain constant, unless some other selection pressure affects the allele. Choice (B) is correct.

**KAPLAN**

2.  C

In the cross of Mouse I with the female, the ratio of the offspring phenotypes is 3:1, indicating a *Bb* × *Bb* cross with *BB* and *Bb* animals black and *bb* animals white. Therefore, mouse I is *Bb*, while the female is *Bb*. In the second cross of mouse II and the female mouse, 100% of the offspring are black. Hence, mouse II must be homozygously dominant.

3.  D

All forms of life, from bacteria to man, have certain things in common. They all have some form of nucleic acid as genetic material as well as proteins, and they are composed largely of water.

4.  D

Osmosis is defined as the diffusion of water through membranes from an area of lesser solute concentration to an area of greater solute concentration.

5.  B

Remember the order of classification: kingdom, phylum, class, order, family, genus, and species. Members of a class are more alike than members of a kingdom or a phylum, but less alike than members of orders, families, genera, and species.

6.  C

The trait is recessive since *Aa* individuals are normal. In an *Aa* × *aa* cross, 50% of the offspring will be *Aa* and the other 50% will be *aa*, and the phenotypes will have the same ratio.

7.  B

A normal sperm will have a haploid (23) number of chromosomes. It could have either an *X* or *Y* chromosome.

8.  B

Stomata are pores in leaves that allow gases in and out of the leaf. The stomata close at night, when there is no light energy to catalyze the light reaction, in order to prevent loss of water through transpiration in the stomata.

9.  D

Meiosis has two divisions that create four haploid cells from one diploid cell, while mitosis results in two diploid cells from one diploid cell. Both mitosis and meiosis replicate DNA during interphase.

10. B

All organisms produce proteins through the triplet code. However, some of them do not need carbon dioxide or oxygen (and, in fact, some, such as tetanus, are poisoned by oxygen). All organisms use ATP as cellular energy.

11. B

Asexual reproduction is more efficient than sexual reproduction in terms of the number of offspring produced per reproduction, the amount of energy invested in this process, and the amount of time involved in the development of the young, both before and after birth. Overall, sexual reproduction is a much more time-consuming, energy-consuming process than its asexual counterpart. Asexual reproduction, however, must rely heavily on mutation to introduce phenotypic variability in future generations, since it almost exclusively produces genetic clones of the parent organism. Sexual reproduction involves the process of meiosis. Recombination and independent assortment during meiosis allows new mixing of alleles that does not occur in asexual reproduction, as well as contributions of alleles from each parent during fertilization. Two genetically unique nuclei, the sperm nucleus and the egg nucleus, fuse to form an equally genetically unique zygote. Phenotypic variability is in this way introduced into individuals in a population, and can allow the population to adapt to a wider variety of conditions.

12. D

DNA is the genetic material for all prokaryotes and eukaryotes.

13. B

The eggs are released from the ovaries and picked up by the fallopian tubes. The fertilized egg will then continue down the fallopian tube until it reaches the uterus, where it will implant. If it implants in the fallopian tube, an ectopic pregnancy results.

## 14. D

Cardiac cells have intercalated disk connections joining the cytoplasm between adjoining cardiac muscle cells. Although they have some striations, they are not voluntary. Smooth muscle, on the other hand, has no striations, is mononuclear, and is involuntary. White blood cells have nuclei. In adult humans, red blood cells lack nuclei, in order to make room for as much hemoglobin as possible.

## 15. D

This question illustrates two types of test cross. A test cross is performed to determine if a particular dominant individual's phenotype is a homozygous or heterozygous genotype. In this case, there are two possible tall genotypes for the tall plant—*TT*, the pure homozygous tall, and *Tt*, the hybrid heterozygous tall. These two individuals would have the same phenotype. To determine the genotype, the unknown tall plant would be mated with a recessive, short plant. If the tall plant and the short plant produce only tall offspring, then it can be assumed that the original tall plant is homozygous *TT*. If the mating of the unknown tall organism and the short organism produces any short offspring at all, then we know that the original unknown tall was heterozygous. This is because short offspring can be produced only when one short gamete is produced from each parent. In I, crossing an unknown with a *Tt* will also give you the information you seek, because if any short progeny are produced at all, your unknown must be heterozygous. If all of the offspring are tall, your unknown must be homozygous dominant.

## 16. D

The medulla monitors blood carbon dioxide levels and pH and adjusts breathing, temperature, and heart rate. It is also the center for reflex activities such as coughing, sneezing, and swallowing, and is not associated with emotional drives. The other answer choices are true.

## 17. D

Fermentation is a process that occurs during anaerobic respiration in organisms such as yeast. Glucose is converted to pyruvic acid, producing ATP. Then pyruvic acid is changed into ethyl alcohol, a waste product of the fermentation process. Fermentation produces energy but does not require oxygen. The oxygen-requiring reactions of respiration occur in aerobic respiration, not in fermentation, and they occur as NADH and FADH2 molecules produced in the Krebs cycle are sent to the electron transport chain for the production of ATP. The final electron acceptor in these reactions is oxygen. In fermentation, there is no aerobic stage, and ATP is never produced through a Krebs cycle and electron transport chain mechanism.

## 18. B

The correct order of classificatory divisions is: kingdom, phylum, subphylum, class, order, family, genus, and species.

## 19. A

The law of segregation states that when gametes are formed, the two alleles for a particular trait will separate or segregate into the gametes, so that each of the gametes only contains one of the alleles for a given trait. So if tall is dominant over short, and both tall and short offspring were produced, then the tall plant is a hybrid or heterozygous plant. This means that the genotype of the tall plant contains both one tall allele and one short allele. The short plant contains two short alleles. When the gametes are formed for this mating, the two alleles in the tall plant, the tall and short, will segregate into the gametes, forming tall-containing gametes and short-containing gametes. When these meet and fertilize the short-containing gametes from the other plant, half the offspring produced will be tall because they are the result of the tall gamete's fertilization of a short gamete, and the other half will be the result of the short gamete's fertilization of the other short gamete.

## 20. D

In a commensal relationship, which is a form of a symbiotic relationship, two organisms live in close association with each other. One benefits from this association, while the other is neither harmed nor benefited (in what is sometimes described as a "+/0" relationship).

## 21. D

Polysomes are defined as a group of ribosomes that attach to a strand of mRNA and simultaneously translate it.

## 22. B

Identical twins are produced when a zygote formed by one egg and one sperm splits during the four- or eight-cell stage to develop into two genetically identical organisms.

**23. C**

The notochord appears as a semi-rigid rod in the dorsal part of all chordates sometime during embryonic development. In lower chordates, this remains as a semi-rigid chord, although in higher chordates it is seen only in the embryo and not as a vestigial organ.

**24. C**

Alveoli are thin air sacs that act as the sites of air exchange between the environment and the blood via passive diffusion.

**25. B**

The Golgi apparatus consists of a stack of membrane-enclosed sacs. The Golgi receives vesicles and their contents from the smooth ER, modifies them (as in glycosylation), repackages them into vesicles, and distributes them. In (A), mitochondria are involved in cellular respiration, and in (C), the ER transports polypeptides around the cell and to the Golgi apparatus for packaging. The ribosome (D) is the site of protein synthesis.

**26. C**

Enzymes are catalysts of biological reactions, increasing the rate of reactions without themselves changing and without changing the final equilibrium. Enzymes are typically proteins (I), although they may rarely be RNA, and they typically act most effectively at a physiological pH of 7–7.4 (except for the enzymes which break down protein in the stomach, which act most effectively in an acidic environment) (II). Enzymes are never changed during a reaction (III). They increase the rate of a reaction, but are not themselves affected by that reaction. Enzymes are found throughout the cell, not just in the nucleus (IV).

**27. C**

The plasma membrane separates the cellular contents from the environment. It is responsible for the permeability of the membrane—in other words, for what is allowed in and out of the cell. The fluid mosaic model of the plasma membrane states that this membrane is a bilayer of phospholipids interspersed with proteins acting as receptors, pores, and channels. The pores and channels cross the entire membrane. The cytochrome chain referred to in the correct answer is actually located in the cristae (the inner membrane) of the mitochondria.

**28. D**

If a homozygous dominant, *TTLL*, is crossed with any genotype, the offspring will be heterozygous and have the dominant phenotype. All the other options have potential for some homozygous recessives.

**29. D**

This question illustrates two test crosses that will determine whether the red plant is homozygous or heterozygous. A test cross is performed to determine if a particular dominant individual's phenotype is caused by a homozygous or heterozygous genotype. In this case, there are two possible red genotypes: RR, the pure homozygous red, and Rr, the hybrid heterozygous red. These two individuals would have the same phenotype. In order to determine the genotype, the unknown red plant would be mated with a recessive, white plant (C) or a known heterozygous red plant (A). If the red plant and the white plant produce only red offspring, then it can be assumed that the original red plant is homozygous. Similarly, if we mate the unknown red plant with a known heterozygous one, and produce only red offspring, then the original plant is homozygous. If the two matings of the unknown red organism produce any white offspring at all, then we know that the original unknown red was heterozygous. This is because white offspring can be produced only through the production of one white gamete by each parent.

**30. B**

A cell that is *n* (haploid) cannot undergo meiosis to become $\frac{1}{2}n$. (A), (C), and (D) are incorrect because there are a number of organisms that are haploid. These organisms undergo mitosis, divide, and grow.

**31. D**

In a *BB* × *bb* cross, 100% of the offspring will be *Bb*. Genotypically, they will be heterozygous, and phenotypically, they will have brown eyes, since brown is dominant.

**32. D**

Chlorophyll is an essential component of an organelle, the chloroplast, but it is a chemical, not an organelle.

### 33. A

In the light reaction, light splits $H_2O$ into excited electrons, $H^+$ and $O_2$. The excited electrons go on to form ATP and the $H^+$ electrons are incorporated into the carbohydrates produced during the dark reaction. $O_2$ is released into the environment as a waste product of this reaction. In (B), $CO_2$ donates the carbon and the oxygen required for carbohydrate formation in the dark reaction. (C) and (D) are end products of photosynthesis.

### 34. B

Lysosomes are membrane-bound organelles containing digestive enzymes. Typically, they have a low pH. Mitochondria (A), on the other hand, are involved in cellular respiration, while (C) the ER synthesizes secreted or membrane-bound proteins and sends them to the Golgi apparatus for packaging. Finally, (D) the ribosome is the site of protein synthesis.

### 35. A

DNA is the only molecule in eukaryotes that contains genes. Proteins may function as hormones (chemical messengers), enzymes (catalysts of chemical reactions), structural proteins (providers of physical support), transport proteins (carriers of important materials), and antibodies (binders of foreign particles).

### 36. D

The electron transport chain directly produces the pH gradient by pumping protons out of the mitochondrial matrix. This proton gradient is used to make ATP.

### 37. D

The average kinetic energy of a gas is proportional to its temperature in K, not °C.

### 38. A

The major portion of an atom's mass consists of neutrons and protons. Electrons, positrons, neutrinos, and other subatomic particles have practically negligible masses.

### 39. A

The nucleus of the element gives off particles. In some instances this release of matter and energy changes the mass of the element by reducing the number of protons and neutrons in the nucleus, thus forming a new element with a lower atomic mass. In other instances it results in the transformation of a neutron into a proton, thereby increasing the atomic number by one while maintaining the same atomic mass.

### 40. C

When you submerge your body into a hot bath the heat from the water will transfer to your body which increases your external skin temperature. After a period of time the bath water becomes cold. This is because your body absorbed the heat and because some of the heat escaped in the form of steam.

### 41. A

All forms of energy may exist either in actualized form, such as the kinetic energy of a falling rock, or in potential form, such as the potential energy of a rock positioned atop a mountain or a certain organic molecules with high-energy bonds, which will release energy when they are broken.

### 42. C

If there is an unequal number of protons and neutrons, the element is considered to be an isotope. An atom is the basic unit of all simple substances (elements). It consists of a positively charged nucleus surrounded by rapidly moving, negatively charged electrons.

### 43. D

The four hydrogen atoms on the reactant side of the equation are transformed into water (product), but there are still only four hydrogen atoms. Now, however, they are bonded to oxygen.

### 44. D

Water at sea level boils at 212° F, 100° C, or 373° K.

### 45. A

Of the subatomic particles listed, the proton has the largest mass. Among subatomic particles, protons and neutrons have the most mass. Electrons, positrons, and neutrinos all have negligible masses.

### 46. A

Diffusion is the transport of substances without using an outside source of energy. Osmosis, (B), includes only the transport of water, and can therefore be eliminated.

Choices (C) and (D), passive and facilitated transport, refer to the transport of substances either down a concentration gradient or using a molecule, respectively.

**47. A**

The Atomic Theory would be utilized to analyze the properties of hydrogen because it deals with the atomic level of matter. Choice (B) would be something that bacteriologists or microbiologists might study and would not be encompassed under the Atomic Theory. Choice (C) is an example of an epidemiological study and choice (D) is a concept studied in physics and theories in that area such as Newton's Laws might be used to analyze it.

**48. B**

As one goes from left to right across a period, electrons are added one at a time; the electrons of the outermost shell experience an increasing amount of nuclear attraction, becoming closer and more tightly bound to the nucleus.

**49. A**

The ionization energy (IE), or ionization potential, is the energy required to completely remove an electron from an atom or ion. Removing an electron from an atom always requires an input of energy, since it is attracted to the positively charged nucleus. The closer and more tightly bound an electron is to the nucleus, the more difficult it will be to remove, and the higher the ionization energy will be.

**50. C**

A compound is a pure substance that is composed of two or more elements in a fixed proportion. Compounds can be broken down chemically to produce their constituent elements or other compounds.

**51. A**

The temperature of a liquid is related to the average kinetic energy of the liquid molecules; however, the kinetic energy of the individual molecules will vary (just as there is a distribution of molecular speeds in a gas). A few molecules near the surface of the liquid may have enough energy to leave the liquid phase and escape into the gaseous phase. This process is known as evaporation (or vaporization).

**52. B**

If five years is one half-life, then 15 years is three half-lives. During the first half-life—the first five years—half of the sample will have decayed. During the second half-life (years six to 10), half of the remaining half will decay, leaving one-fourth of the original. During the third and final period (years 11 to 15), half of the remaining fourth will decay, leaving one-eighth of the original sample. Thus the fraction remaining after three half-lives is $\left(\frac{1}{2}\right)^3$ or $\left(\frac{1}{8}\right)$.

**53. D**

By definition, 1 amu is exactly one-twelfth the mass of the neutral carbon-12 atom. In terms of more familiar mass units:

$$1\ amu = 1.66 \times 10^{-27}\ kg = 1.66 \times 10^{-24}\ g$$

**54. B**

According to Newton's Third Law, a force acting on a body always elicits an equal, opposite force acting against it. Thus, force always acts *in pairs*.

**55. D**

Speed is very different from velocity, in that velocity (a vector quantity) implies both speed and direction.

**56. C**

When current passes through a resistance, a voltage drop will take place. This represents an energy loss, and this energy is normally dissipated in the form of heat.

**57. D**

The coefficient of static friction is always greater than the coefficient of kinetic friction. If a force is applied, but the box does not move, no work has been done ($W = Fd$). The nature of the surface the box rests on will define the coefficient of friction between the box and that surface.

**58. B**

The relationship between force, mass, and acceleration is described using the formula $F = ma$. If mass increases, more force is required to achieve the same acceleration rate.

**59. D**

A vehicle traveling at a constant speed has no net forces acting on it, so its acceleration rate is zero.

**60. C**

Vector quantities express both magnitude and direction. Examples of vector quantities include velocity and force.

**61. A**

Force is a vector quantity. This means that it expresses both magnitude and direction.

**62. A**

An astronaut's mass will be the same no matter where he or she is, but his or her weight will be less in outer space due to his or her increased distance from earth.

**63. A**

Whenever electrical current passes through a resistance, a voltage drop takes place. Areas of high resistance in an electrical circuit will cause a high voltage drop.

**64. C**

Objects at rest still have many forces acting on them (gravity, to name just one). The forces are all counteracted by equal and opposite forces, so the *net force* acting on these objects is zero.

**65. B**

A closed circuit has continuity, and will allow current to flow in it.

# Nursing School Entrance Exams
# Practice Test Two
# Answer Sheet

## Reading Comprehension

| | | | | |
|---|---|---|---|---|
| 1. Ⓐ Ⓑ Ⓒ Ⓓ | 10. Ⓐ Ⓑ Ⓒ Ⓓ | 19. Ⓐ Ⓑ Ⓒ Ⓓ | 28. Ⓐ Ⓑ Ⓒ Ⓓ | 37. Ⓐ Ⓑ Ⓒ Ⓓ |
| 2. Ⓐ Ⓑ Ⓒ Ⓓ | 11. Ⓐ Ⓑ Ⓒ Ⓓ | 20. Ⓐ Ⓑ Ⓒ Ⓓ | 29. Ⓐ Ⓑ Ⓒ Ⓓ | 38. Ⓐ Ⓑ Ⓒ Ⓓ |
| 3. Ⓐ Ⓑ Ⓒ Ⓓ | 12. Ⓐ Ⓑ Ⓒ Ⓓ | 21. Ⓐ Ⓑ Ⓒ Ⓓ | 30. Ⓐ Ⓑ Ⓒ Ⓓ | 39. Ⓐ Ⓑ Ⓒ Ⓓ |
| 4. Ⓐ Ⓑ Ⓒ Ⓓ | 13. Ⓐ Ⓑ Ⓒ Ⓓ | 22. Ⓐ Ⓑ Ⓒ Ⓓ | 31. Ⓐ Ⓑ Ⓒ Ⓓ | 40. Ⓐ Ⓑ Ⓒ Ⓓ |
| 5. Ⓐ Ⓑ Ⓒ Ⓓ | 14. Ⓐ Ⓑ Ⓒ Ⓓ | 23. Ⓐ Ⓑ Ⓒ Ⓓ | 32. Ⓐ Ⓑ Ⓒ Ⓓ | 41. Ⓐ Ⓑ Ⓒ Ⓓ |
| 6. Ⓐ Ⓑ Ⓒ Ⓓ | 15. Ⓐ Ⓑ Ⓒ Ⓓ | 24. Ⓐ Ⓑ Ⓒ Ⓓ | 33. Ⓐ Ⓑ Ⓒ Ⓓ | 42. Ⓐ Ⓑ Ⓒ Ⓓ |
| 7. Ⓐ Ⓑ Ⓒ Ⓓ | 16. Ⓐ Ⓑ Ⓒ Ⓓ | 25. Ⓐ Ⓑ Ⓒ Ⓓ | 34. Ⓐ Ⓑ Ⓒ Ⓓ | 43. Ⓐ Ⓑ Ⓒ Ⓓ |
| 8. Ⓐ Ⓑ Ⓒ Ⓓ | 17. Ⓐ Ⓑ Ⓒ Ⓓ | 26. Ⓐ Ⓑ Ⓒ Ⓓ | 35. Ⓐ Ⓑ Ⓒ Ⓓ | 44. Ⓐ Ⓑ Ⓒ Ⓓ |
| 9. Ⓐ Ⓑ Ⓒ Ⓓ | 18. Ⓐ Ⓑ Ⓒ Ⓓ | 27. Ⓐ Ⓑ Ⓒ Ⓓ | 36. Ⓐ Ⓑ Ⓒ Ⓓ | 45. Ⓐ Ⓑ Ⓒ Ⓓ |

## Vocabulary and Spelling

| | | | | |
|---|---|---|---|---|
| 1. Ⓐ Ⓑ Ⓒ Ⓓ | 14. Ⓐ Ⓑ Ⓒ Ⓓ | 27. Ⓐ Ⓑ Ⓒ Ⓓ | 40. Ⓐ Ⓑ Ⓒ Ⓓ | 53. Ⓐ Ⓑ Ⓒ Ⓓ |
| 2. Ⓐ Ⓑ Ⓒ Ⓓ | 15. Ⓐ Ⓑ Ⓒ Ⓓ | 28. Ⓐ Ⓑ Ⓒ Ⓓ | 41. Ⓐ Ⓑ Ⓒ Ⓓ | 54. Ⓐ Ⓑ Ⓒ Ⓓ |
| 3. Ⓐ Ⓑ Ⓒ Ⓓ | 16. Ⓐ Ⓑ Ⓒ Ⓓ | 29. Ⓐ Ⓑ Ⓒ Ⓓ | 42. Ⓐ Ⓑ Ⓒ Ⓓ | 55. Ⓐ Ⓑ Ⓒ Ⓓ |
| 4. Ⓐ Ⓑ Ⓒ Ⓓ | 17. Ⓐ Ⓑ Ⓒ Ⓓ | 30. Ⓐ Ⓑ Ⓒ Ⓓ | 43. Ⓐ Ⓑ Ⓒ Ⓓ | 56. Ⓐ Ⓑ Ⓒ Ⓓ |
| 5. Ⓐ Ⓑ Ⓒ Ⓓ | 18. Ⓐ Ⓑ Ⓒ Ⓓ | 31. Ⓐ Ⓑ Ⓒ Ⓓ | 44. Ⓐ Ⓑ Ⓒ Ⓓ | 57. Ⓐ Ⓑ Ⓒ Ⓓ |
| 6. Ⓐ Ⓑ Ⓒ Ⓓ | 19. Ⓐ Ⓑ Ⓒ Ⓓ | 32. Ⓐ Ⓑ Ⓒ Ⓓ | 45. Ⓐ Ⓑ Ⓒ Ⓓ | 58. Ⓐ Ⓑ Ⓒ Ⓓ |
| 7. Ⓐ Ⓑ Ⓒ Ⓓ | 20. Ⓐ Ⓑ Ⓒ Ⓓ | 33. Ⓐ Ⓑ Ⓒ Ⓓ | 46. Ⓐ Ⓑ Ⓒ Ⓓ | 59. Ⓐ Ⓑ Ⓒ Ⓓ |
| 8. Ⓐ Ⓑ Ⓒ Ⓓ | 21. Ⓐ Ⓑ Ⓒ Ⓓ | 34. Ⓐ Ⓑ Ⓒ Ⓓ | 47. Ⓐ Ⓑ Ⓒ Ⓓ | 60. Ⓐ Ⓑ Ⓒ Ⓓ |
| 9. Ⓐ Ⓑ Ⓒ Ⓓ | 22. Ⓐ Ⓑ Ⓒ Ⓓ | 35. Ⓐ Ⓑ Ⓒ Ⓓ | 48. Ⓐ Ⓑ Ⓒ Ⓓ | 61. Ⓐ Ⓑ Ⓒ Ⓓ |
| 10. Ⓐ Ⓑ Ⓒ Ⓓ | 23. Ⓐ Ⓑ Ⓒ Ⓓ | 36. Ⓐ Ⓑ Ⓒ Ⓓ | 49. Ⓐ Ⓑ Ⓒ Ⓓ | 62. Ⓐ Ⓑ Ⓒ Ⓓ |
| 11. Ⓐ Ⓑ Ⓒ Ⓓ | 24. Ⓐ Ⓑ Ⓒ Ⓓ | 37. Ⓐ Ⓑ Ⓒ Ⓓ | 50. Ⓐ Ⓑ Ⓒ Ⓓ | 63. Ⓐ Ⓑ Ⓒ Ⓓ |
| 12. Ⓐ Ⓑ Ⓒ Ⓓ | 25. Ⓐ Ⓑ Ⓒ Ⓓ | 38. Ⓐ Ⓑ Ⓒ Ⓓ | 51. Ⓐ Ⓑ Ⓒ Ⓓ | 64. Ⓐ Ⓑ Ⓒ Ⓓ |
| 13. Ⓐ Ⓑ Ⓒ Ⓓ | 26. Ⓐ Ⓑ Ⓒ Ⓓ | 39. Ⓐ Ⓑ Ⓒ Ⓓ | 52. Ⓐ Ⓑ Ⓒ Ⓓ | 65. Ⓐ Ⓑ Ⓒ Ⓓ |

# Mathematics

1. Ⓐ Ⓑ Ⓒ Ⓓ  16. Ⓐ Ⓑ Ⓒ Ⓓ  31. Ⓐ Ⓑ Ⓒ Ⓓ  46. Ⓐ Ⓑ Ⓒ Ⓓ  61. Ⓐ Ⓑ Ⓒ Ⓓ
2. Ⓐ Ⓑ Ⓒ Ⓓ  17. Ⓐ Ⓑ Ⓒ Ⓓ  32. Ⓐ Ⓑ Ⓒ Ⓓ  47. Ⓐ Ⓑ Ⓒ Ⓓ  62. Ⓐ Ⓑ Ⓒ Ⓓ
3. Ⓐ Ⓑ Ⓒ Ⓓ  18. Ⓐ Ⓑ Ⓒ Ⓓ  33. Ⓐ Ⓑ Ⓒ Ⓓ  48. Ⓐ Ⓑ Ⓒ Ⓓ  63. Ⓐ Ⓑ Ⓒ Ⓓ
4. Ⓐ Ⓑ Ⓒ Ⓓ  19. Ⓐ Ⓑ Ⓒ Ⓓ  34. Ⓐ Ⓑ Ⓒ Ⓓ  49. Ⓐ Ⓑ Ⓒ Ⓓ  64. Ⓐ Ⓑ Ⓒ Ⓓ
5. Ⓐ Ⓑ Ⓒ Ⓓ  20. Ⓐ Ⓑ Ⓒ Ⓓ  35. Ⓐ Ⓑ Ⓒ Ⓓ  50 Ⓐ Ⓑ Ⓒ Ⓓ  65. Ⓐ Ⓑ Ⓒ Ⓓ
6. Ⓐ Ⓑ Ⓒ Ⓓ  21. Ⓐ Ⓑ Ⓒ Ⓓ  36. Ⓐ Ⓑ Ⓒ Ⓓ  51. Ⓐ Ⓑ Ⓒ Ⓓ  66. Ⓐ Ⓑ Ⓒ Ⓓ
7. Ⓐ Ⓑ Ⓒ Ⓓ  22. Ⓐ Ⓑ Ⓒ Ⓓ  37. Ⓐ Ⓑ Ⓒ Ⓓ  52. Ⓐ Ⓑ Ⓒ Ⓓ  67. Ⓐ Ⓑ Ⓒ Ⓓ
8. Ⓐ Ⓑ Ⓒ Ⓓ  23. Ⓐ Ⓑ Ⓒ Ⓓ  38. Ⓐ Ⓑ Ⓒ Ⓓ  53. Ⓐ Ⓑ Ⓒ Ⓓ  68. Ⓐ Ⓑ Ⓒ Ⓓ
9. Ⓐ Ⓑ Ⓒ Ⓓ  24. Ⓐ Ⓑ Ⓒ Ⓓ  39. Ⓐ Ⓑ Ⓒ Ⓓ  54. Ⓐ Ⓑ Ⓒ Ⓓ  69. Ⓐ Ⓑ Ⓒ Ⓓ
10. Ⓐ Ⓑ Ⓒ Ⓓ  25. Ⓐ Ⓑ Ⓒ Ⓓ  40. Ⓐ Ⓑ Ⓒ Ⓓ  55. Ⓐ Ⓑ Ⓒ Ⓓ  70. Ⓐ Ⓑ Ⓒ Ⓓ
11. Ⓐ Ⓑ Ⓒ Ⓓ  26. Ⓐ Ⓑ Ⓒ Ⓓ  41. Ⓐ Ⓑ Ⓒ Ⓓ  56. Ⓐ Ⓑ Ⓒ Ⓓ  71. Ⓐ Ⓑ Ⓒ Ⓓ
12. Ⓐ Ⓑ Ⓒ Ⓓ  27. Ⓐ Ⓑ Ⓒ Ⓓ  42. Ⓐ Ⓑ Ⓒ Ⓓ  57. Ⓐ Ⓑ Ⓒ Ⓓ  72. Ⓐ Ⓑ Ⓒ Ⓓ
13. Ⓐ Ⓑ Ⓒ Ⓓ  28. Ⓐ Ⓑ Ⓒ Ⓓ  43. Ⓐ Ⓑ Ⓒ Ⓓ  58. Ⓐ Ⓑ Ⓒ Ⓓ  73. Ⓐ Ⓑ Ⓒ Ⓓ
14. Ⓐ Ⓑ Ⓒ Ⓓ  29. Ⓐ Ⓑ Ⓒ Ⓓ  44. Ⓐ Ⓑ Ⓒ Ⓓ  59. Ⓐ Ⓑ Ⓒ Ⓓ  74. Ⓐ Ⓑ Ⓒ Ⓓ
15. Ⓐ Ⓑ Ⓒ Ⓓ  30. Ⓐ Ⓑ Ⓒ Ⓓ  45. Ⓐ Ⓑ Ⓒ Ⓓ  60. Ⓐ Ⓑ Ⓒ Ⓓ  75. Ⓐ Ⓑ Ⓒ Ⓓ

---

# Science

1. Ⓐ Ⓑ Ⓒ Ⓓ  14. Ⓐ Ⓑ Ⓒ Ⓓ  27. Ⓐ Ⓑ Ⓒ Ⓓ  40. Ⓐ Ⓑ Ⓒ Ⓓ  53. Ⓐ Ⓑ Ⓒ Ⓓ
2. Ⓐ Ⓑ Ⓒ Ⓓ  15. Ⓐ Ⓑ Ⓒ Ⓓ  28. Ⓐ Ⓑ Ⓒ Ⓓ  41. Ⓐ Ⓑ Ⓒ Ⓓ  54. Ⓐ Ⓑ Ⓒ Ⓓ
3. Ⓐ Ⓑ Ⓒ Ⓓ  16. Ⓐ Ⓑ Ⓒ Ⓓ  29. Ⓐ Ⓑ Ⓒ Ⓓ  42. Ⓐ Ⓑ Ⓒ Ⓓ  55. Ⓐ Ⓑ Ⓒ Ⓓ
4. Ⓐ Ⓑ Ⓒ Ⓓ  17. Ⓐ Ⓑ Ⓒ Ⓓ  30. Ⓐ Ⓑ Ⓒ Ⓓ  43. Ⓐ Ⓑ Ⓒ Ⓓ  56. Ⓐ Ⓑ Ⓒ Ⓓ
5. Ⓐ Ⓑ Ⓒ Ⓓ  18. Ⓐ Ⓑ Ⓒ Ⓓ  31. Ⓐ Ⓑ Ⓒ Ⓓ  44. Ⓐ Ⓑ Ⓒ Ⓓ  57. Ⓐ Ⓑ Ⓒ Ⓓ
6. Ⓐ Ⓑ Ⓒ Ⓓ  19. Ⓐ Ⓑ Ⓒ Ⓓ  32. Ⓐ Ⓑ Ⓒ Ⓓ  45. Ⓐ Ⓑ Ⓒ Ⓓ  58. Ⓐ Ⓑ Ⓒ Ⓓ
7. Ⓐ Ⓑ Ⓒ Ⓓ  20. Ⓐ Ⓑ Ⓒ Ⓓ  33. Ⓐ Ⓑ Ⓒ Ⓓ  46. Ⓐ Ⓑ Ⓒ Ⓓ  59. Ⓐ Ⓑ Ⓒ Ⓓ
8. Ⓐ Ⓑ Ⓒ Ⓓ  21. Ⓐ Ⓑ Ⓒ Ⓓ  34. Ⓐ Ⓑ Ⓒ Ⓓ  47. Ⓐ Ⓑ Ⓒ Ⓓ  60. Ⓐ Ⓑ Ⓒ Ⓓ
9. Ⓐ Ⓑ Ⓒ Ⓓ  22. Ⓐ Ⓑ Ⓒ Ⓓ  35. Ⓐ Ⓑ Ⓒ Ⓓ  48. Ⓐ Ⓑ Ⓒ Ⓓ  61. Ⓐ Ⓑ Ⓒ Ⓓ
10. Ⓐ Ⓑ Ⓒ Ⓓ  23. Ⓐ Ⓑ Ⓒ Ⓓ  36. Ⓐ Ⓑ Ⓒ Ⓓ  49. Ⓐ Ⓑ Ⓒ Ⓓ  62. Ⓐ Ⓑ Ⓒ Ⓓ
11. Ⓐ Ⓑ Ⓒ Ⓓ  24. Ⓐ Ⓑ Ⓒ Ⓓ  37. Ⓐ Ⓑ Ⓒ Ⓓ  50. Ⓐ Ⓑ Ⓒ Ⓓ  63. Ⓐ Ⓑ Ⓒ Ⓓ
12. Ⓐ Ⓑ Ⓒ Ⓓ  25. Ⓐ Ⓑ Ⓒ Ⓓ  38. Ⓐ Ⓑ Ⓒ Ⓓ  51. Ⓐ Ⓑ Ⓒ Ⓓ  64. Ⓐ Ⓑ Ⓒ Ⓓ
13. Ⓐ Ⓑ Ⓒ Ⓓ  26. Ⓐ Ⓑ Ⓒ Ⓓ  39. Ⓐ Ⓑ Ⓒ Ⓓ  52. Ⓐ Ⓑ Ⓒ Ⓓ  65. Ⓐ Ⓑ Ⓒ Ⓓ

# Practice Test Two

## READING COMPREHENSION

**Questions 1–2 are based on the following passage.**

Until quite recently, hypnosis has been a specialized—and often controversial—technique used only in marginal areas of medicine. However, hypnosis is now increasingly finding mainstream use. For example, mental health experts have found that the suggestions of a skilled therapist are often remarkably effective in countering anxiety and depression. The benefits of hypnosis, though, are not limited to the emotional and psychological realm. Hypnosis helps burn center patients manage excruciating pain, and a recent research study found that hypnosis can dramatically shorten the time required for bone fractures to heal, often by several weeks.

1. The passage indicates that hypnosis:

    (A) Is the most effective means to manage pain.

    (B) Was formerly regarded with some suspicion.

    (C) Is still a controversial means to treat anxiety and depression.

    (D) Is limited primarily to mental health medicine.

2. In the passage the word *manage* most nearly means:

    (A) Direct

    (B) Administer

    (C) Bring about

    (D) Cope with

GO ON TO THE NEXT PAGE

**KAPLAN**

About 50 miles west of Stonehenge, buried in the peat bogs of the Somerset flatlands in southwestern England, lies the oldest road known to humanity. Dubbed the "Sweet Track" after its discoverer, Raymond Sweet, this painstakingly constructed 1,800-meter road dates back to the early Neolithic period, some 6,000 years ago. Thanks primarily to the overlying layer of acidic peat, which has kept the wood moist, inhibited the growth of decay bacteria, and discouraged the curiosity of animal life, the road is remarkably well preserved. Examination of its remains has provided extensive information about the people who constructed it.

The design of the Sweet Track indicates that its builders possessed extraordinary engineering skills. In constructing the road, they first hammered pegs into the soil in the form of upright X's. Single rails were slid beneath the pegs, so that the rails rested firmly on the soft surface of the bog. Then planks were placed in the V-shaped space formed by the upper arms of the pegs. This method of construction—allowing the underlying rail to distribute the weight of the plank above and thereby prevent the pegs from sinking into the marsh—is remarkably sophisticated, testifying to a surprisingly advanced level of technology.

Furthermore, in order to procure the materials for the road, several different species of tree had to be felled, debarked, and split. This suggests that the builders possessed high quality tools, and that they knew the differing properties of various roundwoods. It appears also that the builders were privy to the finer points of lumbering, maximizing the amount of wood extracted from a given tree by slicing logs of large diameter radially and logs of small diameter tangentially.

Studies of the Sweet Track further indicate a high level of social organization among its builders. This is supported by the observation that the road seems to have been completed in a very short time; tree-ring analysis confirms that the components of the Sweet Track were probably all felled within a single year. Moreover, the fact that such an involved engineering effort could be orchestrated in the first place hints at a complex social structure.

Finally, excavation of the Sweet Track has provided evidence that the people who built it comprised a community devoted to land cultivation. It appears that the road was built to serve as a footpath linking two islands—islands that provided a source of timber, cropland, and pastures for the community that settled the hills to the south. Furthermore, the quality of the pegs indicates that the workers knew enough to fell trees in such a way as to encourage the rapid growth of long, straight, rod-like shoots from the remaining stumps, to be used as pegs. This method is called coppicing and its practice by the settlers is the earliest known example of woodland management.

Undoubtedly, the discovery of the Sweet Track in 1970 added much to our knowledge of Neolithic technology. But while study of the remains has revealed unexpectedly high levels of engineering and social organization, it must be remembered that the Sweet Track represents the work of a single isolated community. One must be careful not to extrapolate sweeping generalizations from the achievements of such a small sample of Neolithic humanity.

3. In the first paragraph, the author claims that which of the following was primarily responsible for the preservation of the Sweet Track until modern times?

(A) It was located in an area containing very few animals.

(B) Its components were buried beneath the peat bog.

(C) It was only lightly traveled during its period of use.

(D) Local authorities prohibited development in the surrounding area.

GO ON TO THE NEXT PAGE ⟶

4. The author's reference to the peat bog as "acidic" primarily serves to:

   (A) Indicate the importance of protecting ancient ruins from the effects of modern pollution.

   (B) Emphasize that the Sweet Track was constructed of noncorrosive materials.

   (C) Distinguish between the effects of acidic and basic conditions on ancient ruins.

   (D) Suggest that acidic conditions were important in inhibiting decay.

5. In the second paragraph, the author describes the construction of the Sweet Track primarily in order to:

   (A) Explain the unusual strength of the structure.

   (B) Show how it could withstand 6,000 years buried underground.

   (C) Prove that its builders cooperated efficiently.

   (D) Indicate its builders' advanced level of technological expertise.

6. The primary focus of the passage is on:

   (A) The high degree of social organization exhibited by earlier cultures.

   (B) The complex construction and composition of the Sweet Track.

   (C) An explanation for the survival of the Sweet Track over 6,000 years.

   (D) Ways in which the Sweet Track reveals aspects of a particular Neolithic society.

7. In the discussion of social organization presented in the fourth paragraph, the author mentions ring analysis primarily as evidence that:

   (A) The road is at least 6,000 years old.

   (B) The Sweet Track was constructed quickly.

   (C) The techniques used in building the road were quite sophisticated.

   (D) The builders knew enough to split thick trees radially and thin trees tangentially.

8. The cited example of "woodland management" is best described as a system in which trees are:

   (A) Lumbered in controlled quantities.

   (B) Planted only among trees of their own species.

   (C) Cultivated in specialized ways for specific purposes.

   (D) Felled only as they are needed.

9. In the last paragraph, the author cautions that the Sweet Track:

   (A) Is not as technologically advanced as is generally believed.

   (B) Should not necessarily be regarded as representative of its time.

   (C) Has not been studied extensively enough to support generalized conclusions.

   (D) Is probably not the earliest road in existence.

GO ON TO THE NEXT PAGE

**KAPLAN**

**Questions 10–11 are based on the following passage.**

In recent years, shark attacks in U.S. waters have received wide attention. Are such attacks a growing threat to swimmers and surfers? Statistics suggest not. The rate of attacks per number of swimmers has not increased over time. What *has* increased is the popularity of aquatic sports, such as surfing, sail boarding, and kayaking. More people are in the water these days, and therefore the chances of a shark encounter increase. Still, to keep the issue in perspective we should remember there were only six fatal shark attacks in U.S. coastal waters from 1990 to 2000.

10. According to the author, which of the following has NOT increased over time?

    (A) The total number of shark attacks in U.S. waters.

    (B) The popularity of aquatic sports.

    (C) The number of fatal shark attacks in U.S. coastal waters.

    (D) The rate of shark attacks per number of people in the water.

11. The author most likely provides the statistic in the final sentence in order to:

    (A) Point out that U.S. coastal waters are safer than those of other countries.

    (B) Illustrate that relatively few fatal shark attacks have occurred in U.S. waters.

    (C) Show that the period 1990–2000 marked a decrease in the number of fatal shark attacks.

    (D) Caution swimmers and surfers against dangers.

GO ON TO THE NEXT PAGE

KAPLAN

**Questions 12–17 are based on the following passage, in which a Nobel Prize–winning scientist discusses ways of thinking about extremely long periods of time.**

There is one fact about the origin of life which is reasonably certain. Whenever and wherever it happened, it started a very long time ago, so long ago that it is extremely difficult to form any realistic idea of such vast stretches of time. The shortness of human life necessarily limits the span of direct personal recollection.

Human culture has given us the illusion that our memories go further back than that. Before writing was invented, the experience of earlier generations, embodied in stories, myths, and moral precepts to guide behavior, was passed down verbally or, to a lesser extent, in pictures, carvings, and statues. Writing has made more precise and more extensive the transmission of such information and, in recent times, photography has sharpened our images of the immediate past. Even so, we have difficulty in contemplating steadily the march of history, from the beginnings of civilization to the present day, in such a way that we can truly experience the slow passage of time. Our minds are not built to deal comfortably with periods as long as hundreds or thousands of years.

Yet when we come to consider the origin of life, the time scales we must deal with make the whole span of human history seem but the blink of an eyelid. There is no simple way to adjust one's thinking to such vast stretches of time. The immensity of time passed is beyond our ready comprehension. One can only construct an impression of it from indirect and incomplete descriptions, just as a blind man laboriously builds up, by touch and sound, a picture of his immediate surroundings.

The customary way to provide a convenient framework for one's thoughts is to compare the age of the universe with the length of a single earthly day. Perhaps a better comparison, along the same lines, would be to equate the age of our earth with a single week. On such a scale the age of the universe, since the Big Bang, would be about two or three weeks. The oldest macroscopic fossils (those from the start of the Cambrian* Period) would have been alive just one day ago. Modern man would have appeared in the last 10 seconds and agriculture in the last one or two.

Odysseus** would have lived only half a second before the present time.

Even this comparison hardly makes the longer time scale comprehensible to us. Another alternative is to draw a linear map of time, with the different events marked on it. The problem here is to make the line long enough to show our own experience on a reasonable scale, and yet short enough for convenient reproduction and examination. But perhaps the most vivid method is to compare time to the lines of print themselves. Let us make a 200-page book equal in length to the time from the start of the Cambrian to the present; that is, about 600 million years. Then each full page will represent roughly three million years, each line about ninety thousand years, and each letter or small space about fifteen hundred years. The origin of the Earth would be about seven books ago and the origin of the universe (which has been dated only approximately) ten or so books before that. Almost the whole of recorded human history would be covered by the last two or three letters of the book.

If you now turn back the pages of the book, slowly reading *one letter at a time*—remember, each letter is fifteen hundred years—then this may convey to you something of the immense stretches of time we shall have to consider. On this scale the span of your own life would be less than the width of a comma.

*Cambrian:* The earliest period in the Paleozoic era, beginning about 600 million years ago.

**Odysseus:* The most famous Greek hero of antiquity; he is the hero of Homer's *The Odyssey*, which describes the aftermath of the Trojan War (ca. 1200 B.C.E.).

12. The phrase "to a lesser extent" indicates that before the invention of writing, the wisdom of earlier generations was:

   (A) Rejected by recent generations when portrayed in pictures, carvings, or statues.
   (B) Passed down orally, or not at all.
   (C) Transmitted more frequently by spoken word than by other means.
   (D) Based on illusory memories that turned fact into fiction.

GO ON TO THE NEXT PAGE ⇨

13. The author most likely describes the impact of writing in order to:

    (A) Illustrate the limitations of human memory.

    (B) Provide an example of how cultures transmit information.

    (C) Indicate how primitive preliterate cultures were.

    (D) Refute an opinion about the origin of human civilization.

14. The analogy of the "blind man" is presented primarily to show that:

    (A) Humans are unable to comprehend long periods of time.

    (B) Myths and legends fail to give an accurate picture of the past.

    (C) Human history is only a fraction of the time since life began.

    (D) Long periods of time can only be understood indirectly.

15. In the passage, the author mentions the Big Bang and the Cambrian Period in order to demonstrate which point?

    (A) The age of the Earth is best understood using the time scale of a week.

    (B) Agriculture was a relatively late development in human history.

    (C) No fossil record exists before the Cambrian Period.

    (D) Convenient time scales do not adequately represent the age of the Earth.

16. According to the passage, one difficulty of using a linear representation of time is that:

    (A) Linear representations of time do not meet accepted scientific standards of accuracy.

    (B) Prehistoric eras overlap each other, making linear representation deceptive.

    (C) The more accurate the scale, the more difficult the map is to copy and study.

    (D) There are too many events to represent on a single line.

17. The author of this passage discusses several kinds of time scales, primarily in order to illustrate the:

    (A) Difficulty of assigning precise dates to past events.

    (B) Variety of choices faced by scientists investigating the origin of life.

    (C) Evolution of efforts to comprehend the passage of history.

    (D) Immensity of time since life began on Earth.

GO ON TO THE NEXT PAGE ▷

**Questions 18–19 are based on the following passage.**

On a stormy June day in 1752, Benjamin Franklin carried out the famous experiment in which he channeled lightning down a kite string and stored the electric charge in a Leyden jar, the precursor to the modern capacitor. The consequences could not have been more pronounced. Franklin proved that electricity was a force of nature, like Newton's gravity, and the subsequent invention of the lightning rod (based on Franklin's theories) sharply reduced risk of fire to tall buildings. Franklin's experiment had cultural repercussions as well. It showed that scientific research could have practical benefits, and it impugned the superstitious belief—widespread at the time—that lightning resulted from divine displeasure.

18. The sentence, "The consequences could not have been more pronounced," conveys:

   (A) That it was difficult to describe the results of the experiment.

   (B) That Franklin became famous because of the experiment.

   (C) The importance of Franklin's findings to the scientific understanding of electricity.

   (D) That Franklin's experiment had far-reaching effects.

19. Based on the passage, Franklin's kite experiment played a part in:

   (A) Promoting superstitious beliefs.

   (B) Explaining the force of gravity.

   (C) The development of the Leyden jar.

   (D) Illustrating the utility of scientific research.

GO ON TO THE NEXT PAGE

**KAPLAN**

**Questions 20–27 are based on the following passage, which was written in 1992 by France Bequette, a writer who specializes in environmental issues.**

The ozone layer, the fragile layer of gas surrounding our planet between 7 and 30 miles above the Earth's surface, is being rapidly depleted. Seasonally occurring holes have appeared in it over the Poles and, recently, over densely populated temperate regions of the northern hemisphere. The threat is serious because the ozone layer protects the Earth from the sun's ultraviolet radiation, which is harmful to all living organisms.

Even though the layer is many miles thick, the atmosphere in it is tenuous and the total amount of ozone, compared with other atmospheric gases, is small. Ozone is highly reactive to chlorine, hydrogen, and nitrogen. Of these, chlorine is the most dangerous since it is very stable and long-lived. When chlorine compounds reach the stratosphere, they bond with and destroy ozone molecules, with consequent repercussions for life on Earth.

In 1958, researchers began noticing seasonal variations in the ozone layer above the South Pole. Between June and October the ozone content steadily fell, followed by a sudden increase in November. These fluctuations appeared to result from the natural effects of wind and temperature. But while the low October levels remained constant until 1979, the total ozone content over the Pole was steadily diminishing. In 1985, public opinion was finally roused by reports of a "hole" in the layer.

The culprits responsible for the hole were identified as compounds known as chlorofluorocarbons, or CFCs. CFCs are compounds of chlorine and fluorine. Nonflammable, nontoxic, and noncorrosive, they have been widely used in industry since the 1950s, mostly as refrigerants and propellants and in making plastic foam and insulation.

In 1989 CFCs represented a sizeable market valued at over $1.5 billion and a labor force of 1.6 million. But with CFCs implicated in ozone depletion, the question arose as to whether we were willing to risk an increase in cases of skin cancer, eye ailments, even a lowering of the human immune defense system—all effects of further loss of the ozone layer. And not only humans would suffer. So would plant life. Phytoplankton, the first link in the ocean food chain and vital to the survival of most marine species, would not be able to

survive near the ocean surface, which is where these organisms grow.

In 1990, 70 countries agreed to stop producing CFCs by the year 2000. In late 1991, however, scientists noticed a depletion of the ozone layer over the Arctic. In 1992 it was announced that the layer was depleting faster than expected and that it was also declining over the northern hemisphere. Scientists believe that natural events are making the problem worse. The Pinatubo volcano in the Philippines, which erupted in June 1991, released 12 million tons of damaging volcanic gases into the atmosphere.

Even if the whole world agreed today to stop all production and use of CFCs, this would not solve the problem. A single chlorine molecule can destroy 10,000–100,000 molecules of ozone. Furthermore, CFCs have a lifespan of 75–400 years and they take ten years to reach the ozone layer. In other words, what we are experiencing today results from CFCs emitted ten years ago. Researchers are working hard to find substitute products. Some are too dangerous because they are highly flammable; others may prove to be toxic and to contribute to the greenhouse effect—to the process of global warming. Nevertheless, even if here is no denying that the atmosphere is in a state of disturbance, nobody can say that the situation will not improve, either in the short or the long term, especially if we ourselves lend a hand.

20. As it is described in the passage, the major function of the ozone layer is closest to that of:

    (A) An emergency evacuation plan for a skyscraper.
    (B) A central information desk at a convention center.
    (C) A traffic light at a busy intersection.
    (D) The filtering system for a city water supply.

GO ON TO THE NEXT PAGE ⟹

21. The passage implies which of the following about the "seasonal variations in the ozone layer" observed by scientists in 1958?

    (A) They were caused by industrial substances other than CFCs.

    (B) They created alarm among scientists but not the public.

    (C) They were least stable in the months between June and November.

    (D) They opened the public's eye to the threat of ozone depletion.

22. In context, the word *constant* means:

    (A) Gentle

    (B) Steady

    (C) Pestering

    (D) Unerring

23. The author mentions market and workforce figures related to CFC production in order to point out that:

    (A) Responsibility for the problem of ozone depletion lies primarily with industry.

    (B) The disadvantages of CFCs are obvious while the benefits are not.

    (C) The magnitude of profits from CFCs has turned public opinion against the industry's practices.

    (D) While the economic stakes are large, they are overshadowed by the effects of CFCs.

24. In the sixth paragraph, the author cites the evidence of changes in the ozone layer over the northern hemisphere to indicate that:

    (A) The dangers of ozone depletion appear to be intensifying.

    (B) Ozone depletion is posing an immediate threat to many marine species.

    (C) Scientists are unsure about the ultimate effects of ozone loss on plants.

    (D) CFCs are not the primary cause of ozone depletion in such areas.

25. Scientists apparently believe which of the following about the "volcanic gases" mentioned in the passage?

    (A) They contribute more to global warming than to ozone loss.

    (B) They pose a greater long-term threat than CFCs.

    (C) They are hastening ozone loss at present.

    (D) They are of little long-term consequence.

26. The author's reference to the long life of chlorine molecules is meant to show that:

    (A) CFCs are adaptable to a variety of industrial uses.

    (B) There is more than adequate time to develop a long-term strategy against ozone loss.

    (C) The long-term effects of ozone loss on human health may never be known.

    (D) The positive effects of actions taken against ozone loss will be gradual.

27. In the final paragraph, the author tries to emphasize that:

    (A) Researchers are unlikely to find effective substitutes for CFCs.

    (B) Human action can alleviate the decline of the ozone layer.

    (C) People must to learn to live with the damaging effects of industrial pollutants.

    (D) Atmospheric conditions are largely beyond human control.

GO ON TO THE NEXT PAGE

**KAPLAN**

**Questions 28–33 are based on the following passage.**

There can be nothing simpler than an elementary particle: It is an indivisible shard of matter, without internal structure and without detectable shape or size. One might expect commensurate simplicity in the theories that describe such particles and the forces through which they interact; at the least, one might expect the structure of the world to be explained with a minimum number of particles and forces. Judged by this criterion of parsimony, a description of nature that has evolved in the past several years can be accounted a reasonable success. Matter is built out of just two classes of elementary particles: the leptons, such as the electron, and the quarks, which are constituents of the proton, the neutron, and many related particles. Four basic forces act between the elementary particles. Gravitation and electromagnetism have long been familiar in the macroscopic world; the weak force and the strong force are observed only in subnuclear events. In principle this complement of particles and forces could account for the entire observed hierarchy of material structure, from the nuclei of atoms to stars and galaxies. An understanding of nature at this level of detail is a remarkable achievement; nevertheless, it is possible to imagine what a still simpler theory might be like. The existence of two disparate classes of elementary particles is not fully satisfying; ideally, one class would suffice. Similarly, the existence of four forces seems a needless complication; one force might explain all the interactions of elementary particles. An ambitious new theory now promises at least a partial unification along these lines. The theory does not embrace gravitation, which is by far the feeblest of the forces and may be fundamentally different from the others. If gravitation is excluded, however, the theory unifies all elementary particles and forces. The first step in the construction of the unified theory was the demonstration that the weak, the strong, and the electromagnetic forces could all be described by theories of the same general kind. The three forces remained distinct, but they could be seen to operate through the same mechanism. In the course of this development a deep connection was discovered between the weak force and electromagnetism, a connection that hinted at a still grander synthesis. The new theory is the leading candidate for accomplishing the synthesis. It incorporates the leptons and the quarks into a single family and provides a means of transforming one kind of particle into the other. At the same time the weak, the strong, and the electromagnetic forces are understood as aspects of a single underlying force. With only one class of particles and one force (plus gravitation), the unified theory is a model of frugality.

28. All of the following are differences between the two theories described by the author EXCEPT:

   (A) The second theory is simpler than the first.

   (B) The first theory encompasses gravitation while the second does not.

   (C) The second theory includes only one class of elementary particles.

   (D) The first theory accounts for only part of the hierarchy of material structure.

29. The primary purpose of the passage is to:

   (A) Correct a misconception in a currently accepted theory of the nature of matter.

   (B) Describe efforts to arrive at a simplified theory of elementary particles and forces.

   (C) Predict the success of a new effort to unify gravitation with other basic forces.

   (D) Explain why scientists prefer simpler explanations over more complex ones.

30. According to the passage, which of the following are true of quarks?

   I. They are the elementary building blocks for neutrons.
   II. Scientists have described them as having no internal structure.
   III. Some scientists group them with leptons in a single class of particles.

   (A) I only

   (B) III only

   (C) I and II only

   (D) I, II, and III

GO ON TO THE NEXT PAGE

**KAPLAN)**

31. The author considers which of the following in judging the usefulness of a theory of elementary particles and forces?

    I. The simplicity of the theory.
    II. The ability of the theory to account for the largest possible number of known phenomena.
    III. The possibility of proving or disproving the theory by experiment.

    (A) I only
    (B) II only
    (C) I and II only
    (D) I and III only

32. It can be inferred that the author considers the failure to unify gravitation with other forces in the theory he describes to be:

    (A) A disqualifying defect.
    (B) An unjustified deviation.
    (C) A needless oversimplification.
    (D) An unavoidable limitation.

33. It can be inferred that the author would be likely to consider a new theory of nature superior to present theories if it were to:

    (A) Account for a larger number of macroscopic structures than present theories.
    (B) Reduce the four basic forces to two more fundamental, incompatible forces.
    (C) Propose a smaller number of fundamental particles and forces than current theories.
    (D) Successfully account for the observable behavior of bodies due to gravity.

GO ON TO THE NEXT PAGE

**KAPLAN**

**Questions 34–37 are based on the following passage.**

A pioneering figure in modern sociology, French social theorist Emile Durkheim examined the role of societal cohesion on emotional well-being. Believing scientific methods should be applied to the study of society, Durkheim studied the level of integration of various social formations and the impact that such cohesion had on individuals within a group. He postulated that social groups with high levels of integration serve to buffer their members from frustrations and tragedies that could otherwise lead to desperation and self-destruction. Integration, in Durkheim's view, generally arises through shared activities and values.

Durkheim distinguished between *mechanical solidarity* and *organic solidarity* in classifying integrated groups. *Mechanical solidarity* dominates in groups in which individual differences are minimized and group devotion to a common aim is high. Durkheim identified *mechanical solidarity* among groups with little division of labor and high rates of cultural similarity, such as among more traditional and geographically isolated groups. *Organic solidarity*, in contrast, prevails in groups with high levels of individual differences, such as those with a highly specialized division of labor. In such groups, individual differences are a powerful source of connection, rather than of division. Because people engage in highly differentiated ways of life, they are by necessity interdependent. In these societies, there is greater freedom from some external controls, but such freedom occurs in concert with the interdependence of individuals, not in conflict with it.

Durkheim realized societies may take many forms and consequently that group allegiance can manifest itself in a variety of ways. In both types of societies outlined above, however, Durkheim stressed that adherence to a common set of assumptions about the world was a necessary prerequisite for maintaining group integrity and avoiding social decay.

34. The author is primarily concerned with:

(A) Supporting a specific approach to the study of the integration of social groups.

(B) Comparing different ways that group dynamics maintain allegiance among group members.

(C) Illustrating how a highly specialized division of labor can protect individuals from depression.

(D) Determining what type of society will best suit an individual's emotional needs.

35. The passage contrasts *mechanical solidarity* with *organic solidarity* along which of the following parameters?

(A) The degree to which each relies on objective measures of group coherence.

(B) The manner and degree to which members are linked to the central group.

(C) The means by which each allows members to rebel against the group norm.

(D) The length of time that each has been used to describe the structure of societies.

36. It can be inferred from the passage that:

(A) Group integration enables societies to mask internal differences to the external world.

(B) Durkheim preferred *organic solidarity* to *mechanical solidarity.*

(C) Individuals from societies with high degrees of *organic solidarity* would be unable to communicate effectively with individuals from societies that rest on *mechanical solidarity.*

(D) The presence of some type of group integration is more important for group perpetuation than the specific form in which it is manifest.

GO ON TO THE NEXT PAGE ⟩

37. The passage states *organic solidarity* predominates in societies with relatively high levels of intragroup dissimilarity because:

    (A) It enables individual differences to be minimized.

    (B) It causes societies to become more highly specialized, thus aiding industrialization.

    (C) Individuals who engage in highly specialized activities must rely on others to ensure that their basic needs are met.

    (D) These societies are at greater risk of being affected by social stressors.

**Questions 38–41 are based on the following passage.**

Migration of animal populations from one region to another is called faunal interchange. Concentrations of species across regional boundaries vary, however, prompting zoologists to classify routes along which penetrations of new regions occur. A corridor, like the vast stretch of land from Alaska to the southeastern United States, is equivalent to a path of least resistance. Relative ease of migration often results in the presence of related species along the entire length of a corridor; bear populations, unknown in South America, occur throughout the North American corridor. A desert or other barrier creates a filter route, allowing only a segment of a faunal group to pass. A sweepstakes route presents so formidable a barrier that penetration is unlikely. It differs from other routes, which may be crossed by species with sufficient adaptive capability. As the name suggests, negotiation of a sweepstakes route depends almost exclusively on chance, rather than on physical attributes and adaptability.

38. It can be inferred from the passage that studies of faunal interchange would probably:

    (A) Fail to explain how similar species can inhabit widely separated areas.

    (B) Be unreliable because of the difficulty of observing long-range migrations.

    (C) Focus most directly on the seasonal movements of a species within a specific geographic region.

    (D) Help to explain how present-day distributions of animal populations might have arisen.

GO ON TO THE NEXT PAGE

**KAPLAN**

39. The author's primary purpose is to show the classification of migratory routes:

    (A) Is based on the probability that migration will occur along a given route.

    (B) Reflects the important role played by chance in the distribution of most species.

    (C) Is unreliable because further study is needed.

    (D) Is too arbitrary, because the regional boundaries cited by zoologists frequently change.

40. The author's description of the distribution of bear populations suggests which of the following conclusions?

    I. The distribution patterns of most other North American faunal species populations are probably identical to those of bears.

    II. There are relatively few barriers to faunal interchange in North America.

    III. The geographic area that links North America to South America would probably be classified as either a filter or a sweepstakes route.

    (A) I only

    (B) II only

    (C) III only

    (D) II and III only

41. According to the passage, in order to negotiate a sweepstakes route an animal species:

    (A) Has to spend at least part of the year in a desert environment.

    (B) Is obliged to move long distances in short periods of time.

    (C) Must sacrifice many of its young to wandering pastures.

    (D) Does not need to possess any special physical capabilities.

**Questions 42–43 are based on the following passage.**

Most people think the Hula Hoop was a fad born in the 1950s, but in fact people were doing much the same thing with circular hoops made from grape vines and stiff grasses all over the ancient world. More than 3,000 years ago, children in Egypt played with large hoops of dried grapevines. The toy was propelled along the ground with a stick or swung around at the waist. During the fourteenth century, a "hooping" craze swept England, and was as popular among adults as kids. The word Hula became associated with the toy in the early 1800s when British sailors visited the Hawaiian Islands and noted the similarity between hooping and Hula dancing. In 1957, an Australian company began making wood rings for sale in retail stores. The item attracted the attention of Wham-O, a fledgling California toy manufacturer. The plastic Hula Hoop was introduced in 1958 and was an instant hit.

42. According to the passage, all of the following statements are true EXCEPT:

    (A) Most people do not appreciate the origins of the Hula Hoop.

    (B) The earliest prototypes of the Hula Hoop were made of grape leaves and stiff grasses.

    (C) Early precursors Hula Hoop were primarily children's toys.

    (D) The Hula Hoop was an early success for the toy maker Wham-O.

43. The author's primary purpose in this passage is to:

    (A) Describe the way that fads like the Hula Hoop come and go.

    (B) Discuss the origins of the Hula Hoop.

    (C) Explain how the Hula Hoop got its name.

    (D) Question the reasons for the Hula Hoop's popularity.

GO ON TO THE NEXT PAGE

**KAPLAN**

**Questions 44–45 are based on the following passage.**

Both alligators and crocodiles can be found in southern Florida, particularly in the Everglades National Park. Alligators and crocodiles do look similar but there are several physical characteristics that differentiate the two giant reptiles. The most easily observed difference between alligators and crocodiles is the shape of the head. A crocodile's skull and jaws are longer and narrower than an alligator's. When an alligator closes its mouth, its long teeth slip into sockets in the upper jaw and disappear. When a crocodile closes its mouth, its long teeth remain visible, protruding outside the upper jaw. In general, if you can still see a lot of teeth even when the animal's mouth is closed, you are looking at a crocodile.

44.  One can distinguish a crocodile from an alligator:

  (A)  Only when the animal's mouth is closed.

  (B)  By the location in Florida where the animal is found.

  (C)  By its thick, heavily armored skin.

  (D)  By the narrower snout found on a crocodile.

45.  It can be inferred from the passage that:

  (A)  The Everglades National Park is in southern Florida.

  (B)  Scientific tests are required to differentiate between alligators and crocodiles.

  (C)  Alligators are more deadly than crocodiles.

  (D)  There is no difference between alligators and crocodiles.

GO ON TO THE NEXT PAGE

KAPLAN

## VOCABULARY AND SPELLING

1. *Noble* most nearly means:

   (A) Comely
   (B) Loose
   (C) Majestic
   (D) Lackadaisical

2. *Judicious* most nearly means:

   (A) Accessible
   (B) Cold
   (C) Fair
   (D) Talkative

3. *Prerequisite* most nearly means:

   (A) Required
   (B) Tiny
   (C) Gleeful
   (D) Tasteful

4. *Coax* most nearly means:

   (A) Advise
   (B) Trade
   (C) Plead
   (D) Grace

5. *Terminal* most nearly means:

   (A) Easy
   (B) Glittering
   (C) Busy
   (D) Final

6. *Augment* most nearly means:

   (A) Craft
   (B) End
   (C) Throw away
   (D) Enhance

7. *Tactile* most nearly means:

   (A) Ghastly
   (B) Easy
   (C) Patient
   (D) Tangible

8. *Germinate* most nearly means:

   (A) Seed
   (B) Oppress
   (C) Adulate
   (D) Foster

9. *Restore* most nearly means:

   (A) Trip up
   (B) Invigorate
   (C) Care for
   (D) Toughen

10. *Filament* most nearly means:

    (A) Horse
    (B) Triage
    (C) Nightmare
    (D) Thread

11. *Congeal* most nearly means:

    (A) Fade
    (B) Swirl
    (C) Harden
    (D) Undulate

12. *Impose* most nearly means:

    (A) Create
    (B) Force
    (C) Damage
    (D) Trade

**GO ON TO THE NEXT PAGE**

**KAPLAN**

13. *Stunted* most nearly means:

    (A) Halted

    (B) Daring

    (C) Loose

    (D) Blatant

14. *Longevity* most nearly means:

    (A) Training

    (B) Lifetime

    (C) Girth

    (D) Lifestyle

15. *Mutable* most nearly means:

    (A) Changing

    (B) Silent

    (C) Big-hearted

    (D) Calm

16. *Virtuoso* is the opposite of:

    (A) Malefactor

    (B) Gnome

    (C) Incompetent

    (D) Lackey

17. *Polarize* is the opposite of:

    (A) Delay

    (B) Welcome

    (C) Cancel

    (D) Unite

18. *Whimsical* is the opposite of:

    (A) Grave

    (B) Dull

    (C) Proud

    (D) Thought-provoking

19. *Dandy* is the opposite of:

    (A) Rogue

    (B) Fatalist

    (C) Careless dresser

    (D) Dull conversationalist

20. *Mar* is the opposite of:

    (A) Deaden

    (B) Flatter

    (C) Praise

    (D) Enhance

21. *Disperse* means the opposite of:

    (A) Gather

    (B) Display

    (C) Reverse

    (D) Handle

22. *Hamper* means the opposite of:

    (A) Relax

    (B) Hinder

    (C) Seize

    (D) Assist

23. *Aptitude* means the opposite of:

    (A) Inability

    (B) Height

    (C) Peak

    (D) Talent

24. *Gullible* means the opposite of:

    (A) Dirty

    (B) Cosmopolitan

    (C) Incredulous

    (D) Immaculate

GO ON TO THE NEXT PAGE

**KAPLAN**

25. *Replenish* is the opposite of:

    (A) Reward

    (B) Supply

    (C) Increase

    (D) Deplete

26. *Abundant* is the opposite of:

    (A) Scarce

    (B) Lush

    (C) Collect

    (D) Loyal

27. *Wary* means the opposite of:

    (A) Forgetful

    (B) Wise

    (C) Hopeful

    (D) Careless

28. *Sedentary* means the opposite of:

    (A) Optimistic

    (B) Calm

    (C) Active

    (D) Loyal

29. *Rudimentary* is the opposite of:

    (A) Advanced

    (B) Polite

    (C) Regulated

    (D) Essential

30. *Convoke* is the opposite of:

    (A) Pacify

    (B) Disperse

    (C) Arc

    (D) Forswear

31. Shard : Glass ::

    (A) Grain : Sand

    (B) Strand : Rope

    (C) Scrap : Quilt

    (D) Splinter : Wood

32. Filter : Impurity ::

    (A) Expurgate : Obscenity

    (B) Whitewash : Infraction

    (C) Testify : Perjury

    (D) Perform : Penance

33. Cut : Laceration ::

    (A) Park : Place

    (B) Slit : Gap

    (C) Knife : Separation

    (D) Hole : Puncture

34. Realist : Quixotic ::

    (A) Scholar : Pedantic

    (B) Fool : Idiotic

    (C) Idler : Lethargic

    (D) Tormentor : Sympathetic

35. Badge : Policeman ::

    (A) Placard : Demonstrator

    (B) Tattoo : Sailor

    (C) Dog-Tag : Soldier

    (D) Pedigree : Dog

36. Scrutinize : Observe ::

    (A) Excite : Pique

    (B) Beseech : Request

    (C) Search : Discover

    (D) Smile : Grin

GO ON TO THE NEXT PAGE

37. Indulge : Epicurean ::

    (A) Frighten: Ugly
    (B) Retract : Revocable
    (C) Hesitate : Unproductive
    (D) Revenge : Vindictive

38. Stare : Look ::

    (A) Peek : Glare
    (B) Want : Crave
    (C) Befriend : Alienate
    (D) Despair : Worry

39. Pancreas : Organ ::

    Knee : Joint
    Stomach : Obesity
    Artery : Vein
    Tooth : Molar

40. Enunciate : Pronounce ::

    Recite : Impress
    Reiterate : Bother
    Inquire : Ask
    Elaborate : Explain

41. Meander : Walk ::

    (A) Prattle : Talk
    (B) Mutilate : Destroy
    (C) Legislate : Mandate
    (D) Draw : Write

42. Flood : Diluvial ::

    (A) Punishment : Criminal
    (B) Bacteria : Biological
    (C) Verdict : Judicial
    (D) Heart : Cardiac

43. Penitent : Regret ::

    (A) Imperceptible : Detect
    (B) Zealous : Doubt
    (C) Exuberant : Socialize
    (D) Querulous : Quibble

44. Vegetate : Active ::

    (A) Resist : Beaten
    (B) Mope : Gloomy
    (C) Grow : Small
    (D) Accept : Questioning

45. Debilitate : Weak ::

    (A) Empower : Strong
    (B) Countermand : Illegal
    (C) Abominate : Absent
    (D) Instigate : Guilty

**Choose the word that is misspelled.**

46. (A) Regulated
    (B) Insignificant
    (C) Ambiguous
    (D) Apalling

47. (A) Desperation
    (B) Recognizible
    (C) Extensive
    (D) Potential

48. (A) Acknowledgment
    (B) Distinguished
    (C) Identified
    (D) Hieght

GO ON TO THE NEXT PAGE

KAPLAN

49. (A) Approachable
    (B) Irational
    (C) Summon
    (D) Attempted

50. (A) Avoidible
    (B) Simultaneous
    (C) Stagnant
    (D) Invitation

51. (A) Contentious
    (B) Sufficient
    (C) Discussion
    (D) Limitted

52. (A) Companion
    (B) Various
    (C) Indication
    (D) Emphisize

53. (A) Obsessed
    (B) Trauma
    (C) Appearence
    (D) Definitely

54. (A) Development
    (B) Vaccuum
    (C) Elective
    (D) Ostentatious

55. (A) Literally
    (B) Unobtrusive
    (C) Except
    (D) Campain

**Choose the sentence that contains a misspelled word. If there are no mistakes, choose (D).**

56. (A) My grandmother used allot of raisins in her oatmeal cookies.
    (B) The task seemed daunting at first.
    (C) The entire scene was unscripted.
    (D) No mistake.

57. (A) He would rather walk than hail a taxi.
    (B) She was unprepared for the new responsibility.
    (C) Johann gives great advise.
    (D) No mistake.

58. (A) The shirt was the perfect complement to the pants.
    (B) He ensured me that the meat was fresh.
    (C) Yuri is an avid skater.
    (D) No mistake.

59. (A) Walter was ready for some amusement.
    (B) It was fitting that Juana was quick to reply.
    (C) Typically, it takes several weeks to receive results.
    (D) No mistake.

60. (A) He apologized for the oversite.
    (B) Sarah unintentionally locked herself out.
    (C) The corporate offices are relocating this week.
    (D) No mistake.

61. (A) Whether or not you agree, it is true.
    (B) His car insurance rates are ghastly.
    (C) He finished painting and than he started cleaning up.
    (D) No mistake.

GO ON TO THE NEXT PAGE

62. (A) I need an accurate account of the situation.

    (B) Nicholas declined my offer.

    (C) She was very good at keeping up her correspondance

    (D) No mistake.

63. (A) It took all afternoon to polish the furniture.

    (B) Much to Joe's amazment, there was a raccoon in his kitchen.

    (C) His attempt at flattery was pointless.

    (D) No mistake.

64. (A) Jikja wilingly offered her seat to the elderly lady.

    (B) Julius was bored by unemployment.

    (C) I found all the food delicious.

    (D) No mistake.

65. (A) She was very fond of her antiques.

    (B) There was no way to estimate the damage.

    (C) Her likeability was a factor in getting her the job.

    (D) No mistake.

GO ON TO THE NEXT PAGE

KAPLAN

## MATHEMATICS

1. Which of the following is 53,298 rounded off to the nearest 100?

   (A) 53,290
   (B) 52,000
   (C) 53,300
   (D) 53,000

2. A worker earns $16 for the first 40 hours she works each week, and one and a half times this much for every hour over 40 hours. If she earned $700 for one week's work, how many hours of overtime did she work?

   (A) 3.3
   (B) 3
   (C) 2.5
   (D) 4

3. Liza has 40 less than 3 times the number of books that Janice has. If $B$ is equal to the number of books that Janice has, which of the following expressions shows the total number of books that Liza and Janice have together?

   (A) $4B - 40$
   (B) $3B - 40$
   (C) $4B$
   (D) $4B + 40$

4. If $x$ is an even integer and $8 < x < 17$, what is the mean of all possible values of $x$?

   (A) 10
   (B) 11
   (C) 13
   (D) 12

5. If $x$ is an odd integer and $y$ is an even integer, which of the following expressions MUST be odd?

   (A) $2x + y$
   (B) $2(x + y)$
   (C) $x^2 + y^2$
   (D) $xy + y$

6. All of the following can be a product of a negative integer and a positive integer EXCEPT:

   (A) $-6$
   (B) $1$
   (C) $-1$
   (D) $-2$

7. The Tigers had 5 times as many losses as they had ties in a season. If the Tigers did not win any of their games, which could be the total number of games they played in the season?

   (A) 16
   (B) 5
   (C) 10
   (D) 12

8. $2^3(3 - 1)^2 + (-4)^2 = ?$

   (A) 48
   (B) 32
   (C) 136
   (D) $-48$

9. Ruth has finished 3 chapters of an 8-chapter novel in just one evening of reading. If she reads an additional $\frac{1}{10}$ of the novel tomorrow night, what part of the novel will she have finished?

   (A) $\frac{4}{10}$
   (B) $\frac{1}{2}$
   (C) $\frac{19}{40}$
   (D) $\frac{36}{80}$

GO ON TO THE NEXT PAGE

**KAPLAN**

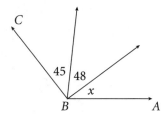

10. If the measure of angle *ABC* is 145°, what is the value of *x*?

    (A) 39
    (B) 45
    (C) 52
    (D) 62

11. If $90 \div x = 9n$, then what is the value of *nx*?

    (A) 10
    (B) 9x
    (C) 900
    (D) 90xn

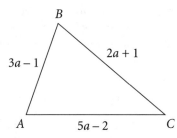

12. If the perimeter of triangle *ABC* is 28 meters, what is the number of meters in the length of *AC*?

    (A) 28
    (B) 13
    (C) 10
    (D) 12 .

13. A student finishes the first half of an exam in $\frac{2}{3}$ the time it takes him to finish the second half. If the entire exam takes him an hour, how many minutes does he spend on the first half of the exam?

    (A) 20
    (B) 24
    (C) 27
    (D) 36

14. A machine labels 150 bottles in 20 minutes. At this rate, how many minutes does it take to label 60 bottles?

    (A) 2
    (B) 4
    (C) 6
    (D) 8

15. For what value of *y* is $4(y - 5) = 2(y + 3)$?

    (A) −13
    (B) 13
    (C) 7
    (D) −8

16. If a man earns $200 for his first 40 hours of work in a week and then is paid one-and one-half times his regular rate for any additional hours, how many hours must he work to make $230 in a week?

    (A) 43
    (B) 44
    (C) 45
    (D) 46

17. In a group of 25 students, 16 are female. What percent of the group is female?

    (A) 16%
    (B) 40%
    (C) 60%
    (D) 64%

GO ON TO THE NEXT PAGE

**KAPLAN**

18. What is the average (arithmetic mean) of $\frac{1}{20}$ and $\frac{1}{30}$?

    (A) $\frac{1}{25}$

    (B) $\frac{1}{24}$

    (C) $\frac{2}{25}$

    (D) $\frac{1}{12}$

19. If a barrel has the capacity to hold 75 gallons, how many gallons does it contain when it is $\frac{3}{5}$ full?

    (A) 45

    (B) 48

    (C) 54

    (D) 60

20. If an angle measures $y°$, what will its supplement measure in terms of $y$?

    (A) $90 - y$

    (B) $90 + y$

    (C) $180 - y$

    (D) $180 + y$

21. If a tree grew 5 feet in $n$ years, what was the average rate at which the tree grew, in inches per year?

    (A) $\frac{60}{n}$

    (B) $\frac{5}{12n}$

    (C) $\frac{12n}{5}$

    (D) $\frac{n}{60}$

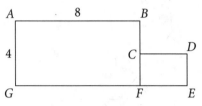

22. In the above diagram, $ABFG$ and $CDEF$ are rectangles, $C$ bisects $BF$, and $EF$ has a length of 2 cm. What is the area, in cm$^2$, of the entire figure?

    (A) 36

    (B) 32

    (C) 16

    (D) 72

23. If $13 + a = 25 + b$, then $b - a = ?$

    (A) 38

    (B) 12

    (C) 8

    (D) −12

24. If a kilogram is equal to approximately 2.2 pounds, which of the following is the best approximation of the number of kilograms in one pound?

    (A) $\frac{5}{11}$

    (B) $\frac{3}{7}$

    (C) $\frac{3}{8}$

    (D) $\frac{1}{3}$

GO ON TO THE NEXT PAGE

**KAPLAN**

25. What is the average weight, in pounds, of the 5 people whose weights are listed in the following table ?

| Name | Weigh in Pounds |
|---|---|
| Chris | 150 |
| Anne | 153 |
| Malcolm | 154 |
| Paul | 157 |
| Sam | 151 |

(A) 153

(B) $153\frac{1}{2}$

(C) 154

(D) 155

26. Brad bought a radio on sale at a 20% discount from its regular price of $118. If there is an 8% sales tax that is calculated on the sale price, how much did Brad pay for the radio?

(A) $86.85

(B) $94.40

(C) $101.95

(D) $127.44

27. $\sqrt{104,906}$ is between

(A) 100 and 200

(B) 200 and 300

(C) 300 and 400

(D) 400 and 500

28. If the ratio of males to females in a group of students is 3:5, which of the following could be the total number of students in the group?

(A) 148

(B) 150

(C) 152

(D) 154

29. If 48 of the 60 seats on a bus were occupied, what percent of the seats were not occupied?

(A) 12%

(B) 15%

(C) 20%

(D) 25%

30. 36% of 18 is 18% of what number?

(A) 9

(B) 36

(C) 72

(D) 200

31. A delivery service charges $25.00 per pound for making a delivery. If there is an additional 8% sales tax, what is the cost of delivering an item that weighs $\frac{4}{5}$ of a pound?

(A) $20.00

(B) $21.60

(C) $22.60

(D) $24.00

32. A truck going at a rate of 20 miles per hour takes 6 hours to complete a trip. How many fewer hours would the trip have taken if the truck were traveling at a rate of 30 miles per hour?

(A) 4

(B) 3

(C) 2

(D) 1

GO ON TO THE NEXT PAGE

**KAPLAN**

49

A      B   C   D      E

33. In the figure above, $AB$ is twice the length of $BC$, $BC = CD$, and $DE$ is three times the length of $CD$. If $AE = 49$ cm, what is the length, in cm, of $BD$?

(A) 14

(B) 20

(C) 22

(D) 29

34. Ed has $100 more than Robert. After Ed spends $20 on groceries, he now has 5 times as much money as Robert. How much money does Robert have?

(A) $16

(B) $20

(C) $24

(D) $30

35. If $2m > 24$ and $3m < 48$, which of the following could NOT be a possible value for $m$?

(A) 13

(B) 14

(C) 15

(D) 16

36. What is the value of $x$ in the equation $(\frac{1}{2} + x = 6.5)$?

(A) 3.5

(B) 3.25

(C) 5.5

(D) 6

37. For all $x$, $3x^2 \times 5x^3 = ?$

(A) $8x^5$

(B) $8x^6$

(C) $15x^5$

(D) $15x^6$

38. Which of the following is not a prime number?

(A) 2

(B) 37

(C) 51

(D) 67

39. After a 5-hour flight from Newark, Harry arrives in Denver at 2:30 P.M. If the time in Newark is 2 hours later than the time in Denver, what was the time in Newark when Harry began the flight?

(A) 10:30 A.M.

(B) 11:30 A.M.

(C) 3:30 P.M.

(D) 5:30 P.M.

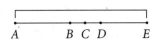

A      B   C   D      E

40. In the diagram above, if $AD = BE = 6$, $AE = 8$ and $CD = 3(BC)$, then $BC = ?$

(A) 4

(B) 3

(C) 2

(D) 1

41. If 75% of $x$ is 150, what is the value of $x$?

(A) 150

(B) 175

(C) 200

(D) 250

42. If $\dfrac{\sqrt{n}}{3}$ is an even integer, which of the following could be the value of $n$?

(A) 27

(B) 48

(C) 81

(D) 144

GO ON TO THE NEXT PAGE

43. If $2(a + m) = 5m - 3 + a$, what is the value of $a$, in terms of $m$?

    (A) $\dfrac{3m}{2}$

    (B) 3

    (C) $4m + 33$

    (D) $3m - 3$

44. If the product of 3 and $x$ is equal to 2 less than $y$, which of the following must be true?

    (A) $3x - \dfrac{2}{y} = 0$

    (B) $3x - y - 2 = 0$

    (C) $3x + y - 2 = 0$

    (D) $3x - y + 2 = 0$

45. Carla drove her truck 414 miles on 18 gallons of gasoline. How many miles did she drive per gallon?

    (A) 18

    (B) 23

    (C) 74

    (D) 95

46. In triangle $ABC$, the degree measures of the three interior angles are in the ratio of 1:2:3. What is the difference in the degree measures between the largest and the smallest angles?

    (A) 30

    (B) 60

    (C) 90

    (D) 120

47. If $5^n > 10,000$ and $n$ is an integer, what is the smallest possible value of $n$?

    (A) 8

    (B) 7

    (C) 6

    (D) 5

48. A carpenter is cutting wood to make a new bookcase with a board that is 12 feet long. If the carpenter cuts off 3 pieces, each of which is 17 inches long, how many inches long is the remaining board?

    (A) 36

    (B) 51

    (C) 93

    (D) 108

49. In 2000, the population of Town A was 9,400 and the population of Town B was 7,600. Since then, each year the population of Town A has decreased by 100 and the population of Town B has increased by 100. Assuming that in each case the rate continues, in what year will the two populations be equal?

    (A) 2009

    (B) 2010

    (C) 2017

    (D) 2018

50. If $x = \sqrt{5}$, $y = \dfrac{1}{3}$, and $z = 3$, then $x^2 - 4yz + z^2 = ?$

    (A) 30

    (B) 10

    (C) 2

    (D) 1

GO ON TO THE NEXT PAGE ⟹

**KAPLAN**

51. A total of 9 temperature readings were taken, one reading every 4 hours, with the first reading taken at 12 P.M. What will be the time when the final reading is taken?

    (A) 4 P.M.
    (B) 8 P.M.
    (C) 12 A.M.
    (D) 4 A.M.

52. A certain room measures 18 feet by 24 feet. What is the square yardage of a wall-to-wall carpet that covers the floor of the room?

    (A) 24 square yards
    (B) 32 square yards
    (C) 42 square yards
    (D) 48 square yards

53. If the minute hand of a properly functioning clock moves 45°, how many minutes have passed?

    (A) 6
    (B) 7.5
    (C) 12
    (D) 15

54. How many minutes are there in one week?

    (A) 3,600
    (B) 7,200
    (C) 10,080
    (D) 86,400

55. Rachel's average score after 6 tests is 83. If Rachel earns a score of 97 on the 7th test, what is her new average?

    (A) 85
    (B) 86
    (C) 87
    (D) 88

56. When 7.6 is divided by 0.019, the quotient is:

    (A) 4,000
    (B) 400
    (C) 40
    (D) 4

57. If $a < b$ and $b < c$, which of the following must be true?

    (A) $b + c < 2a$
    (B) $a + b < c$
    (C) $a - b < b - c$
    (D) $a + b < 2c$

58. A stock decreases in value by 25%. By what percent must the stock price increase to reach its former value?

    (A) 15%
    (B) 20%
    (C) $33\frac{1}{3}\%$
    (D) 40%

59. What is the radius of a circle whose circumference is $18\pi$ inches?

    (A) 3 in
    (B) 6 in
    (C) 18 in
    (D) 9 in

60. There are 587 people traveling by bus for a field trip. If each bus seats 48 people and all of the buses but one are filled to capacity, how many people sit in the unfilled bus?

    (A) 37
    (B) 36
    (C) 12
    (D) 11

GO ON TO THE NEXT PAGE

61. If $3^{n-7} = 81$, then $n = ?$

    (A)   4
    (B)   9
    (C)   11
    (D)   18

62. What is the area of a circle with a circumference of 8?

    (A)   $\dfrac{16}{\pi}$
    (B)   $4\pi$
    (C)   16
    (D)   $16\pi$

63. For what value of $y$ is $4(y-1) = 2(y+2)$ ?

    (A)   0
    (B)   2
    (C)   4
    (D)   6

64. Joan can shovel a certain driveway in 50 minutes. If Mary can shovel the same driveway in 20 minutes, how long will it take them, to the nearest minute, to shovel the driveway if they work together?

    (A)   12
    (B)   13
    (C)   14
    (D)   15

65. If the sides of a square increase in length by 10%, the area of the square increases by?

    (A)   10%
    (B)   15%
    (C)   20%
    (D)   21%

66. If the sum of 3 different prime numbers is an even number, what is the smallest of the 3?

    (A)   2
    (B)   3
    (C)   5
    (D)   It cannot be determined from the information given.

67. What is the number of rectangular tiles, each 12 centimeters by 18 centimeters, needed to completely cover 4 flat rectangular surfaces, each 60 centimeters by 180 centimeters?

    (A)   50
    (B)   100
    (C)   200
    (D)   400

68. If $\dfrac{c}{d} = 3$ and $d = 1$, then $3c + d = ?$

    (A)   4
    (B)   7
    (C)   9
    (D)   10

69. The average of 2 numbers is equal to twice the positive difference between the 2 numbers. If the larger number is 35, what is the smaller number?

    (A)   9
    (B)   15
    (C)   21
    (D)   27

GO ON TO THE NEXT PAGE

**KAPLAN**

70. Phil is making a 40-kilometer canoe trip. If he travels at 30 kilometers per hour for the first 10 kilometers, and then at 15 kilometers per hour for the rest of the trip, how many minutes more will it take him than if he travels the entire trip at 20 kilometers per hour?

   (A) 20
   (B) 24
   (C) 30
   (D) 40

71. What is the complete factorization of $2x + 3x^2 + x^3$?

   (A) $x(x-2)(x+3)$
   (B) $x(x-1)(x+2)$
   (C) $x(x+1)(x+2)$
   (D) $x(x+2)(x+3)$

72. A Ferris wheel has 12 cars that can seat up to 3 people each. If every car on the Ferris wheel is full except for 2 that contain 2 people and one that is empty, how many people are currently riding on the Ferris wheel?

   (A) 31
   (B) 32
   (C) 34
   (D) 35

73. A person 4 feet tall casts a 9-foot shadow at the same time that a nearby tree casts a 21-foot shadow. What is the height of this tree?

   (A) 7
   (B) $8\frac{1}{2}$
   (C) $9\frac{1}{3}$
   (D) 10

74. June's weekly salary is $70 less than Kelly's. Kelly's salary is $50 more than Eileen's. If Eileen earns $280 per week, how much does June earn per week?

   (A) $160
   (B) $260
   (C) $280
   (D) $300

75. Jim can run at a rate of 1 mile per 5 minutes and Rebecca can run at a rate of 1 mile per 8 minutes. If they both start at Point A at the same time and run in the same direction at their respective rates, how far ahead will Jim be from Rebecca in 40 minutes?

   (A) 3 miles
   (B) 5 miles
   (C) 8 miles
   (D) 15 miles

GO ON TO THE NEXT PAGE ⟶

## Science

1. If one parent is homozygous dominant and the other is homozygous recessive, which of the following might appear in an F2 generation, but not in an F1 generation?

    I. Heterozygous genotype
    II. Dominant phenotype
    III. Recessive phenotype

(A) I only
(B) II only
(C) III only
(D) I and II

2. Which of the following is a function of bone?

    I. Formation of blood cells.
    II. Protection of vital organs.
    III. Framework for movement.

(A) I only
(B) II only
(C) III only
(D) I, II, and III

3. The rate of breathing is controlled by involuntary centers in the:

(A) Cerebrum
(B) Cerebellum
(C) Medulla oblongata
(D) Spinal cord

4. Which of the following occurs in the cell nucleus?

    I. RNA synthesis
    II. Protein synthesis
    III. DNA synthesis

(A) I only
(B) II only
(C) III only
(D) I and III

5. In fruit flies, the gene for wing type is located on an autosomal chromosome. The allele for wild-type wings is dominant over the allele for vestigial wings. If a homozygous dominant male fly is crossed with a female with vestigial wings, what percentage of their female progeny are expected to have wild-type wings?

(A) 0%
(B) 25%
(C) 50%
(D) 100%

6. Members of an order are more alike than members of a:

(A) Class
(B) Family
(C) Genus
(D) Species

7. The process by which plants convert carbon dioxide and water into sugar and oxygen is called:

(A) Decomposition
(B) Photosynthesis
(C) Oxidation
(D) Respiration

8. Which of the following accurately describes the function of the hormone oxytocin?

(A) Increases uterine contractions during childbirth.
(B) Stimulates the release of glucose to the blood.
(C) Induces water resorption in the kidneys.
(D) Prepares the uterus for implantation of the fertilized egg.

GO ON TO THE NEXT PAGE

**KAPLAN**

9. Which blood type can be donated to anyone?

   (A) A
   (B) B
   (C) O
   (D) AB

10. A typical human gamete contains:

   (A) A total of 2 chromosomes.
   (B) A total of 23 chromosomes.
   (C) A total of 46 chromosomes.
   (D) A total of 92 chromosomes.

11. Color-blindness is a sex-linked recessive trait found on the X chromosome. If the incidence of color-blindness in a certain male population is 1 in 20, what would be the predicted incidence of colorblindness among females in the same population?

   (A) 1 in 20
   (B) 1 in 40
   (C) 1 in 200
   (D) 1 in 400

12. Most human digestion takes place in the:

   (A) Esophagus
   (B) Stomach
   (C) Small intestine
   (D) Large intestine

13. The order that includes man is called:

   (A) Chordata
   (B) Mammalia
   (C) Primate
   (D) Homidae

14. Insulin is created in the body's:

   (A) Adrenal glands
   (B) Kidneys
   (C) Pancreas
   (D) Thymus

15. If 2 brown-eyed parents have a blue-eyed child, the probability that their next child will have blue eyes is:

   (A) Zero
   (B) 1 in 2
   (C) 1 in 3
   (D) 1 in 4

16. Tough elastic tissues found in the joints that connect bones to bones are called:

   (A) Ligaments
   (B) Tendons
   (C) Cartilage
   (D) Muscles

17. Marsupial mammals differ from placental mammals in that:

   (A) Marsupials lay eggs.
   (B) Marsupial eggs contain very little yolk matter.
   (C) Marsupial umbilical cords do not contain blood vessels.
   (D) Marsupials bear premature embryos that complete development in their mothers' pouches.

18. Rods and cones are light-sensitive cells inside the eye's:

   (A) Cornea
   (B) Iris
   (C) Pupil
   (D) Retina

GO ON TO THE NEXT PAGE

19. Which of the following muscles are controlled by conscious thought?

    (A) Smooth

    (B) Striated

    (C) Cardiac

    (D) All of the above

20. The study of interactions between organisms and their interrelationships with the physical environment is known as:

    (A) Cytology

    (B) Ecology

    (C) Physiology

    (D) Embryology

21. Most of the nutrients in food are absorbed in the body's:

    (A) Stomach

    (B) Pylorus

    (C) Small intestine

    (D) Large intestine

22. Carbohydrates include:

    (A) Starches

    (B) Sugars

    (C) Both A and B are correct.

    (D) Neither A nor B is correct.

23. Which of the following is the phylum that includes man?

    (A) Animalia

    (B) Chordata

    (C) Mammalia

    (D) Primata

24. Which statement regarding protein synthesis is false?

    (A) tRNA molecules help incorporate the correct amino acids into proteins.

    (B) Proteins are formed on the ribosomes.

    (C) mRNAis not necessary for proper protein synthesis.

    (D) Ribosomal RNAis needed for proper binding of the mRNA message.

25. A typical human gamete:

    I. Contains a haploid number of genes.
    II. Will always contain an $X$ or a $Y$ chromosome.
    III. Is a result of mitosis.
    IV. Has undergone genetic recombination.

    (A) I and II

    (B) I and III

    (C) II and III

    (D) I, II, and IV

26. In adult humans, red blood cells:

    (A) Have no nucleus.

    (B) Are replaced in the liver.

    (C) Are outnumbered by white blood cells in the circulatory system.

    (D) Are made in the spleen.

27. Which of the following best describes tRNA?

    (A) Site of rRNA synthesis.

    (B) Product of transcription, encoding translated proteins.

    (C) Binds specific amino acids and carries them to the ribosomes during protein synthesis.

    (D) Contains the genome and is the site at which genes are used to make mRNA.

GO ON TO THE NEXT PAGE

**KAPLAN)**

28. Which statement about human gamete production is false?

    (A) In the testes, sperm develop in the seminiferous tubules.

    (B) In the ovaries, eggs develop in the ovarian follicles.

    (C) FSH stimulates gamete production in both sexes.

    (D) The result of meiosis in females is the production of four egg cells from each diploid precursor cell.

29. If a diabetic accidentally overdosed on insulin, which of the following would be likely to occur?

    (A) Increased levels of glucose in the blood.

    (B) Increased glucose concentration in urine.

    (C) Dehydration due to increased urine excretion.

    (D) Increased conversion of glucose to glycogen.

30. Saliva in the mouth begins the process of breaking down:

    (A) Starch

    (B) Fat

    (C) Protein

    (D) All of the above

31. Spermatogenesis and oogenesis differ in that:

    I. Meiosis proceeds continually without pausing in spermatogenesis, while oogenesis involves a meiotic pause.
    II. Spermatogenesis only occurs at puberty.
    III. Spermatogenesis produces four haploid sperm cells from each diploid precursor cell, while oogenesis produces one egg cell and two or more polar bodies.

    (A) I only

    (B) II only

    (C) III only

    (D) I and III

32. An individual that has only one $X$ chromosome is genotypically *XO*. This person:

    (A) Cannot survive.

    (B) Will have immature, ambiguous (both male and female) reproductive systems.

    (C) Will be phenotypically female but sterile.

    (D) Does not produce steroid hormones.

33. The first organisms on Earth were thought to be:

    (A) Autotrophs

    (B) Chemosynthetic

    (C) Heterotrophs

    (D) Oxygen producing

34. In an emergency, an individual with type *AB* antigen in his red blood cells may receive a transfusion of:

    I. Type O blood
    II. Type A blood
    III. Type B blood

    (A) I only

    (B) II only

    (C) II and III only

    (D) I, II, and III

35. Which of the following accurately describes the function of the hormone progesterone?

    (A) Increases human growth.

    (B) Stimulates the release of glucose to the blood.

    (C) Induces water resorption in the kidneys.

    (D) Prepares the uterus for implantation of the fertilized egg.

GO ON TO THE NEXT PAGE

**KAPLAN)**

36. The gene for color blindness is *X*-linked. If normal parents have a color-blind son, what is the probability that he inherited the gene for color blindness from his mother?

    (A)  0%

    (B)  25%

    (C)  50%

    (D) 100%

37. Which of the following depicts a chemical process?

    (A) Helium is combined with neon.

    (B) Iron forms rust.

    (C) Water causes soil erosion.

    (D) Ice melts.

38. The major portion of an atom's mass consists of:

    (A) Neutrons and protons

    (B) Electrons and protons

    (C) Electrons and neutrons

    (D) Neutrons and positrons

39. Orbiting around the nucleus of an atom are:

    (A) Anions

    (B) Electrons

    (C) Positrons

    (D) Photons

40. In degrees Kelvin, the freezing pointing of water is:

    (A) −273°

    (B)    0°

    (C)  100°

    (D)  273°

41. The atom of an element with an atomic number of 17 must have:

    (A) 17 electrons

    (B) 17 protons

    (C) 17 neutrons

    (D) An atomic mass of 17

42. An atom that is not electrically neutral is called:

    (A) An isotope

    (B) A positron

    (C) An ion

    (D) An allotrope

43. The sun's core consists primarily of $^1$H and $^4$He, as well as various other trace elements and isotopes. Which of the following statements is NOT true regarding the fusion reaction that occurs within the core?

    (A) Electrons are released as a product of the fusion reaction.

    (B) The mass of the products is less than the mass of the reactants in the balanced fusion equation.

    (C) Six photons are emitted as a product of the fusion reaction.

    (D) Four hydrogen atoms combine to form a single helium atom.

44. The greater the electronegativity of an atom:

    (A) The lesser its attraction for bonding electrons is.

    (B) The lesser its electron affinity is.

    (C) The greater its attraction for bonding electrons is.

    (D) The lesser its ionization energy is.

GO ON TO THE NEXT PAGE

**KAPLAN**

45. Noble gases:

   (A) Have low boiling points.

   (B) Are all gases at room temperature.

   (C) Are also called inert gases.

   (D) All of the above.

46. A pH below 7 indicates:

   (A) A relative excess of $OH^-$ ions.

   (B) A basic solution.

   (C) A relative shortage of $H^+$ ions.

   (D) None of the above.

47. Which of the following is NOT a classification of hydrocarbons?

   (A) Alkanes

   (B) Aromatics

   (C) Alkones

   (D) Alkenes

48. Electron affinity:

   (A) Is the energy that is released when an electron is added to a gaseous atom.

   (B) Represents the ease with which an atom can accept an electron.

   (C) Both A and B are correct.

   (D) Neither A nor B is correct.

49. The ability of a metal to be hammered into shapes is called:

   (A) Conductibility

   (B) Malleability

   (C) Reactivity

   (D) Resolvability

50. In the kinetic molecular theory of gases, which of the following statements concerning average speeds is true?

   (A) Most of the molecules are moving at the average speed.

   (B) Any given molecule moves at the average speed most of the time.

   (C) When the temperature increases, more of the molecules will move at the new average speed.

   (D) When the temperature increases, fewer molecules will move at the new average speed.

51. At high altitudes, the boiling point of water:

   (A) Is higher than at sea level.

   (B) Is lower than at sea level.

   (C) Is the same as at sea level.

   (D) Cannot be determined.

52. Which of the following is NOT true of an element that is very highly electronegative?

   (A) Its electron affinity is likely to be near zero.

   (B) It is likely to have a high level of ionization energy.

   (C) It is likely to have a small atomic radius.

   (D) It is likely to be located in the upper right hand corner of the periodic table.

53. Which of the following represents Avogadro's number?

   (A) $1.66 \times 10^{-24}$

   (B) $1.0 \times 10^{24}$

   (C) $6.022 \times 10^{23}$

   (D) $3.011 \times 10^{23}$

GO ON TO THE NEXT PAGE ⇨

**KAPLAN**

54. In electricity, a unit of resistance is called a(n):

    (A) Ampere

    (B) Ohm

    (C) Volt

    (D) Watt

55. As an ambulance passes, its pitch seems to change. This perception is best explained by:

    (A) Convection

    (B) Refraction

    (C) The Doppler effect

    (D) Momentum

56. Which of the following states of electromagnetic radiation has the longest wavelength and lowest frequency?

    (A) Radio waves

    (B) Microwaves

    (C) Gamma rays

    (D) Visible light

57. All of the following statements about weight are true EXCEPT:

    (A) Weight increases closer to Earth's surface.

    (B) Weight is not dependent on mass.

    (C) Weight is greater on planets with greater mass.

    (D) Weight varies from location to location.

58. Resistance is measured in:

    (A) Amperes

    (B) Ohms

    (C) $\Omega$

    (D) B and C are correct.

59. One pound of force is applied to move an object a distance of one foot. The amount of work that has been done is _____ .

    (A) 1 foot-pound

    (B) 1 watt

    (C) 1 joule

    (D) Both B and C are correct.

60. A material that will not conduct electricity is known as:

    (A) A conductor

    (B) A semiconductor

    (C) An insulator

    (D) None of the above

61. All of the following statements about energy are true EXCEPT:

    (A) Energy cannot be created.

    (B) The amount of energy in the universe is slowly diminishing.

    (C) Energy cannot be destroyed.

    (D) Energy can be converted from one form into another.

62. A boulder that begins to roll down a hill is an example of an energy conversion from:

    (A) Potential to thermal.

    (B) Potential to kinetic.

    (C) Kinetic to thermal.

    (D) Kinetic to potential.

GO ON TO THE NEXT PAGE

**KAPLAN**

63. A policeman fires a handgun during target practice. His weapon recoils slightly as he fires because:

   (A) For every action, there is an equal but opposite reaction.

   (B) The bullet exerts a smaller force on the gun than the gun exerts on the bullet.

   (C) The policeman slipped as the gun was fired.

   (D) None of the above.

64. Meters per second is a measure of:

   (A) Acceleration

   (B) Speed

   (C) Gravity

   (D) All of the above

65. The energy of movement is known as:

   (A) Potential energy

   (B) Chemical energy

   (C) Electromotive energy

   (D) Kinetic energy

END OF TEST. STOP

THE ANSWER KEY APPEARS ON THE FOLLOWING PAGE.

# Practice Test Two: **Answer Key**

| Reading Comprehension | | Vocabulary and Spelling | | Mathematics | | | Science | |
|---|---|---|---|---|---|---|---|---|
| 1. B | 24. A | 1. C | 34. D | 1. C | 26. C | 51. B | 1. C | 34. D |
| 2. D | 25. C | 2. C | 35. C | 2. C | 27. C | 52. D | 2. D | 35. D |
| 3. B | 26. D | 3. A | 36. B | 3. A | 28. C | 53. B | 3. C | 36. D |
| 4. D | 27. B | 4. C | 37. D | 4. C | 29. C | 54. C | 4. D | 37. B |
| 5. D | 28. D | 5. D | 38. D | 5. C | 30. B | 55. A | 5. D | 38. A |
| 6. D | 29. B | 6. D | 39. A | 6. B | 31. B | 56. B | 6. A | 39. B |
| 7. B | 30. D | 7. D | 40. D | 7. D | 32. C | 57. D | 7. B | 40. D |
| 8. C | 31. C | 8. A | 41. A | 8. A | 33. A | 58. C | 8. A | 41. B |
| 9. B | 32. D | 9. B | 42. D | 9. C | 34. B | 59. D | 9. C | 42. C |
| 10. D | 33. C | 10. D | 43. D | 10. C | 35. D | 60. D | 10. B | 43. A |
| 11. B | 34. B | 11. C | 44. D | 11. A | 36. D | 61. C | 11. D | 44. C |
| 12. C | 35. B | 12. B | 45. A | 12. B | 37. C | 62. A | 12. C | 45. D |
| 13. B | 36. D | 13. A | 46. D | 13. B | 38. C | 63. C | 13. C | 46. D |
| 14. D | 37. C | 14. B | 47. B | 14. D | 39. B | 64. C | 14. C | 47. C |
| 15. A | 38. D | 15. A | 48. D | 15. B | 40. D | 65. D | 15. D | 48. C |
| 16. C | 39. A | 16. C | 49. B | 16. B | 41. C | 66. A | 16. A | 49. B |
| 17. D | 40. D | 17. D | 50. A | 17. D | 42. D | 67. C | 17. D | 50. D |
| 18. D | 41. D | 18. A | 51. D | 18. B | 43. D | 68. D | 18. D | 51. B |
| 19. D | 42. C | 19. C | 52. D | 19. A | 44. D | 69. C | 19. B | 52. A |
| 20. D | 43. B | 20. D | 53. C | 20. C | 45. B | 70. A | 20. B | 53. C |
| 21. C | 44. D | 21. A | 54. B | 21. A | 46. B | 71. C | 21. C | 54. B |
| 22. B | 45. A | 22. D | 55. D | 22. A | 47. C | 72. A | 22. C | 55. C |
| 23. D | | 23. A | 56. A | 23. D | 48. C | 73. C | 23. B | 56. A |
| | | 24. C | 57. C | 24. A | 49. A | 74. B | 24. C | 57. B |
| | | 25. D | 58. B | 25. A | 50. B | 75. A | 25. D | 58. D |
| | | 26. A | 59. D | | | | 26. A | 59. A |
| | | 27. D | 60. B | | | | 27. C | 60. C |
| | | 28. C | 61. C | | | | 28. D | 61. B |
| | | 29. A | 62. C | | | | 29. D | 62. B |
| | | 30. B | 63. B | | | | 30. A | 63. A |
| | | 31. D | 64. A | | | | 31. D | 64. B |
| | | 32. A | 65. A | | | | 32. C | 65. D |
| | | 33. B | | | | | 33. C | |

# Answers and Explanations

## Reading Comprehension

**1.    B**

There's no way to predict an answer here, so jump right into the answer choices. But read carefully! Tempting choices like (C) can be wrong because of a single word. (A) is too extreme. The passage states that hypnosis is useful for managing pain, but it's never implied that it is the *most* effective means. (C) is incorrect because it was controversial, *until recently*. (D) is the opposite case. Hypnosis is also used to speed the healing of bones. (B) is correct. Until recently, hypnosis was "marginal" and "controversial." It makes sense to say that it was regarded with some suspicion.

**2.    D**

Watch out for common meanings that are not appropriate in the sentence. Here, the word *excruciating,* which means "agonizing" or "extremely intense," suggests that patients may live with, but not get rid of, the pain. Your answer should reflect this shade of meaning. Burn victims are unlikely to be able to *direct* pain, so (A) is out. *Administer,* (B), makes no sense here, even tough it is one meaning of manage. (C) is the opposite case: Patients want to minimize pain, not bring it about. The pain is not fixed; it is only "coped with," choice (D).

**3.    B**

This question sends you back to the first paragraph. What accounts for the road's being so well preserved? The remains were buried under a layer of acidic peat, which kept the wood moist, prevented decay from bacteria, and kept nosy animals away. (A) may have given you pause, since a lack of interfering animals is mentioned in the first paragraph. But it wasn't the location of the road that kept animals away; it was the fact that the road was buried, so the animals couldn't get to it. (C) and (D) might seem to offer reasonable explanations for the road's good condition, but the passage never mentions light travel patterns or development prohibitions.

**4.    D**

Reread the sentence in which *acidic* is mentioned. It says that the "acidic peat" allowed for three conditions that caused the road to be preserved: It kept it moist, relatively free of bacteria, and free from animal interference. So the fact that the bog was "acidic" must have something to do with causing those conditions. Only (D) mentions one of these three conditions, so it's the answer. (A) and (C) bring in unmentioned issues, and (B) is incorrect because the author never mentions noncorrosive materials as a factor that kept the road in such good shape.

**5.    D**

You're asked why the author describes the construction of the Sweet Track. In the last sentence, it says that method of construction "is remarkably sophisticated, testifying to a surprisingly advanced level of technology, which is (D). (B) and (C) point to conclusions the author makes elsewhere in the passage. (A) talks about the *unusual strength* of the road, which the author never discusses.

**6.    D**

The key to this question is in the last sentence of the first paragraph. The author discusses how Sweet Track's remains tell us a great deal about the Neolithic people who built it—a focus best summed up by (D). (B) is probably the closest wrong choice, but it's only half of the main focus. The author does focus on the complex construction and composition of the road, but for a purpose—to discuss what that construction and composition tells us about the builders of the road. (A) is too broad. (C) is too narrow. The survival of the road over 6,000 years (C) is the purpose of just the end of the first paragraph.

**7.    B**

To find out why the author brings up *ring analysis,* re-read the fourth paragraph. The road "seems to have been completed in a very short time." How do we know? Because "tree-ring analysis," the topic of this question, confirms that the trees used to build the road were all felled within a single year. So tree-ring analysis offers evidence to support the claim that the Sweet Track was built quickly; choice (B). Choice (A) may seem plausible, because we usually count tree-rings to find out how old trees are. But in the fourth paragraph, tree-ring analysis was used for another purpose. The other choices raise issues discussed elsewhere. Those *sophisticated building techniques*, (C), were the subject of the second paragraph, while the fancy lumbering technique mentioned in (D) were brought up in the third paragraph and have nothing to do with the tree-ring analysis mentioned in the fourth paragraph.

**8. C**

What is the cited example of "woodland management" that the question refers to? When you go to the passage, you'll find it's called "coppicing." Coppicing is described as the process of felling trees "in such a way as to encourage the rapid growth of long, straight, rod-like shoots from the remaining stumps, to be used as pegs." In other words, trees are grown in a special way in order to yield *special* materials—that is, the rod-like shoots. (A) and (D) have nothing to do with the paragraph. (B) may sound plausible, but the process described here focuses not on the *kind* of trees being planted, but rather the *way* they are planted.

**9. B**

This question directs you to that interesting last paragraph we discussed above—the one that cautions not to form too many generalized opinions relating to the Sweet Track. The author says the Sweet Track represents "the work of a single isolated community," and that therefore we shouldn't use it to make conclusions about all Neolithic communities. (A) and (D) are not the subject of the last paragraph; besides, they're just plain incorrect. (C) is a distortion. The reason we shouldn't draw generalized conclusions from the Sweet Track is because it's the work of just one small community, not because the road has been studied too little.

**10. D**

From the word *NOT* in the question stem, you know to look for something that has either remained constant or decreased. The *rate* of attacks hasn't increased, though the total number *has* increased. That's because the total number of swimmers has increased. Think of it this way: If the number of total swimmers was 5 and there was 1 attack, that would be a rate of 1-in-5. If later, there were 15 swimmers and 3 attacks, the rate would still be 1-in-5, though the total number of attacks increased from 1 to 3. The rate hasn't increased, but this doesn't mean that the total number hasn't increased. (A) is incorrect. (B) is contradicted in the text. With (C), the text distinguishes

between fatal attacks and other attacks only in the last sentence. Since only one period is cited 1990–2000, you don't know if this is an increase or not.

**11. B**

Before citing the number of fatal attacks, the author says to "keep the issue in perspective." So, the statistic should show that the total number of attacks is fairly small. The correct answer choice should be consistent with this moderate, balanced approach. (A) and (D) are never mentioned. As for (C), you don't know if this is a decrease, since no other statistics are given for comparison.

**12. C**

Before writing, we're told, the wisdom of generations was passed down in two ways—verbally, and *to a lesser extent*, in pictures, carvings, and statues. This means that the wisdom of the past was transmitted less frequently by nonverbal means and thus (C) *more frequently by the spoken word than by other means.* Choices (A) and (B) *distort* this idea. Nowhere are we told that wisdom was rejected, and since spoken words *and* pictures were both used, it was obviously not an all or nothing proposition. (D), finally, makes no sense at all—the author never says that all ancient wisdom was fiction.

**13. B**

The question asks why the author discusses the impact of writing. In the passage, we're told that writing has made the transmission of information about the past a lot more precise and extensive. Pictures and photography are also mentioned as ways in which the experience of the past has been passed down. So choice (B) is correct here—writing is mentioned as an *example* of how cultures record knowledge about the past. (A) is a distortion—the author is showing us something about the past, not why we remember hardly anything. He never implies any criticism of preliterate cultures, so choice (C) is incorrect too. Choice (D) is incorrect because the author never mentions it in the context referred to or in the whole passage.

**14. D**

Give the context a quick scan. Once again, the author is talking about how difficult it is to understand vast stretches of time. We're told that it's like a blind man building up a sensory picture of his surroundings. This is an *indirect* process, so choice (D) is right. Choice (C) is dealt with later in the fourth paragraph, so you can eliminate it right away. (A) is too sweeping. The author never says that human beings are *completely unable to comprehend time.* (B) has nothing to do with the passage.

**15. A**

Inference skills are required here. What is the author's underlying point in mentioning the Big Bang and the Cambrian Period? The author *introduces* this discussion in the cited passage by saying that *a week* provides a better yardstick for the age of the Earth than a day. The Big Bang and the Cambrian Period are used as examples to support this point. So (A) is right—it's the point about the time scale that the author's trying to demonstrate. Choice (D) distorts the point in a different way. The author is suggesting that the week is a better scale. The development of *agriculture,* as presented in choice (B), is another supporting example like the Big Bang and the Cambrian Period, but it's not the author's central point. Finally, *fossils* have nothing to do with the question at hand, so (C) is easily eliminated.

**16. C**

A more straightforward comprehension question this time. When we go back to the passage, we're told about the problem with linear maps: When one is produced that's big enough to show our place on it, the map becomes too big to study and reproduce conveniently. (C) gets the right paraphrase here. Notice especially the match up in synonyms for *convenient reproduction* and *examination*. (A) and (B) aren't supported here. (D) doesn't address the problem. The question is about getting our human experience on the map.

**17. D**

What's the overall point the author is trying to prove? The big picture is that life started on Earth so long ago that it is difficult for us to comprehend. Everything that follows is meant to illustrate this point, including the time scales. Don't let the material confuse you. The point is (D)—*the immensity of time* since the origin of *life.* (C) is tricky to reject because it's an aspect of the larger argument, but it's not the whole point. The other wrong choices mention issues that the author hardly touches on. In paragraphs 4–6, the author's *not* concerned with getting dates right (A), or the question of how life actually began (B).

**18. D**

After the cited sentence, the author describes many effects that Franklin's experiment had. The sentence sets up this idea, conveying that the experiment was important. (A) assumes that *pronounced* takes on the meaning of *declared* or *stated*, but that isn't appropriate for the text. There's nothing in the text to indicate that the experiment was *stated*. (B) is out of scope. The experiment itself was famous, but we don't know that Franklin was. (Be careful here; even though we know from history that Benjamin Franklin was quite famous indeed, there is nothing in the text that tells us that. On the test, you should not use your previous knowledge of a topic; you should use only the information presented on the test. That is all that will be necessary to answer the question.) (C) is tempting. It's close, but it's not entirely complete. The effects of Franklin's experiment also included practical and cultural effects—lightning rods, and dispelling a misunderstanding of lightning. True, it had a large impact in the scientific world, but those were not the only consequences.

**19. D**

You can't make a prediction, so jump into the answer choices. (A) is the opposite case: The experiment helped to *dispel* a superstitious belief, not promote it, (B) and (C) are misused details. The text doesn't say that Franklin studied gravity; gravity is simply mentioned as an example of another natural force. And though Franklin used a Leyden jar, we don't know he helped to develop it. (D) makes sense. The experiment had a cultural effect in "show[ing] that scientific research could have practical benefits."

**20. D**

The author describes the *function* of the ozone layer. We're told that the ozone layer "protects the Earth from UV radiation," which is "harmful to all living organisms." Choice (D) is the closest analogy here. It captures the idea of something which constantly provides protection against a life-threatening force. The *evacuation plan* mentioned in (A) only helps in *emergencies.* None of the other choices—(B) *information desks* nor (C) *traffic lights* are facilities designed to provide protection against specific threats.

**21. C**

The "seasonal variations" noticed in 1958 were initially regarded as the "natural effects of wind and temperature."

According to the passage, it was only much later that the connection between CFCs and ozone depletion became known. Therefore, we can infer that in 1958, these seasonal variations *were not regarded as a threat,* making (C) correct and (B) and (D) incorrect. No other items that lead to *ozone depletion* are mentioned (A).

**22. B**

The key word is *while,* because it indicates a contrast. We're told that *while* the low October levels stayed *constant,* ozone levels as a whole *diminished,* or fell. *Unlike* the overall figures, in other words, the October levels did not fluctuate—they remained (B) *steady.* (A), *gentle,* and (C), *pestering,* are unlikely words to use to describe atmospheric measurements. (D), *unerring* suggests that the accuracy of scientists' measurements is the issue.

**23. D**

The author's point is implied in the first two lines of the paragraph. We're told that CFCs represent a sizeable market. Then we're told that in spite of this, people began to question the risks to human health when CFCs were implicated in ozone depletion. So the author's point in mentioning the CFC market is that the dangers of using CFCs *overshadowed* the *economic* considerations (D). (A) can't be inferred from the context. The author doesn't explicitly blame industry for the problem. (B) is incorrect because the author makes no mention of *benefits.* (C) gets the issue wrong; it was the health risks, not *industry profits,* that *turned public opinion.*

**24. A**

Here the author's giving us a progress report on ozone depletion in the 1990s. We're told the layer was "depleting faster than expected" in addition to natural events "making the problem worse." (A) summarizes this idea that the situation is worsening. The sixth paragraph describes the problem as a whole, without relating it to any particular species, even though threats to *marine species* (B) and *plant life* (C) are mentioned elsewhere. (D) goes against the gist of the passage, which basically identifies CFCs as the main culprits.

**25. C**

The passage says that scientists believe that natural events are "making the problem worse," and the volcanic gases emitted by the Pinatubo volcano are mentioned as one

example. (C) is the correct answer. (A) *global warming* isn't mentioned until the eighth paragraph. (B) distorts the author's point; *CFCs* are still the biggest *threat.* Since the gases are adding to a *long-term* problem, (D) must be incorrect.

**26. D**

Even stopping all CFC production today wouldn't solve the problem, we're told, because CFCs can live for up to 400 years. (D) captures the underlying point here; measures against ozone depletion may take years to have an effect. Choice (A) doesn't fit with the passage at all. (B) is too positive; the author's saying the problem's going to take years to fix, not that there's plenty of time to deal with it. There's no mention of the implications for *human health,* (C), in the seventh paragraph.

**27. B**

The last paragraph focuses on what scientists are doing about the problem. Even if things are bad, the author says, "nobody can say that the situation will not improve" if people lend a hand. (B) captures this positive note. (A) exaggerates the obstacles to research discussed at the beginning of the paragraph. Choices (C) and (D) just accept ozone depletion as a fact of life, which is not the author's position at all.

**28. D**

We need either a choice that describes the similarity between the theories, or one that falsifies information about them. (D) should raise your suspicions. The author acknowledged at the end of the first paragraph that the first theory could account for the entire observed hierarchy of material structure. (D) is right, but let's look at the others. (A) is a valid difference between the two theories—the second is presented as a simpler alternative to the first. (B) is also a real difference. The first theory encompasses gravitation and the second unifies three of the four forces, which makes it a better theory, but it doesn't account for gravitation. The first theory includes leptons and quarks, while the second combines these two classes into just one, so (C) is valid.

**29. B**

This question asks for the primary purpose, and we know that the author is concerned with theories that describe, simply and precisely, particles and their forces. The author's primary purpose is to describe attempts to develop a simplified theory of nature. Skimming through the choices, (B) looks good. As for (A), the author doesn't cite a misconception in either of the theories he describes. At most, he mentions ways in which the first could be simplified but this doesn't imply that there's a misconception. The author does refer to the second theory as a leading candidate for achieving unification, but predicting its success, (C), is far from his primary purpose. As for (D), although it's implied that scientists in general do prefer simpler theories, their reasons for this preference are never discussed.

## 30. D

In the first paragraph we're told that quarks are constituents of the proton and the neutron. It's reasonable, then, to say that quarks are the elementary building blocks of protons and neutrons, option I. Since option I is correct, we can eliminate the choice that excludes it, (B). The remaining choices are either I only, I and II only, or I, II, and III. You could skip II and go to III. If you're sure III is right, you can assume that II is also and pick (D). It turns out that III can be easily checked at the end of the third paragraph, where the author states that a new theory incorporates the leptons and quarks into a single family or class, so option III is correct. For a complete list, let's look at option II. In the very first sentence the author tells us that elementary particles don't have an internal structure and since quarks are elementary particles, option II is indeed correct, and (D) is our answer.

## 31. C

It should be clear the author has some very definite criteria for judging the usefulness or worth of various theories of nature. As for option I, *simplicity* should leap off the page at you—it's what this passage is all about. We can eliminate (B). The author also takes the theory's completeness into consideration. He commends the first theory he describes because it accounts for the entire observed hierarchy of material structure and therefore option II is correct. We know that (C) must be correct because there is no I, II, and III choice. But let's look at III anyway. Does the author ever mention proving either of those two theories he describes? Proof is of no concern to him—there's no mention in the passage of any experiments, or of wanting to find experimental proof. So III is incorrect.

## 32. D

We've mentioned the second theory doesn't include gravitation in its attempt to unify the four basic forces. We need the author's opinion about this omission. The author introduces the theory in the second paragraph, describing it as an ambitious theory that promises at least a partial unification of elementary particles and forces. The failure to include gravitation and achieve complete unification doesn't dampen the author's enthusiasm and he seems to suggest that gravitation's omission can't be helped, at least at this stage. So, although the omission is a limitation—it prevents total unification—it is also unavoidable. It looks like (D) does the trick. You could see the limitation as a defect, (A), but the author never gives the impression that the omission of gravitation disqualifies the theory. As for (B), *deviation* is a funny word—deviation from what? More important, we've already seen that the author doesn't consider the omission to be unjustified. For the same reason, (C) can be eliminated. If the omission of gravitation can't be avoided, then it certainly isn't a needless oversimplification.

## 33. C

This question shouldn't be difficult. It asks us to put ourselves in the author's shoes and figure out what sort of theory he would find superior to present theories. We already know—a simpler theory. The author's criteria for judging a theory are its simplicity and its ability to account for the largest possible number of known phenomena. Which choice represents a theory with one or both of these characteristics? (A) misrepresents the two theories described in the passage. The author says that the first theory could account for the entire observed hierarchy of material structure. The second does also, even though gravitation must be thrown in as a separate force. A theory that could account for a larger number of structures isn't what's needed. As for (B), why would the author approve of a theory that reduces the four basic forces to two which are incompatible? (C) is on the right track. The author would prefer a theory that accounts for all matter with the fewest particles and forces and this is offered by (C), the correct answer. (D) is incorrect because it wouldn't represent an improvement on currently existing theories. They account for gravitation, although they haven't yet unified it with the other three forces.

**34. B**

The topic of this passage is Emile Durkheim's study of social cohesion in society and the author's purpose might be summed up as describing two different ways that societies can maintain social integration among their members. A road map of the paragraph structure might look like this: The first paragraph introduces Durkheim and his study of social groups; the second paragraph discusses two ways societies can maintain social integration; the third paragraph offers a broader context for interpreting the evidence in the second paragraph. The final paragraph gives you the key to answering this global question. The author is describing different ways societies can function without choosing a side or advocating a specific position. You can rule out (A) immediately for its strong stand. (C) distorts a detail beyond its acceptable scope. While the passage does discuss how social cohesion can function in societies with high degrees of labor specialization, this is not the author's main goal. (D) takes a prescriptive stance, and the author never tells us how to live our lives.

**35. B**

What is the crucial difference between *mechanical solidarity* and *organic solidarity*? The level of homogeneity in the group in which each functions. Neither one relies on any measure, objective or otherwise, of group coherence. Rather, they describe the way societies function naturally, ruling out (A). (C) introduces the notion of rebellion, a concept that is not mentioned in the passage and hence, cannot be correct. (D) is incorrect because the two types of solidarity were developed at the same time by Durkheim; we do not have a traditional view and a more recent view of the same phenomenon, but rather two different ways that societies can function within the same worldview.

**36. D**

In this inference question, you will need to think about the author's opinion as you approach the answer choices. (A) is outside the scope, as the relationship of individual societies to the world-at-large is not an issue that concerns the author. (B) makes a subjective statement about Durkheim that is never suggested by the passage. (C) makes a comparison between the two types of social groups that is not supported by the passage. (D), however, is basically a close paraphrase of the final paragraph of the passage. The particular type of integration that exists within a given society is less important than that it is present in some form.

**37. C**

In this detail question, you should research the second paragraph, where *organic solidarity* is discussed. There you'll find Durkheim's reasoning for why it exists in societies with high levels of heterogeneity. *Organic solidarity* prevails in societies with fewer similarities among members because when a society is highly specialized its members rely on each other out of necessity—as a way to ensure that everyone's needs are met. Reading through the answers, (C) should jump out at you as conveying this sentiment. (A) is the opposite of what we want. In societies in which *organic solidarity* dominates, individual differences are relatively high. (B) implies a causal relationship between *organic solidarity* and the way a society is organized, but *organic solidarity* is simply a term to describe the way a society *is* functioning; it is not an active agent of anything. (D) uses information that was never mentioned in the passage—namely, that some societies are more likely to be affected by social stressors.

**38. D**

The passage gives the example of the corridor of land from Alaska to the southeastern United States to show how bears easily distributed themselves throughout the region. Thus, it can be inferred that the studies of faunal interchange help explain how animal populations arose.

**39. A**

The passage describes each of the migratory routes in terms of the difficulty of passing them, or the probability that migration will occur. Choice (A) is correct.

**40. D**

There is no support for statement I in the passage, so choice (D) is the correct answer.

**41. D**

The last sentence of the passage gives the answer to the question: *As the name suggests, negotiation of a sweepstakes route depends almost exclusively on chance, rather than on physical attributes and adaptability.* Choice (D) is the correct answer.

**42. C**

In an "all are true EXCEPT" question, concentrate on eliminating any answer choices that are true according to the passage. Eliminate choice (A) because it is true according to the first sentence. The second sentence says that choice (B) is true, so eliminate it too. Sentence four says that adults enjoyed the early Hula Hoops, so (C) must be false. (C) is the correct answer. The last two sentences of the passage show how (D) must be true since they describe how the Hula Hoop was a hit for the "fledgling" toy company.

**43. B**

Eliminate answer choices that are too broad, too narrow, or not mentioned in the passage. (A) is too broad—the passage doesn't include any information on fads besides the Hula Hoop. (B) is the correct answer: The passage starts with the earliest origins of the hoop toy and ends up with the popularization of the Hula Hoop. (C) is too narrow: only one sentence in the passage explains how the name came about. The passage says that the Hula Hoop is popular, (D), but doesn't address why.

**44. D**

The passage discusses a few ways to distinguish a crocodile from an alligator. The first and most easily observed of these is the fact that the crocodile's head and jaws are longer and narrower; in other words, it has a narrower snout, choice (D). (A) is incorrect, because the animals' mouths do not necessarily have to be closed to distinguish one from the other. Choice (B) is incorrect because both animals can be found in the Everglades National Park, and (C) is never discussed as one of the ways to distinguish one giant reptile from the other.

**45. A**

The passage says that *both alligators and crocodiles can be found in southern Florida, particularly in the Everglades National Park.* From this you can infer the Everglades are in southern Florida.

## Vocabulary and Spelling

**1. C**

*Noble* means *appearing in a majestic or royal fashion.*

**2. C**

Judicious means *possessing or displaying good judgment,* or in other words, being *fair.*

**3. A**

Note that choice (A) is the word *required*, which has the same root as the given word. In this case, those roots are the same.

**4. C**

The verb *to coax* means *to try to persuade*.

**5. D**

*Terminal* means *relating to an end, limit or boundary.*

**6. D**

*Augment* means *to enhance something already developed.*

**7. D**

*Tactile* means *relating to the sense of touch*. Of the answer choices, (D), *tangible*, is the most similar in meaning to the original word.

**8. A**

To *germinate* means to *sprout, seed, or bud.*

**9. B**

*Restore* has the prefix "re-", meaning *again*. Thus, restore means *bring back something that had been lost*. Of the choices given, both (B) and (D) refer to affecting change on something. But of the two, only (B), *invigorate*, means to renew.

**10. D**

A *filament* is any *thread or string that is very thin.*

**11. C**

*Congeal* means to *solidify, coagulate, or harden.*

**12. B**

*Impose* as a verb means to *establish by authority*. Of the answer choices given, only one seems to imply one person dictating to another. *Force* as a verb can be construed as *imposing*. Thus, answer choice (B) is correct.

**13. A**

*Stunted* means *stopped short* or *cancelled abruptly*. Answer choice (A), *halted*, also means stopped short.

**14. B**

*Longevity* means *length of life*, so choice (B), *lifetime*, is correct.

**15. A**

*Mutable* means *prone to change*. Choice (A), *changing*, is the best answer.

**16. C**

A *virtuoso* has great skill. An *incompetent* describes one who can't do something adequately.

**17. D**

To *polarize* is to cause to concentrate around two conflicting positions. *Unite* means "bring together as one."

**18. A**

*Whimsical* means playful. *Grave* means very serious, so it is correct.

**19. C**

A *dandy* is one who is very elegant in dress or manners. *Careless dresser* is the opposite.

**20. D**

To *mar* is to damage in a way that makes something less attractive or perfect. *Enhance* means "to increase the value or beauty" of something. If you needed to guess, you could eliminate *flatter* and *praise* because they're synonyms.

**21. A**

To *disperse* means to scatter; the opposite is gather.

**22. D**

To *hamper* means hinder or interfere with; the opposite is assist.

**23. A**

*Aptitude* is ability; the opposite is inability.

**24. C**

*Gullible* means naïve or easily deceived; the opposite is incredulous.

**25. D**

To *replenish* means to provide more; the opposite is deplete.

**26. A**

*Abundant* means plenty, so the opposite is scarce.

**27. D**

*Wary* means careful; the opposite is careless.

**28. C**

*Sedentary* means seated or inactive; the opposite is active.

**29. A**

*Rudimentary* means basic; the opposite is advanced.

**30. B**

To *convoke* is to assemble in a group; the opposite is disperse.

**31. D**

A *shard* is a broken fragment of *glass* or crockery. Glass, when it shatters, creates shards, so a shard is a piece of broken glass. (D) shows the same analogy—a *splinter* is a piece of broken *wood*. As for the incorrect choices, in (A), a *grain* is the basic unit that *sand* comes in, but you can't talk about breaking sand. In (B), a *rope* is composed of *strands,* and in (C), a *quilt* is made from *scraps*. The correct answer is (D).

**32. A**

The word *filter* is used as a verb. When you use a filter, an *impurity* is removed, so you *filter* to remove an *impurity*. The word *expurgate* in (A) means to censor, to remove *obscenities*—you *expurgate* to remove an *obscenity*. To *whitewash*, (B), is to misrepresent a bad thing to make it look better. An *infraction* isn't removed by *whitewashing* it, it's only covered up, so (B) isn't parallel. In (C), *perjury* is the crime of lying under oath. To *testify* doesn't mean to remove a false statement. In (D), *penance* is something you do to atone for a sin, but you don't *perform* to remove *penance*.

**33. B**

A *laceration* is a large *cut,* especially as it pertains to a wound. Or you could say a cut is an especially small or minor laceration. Similarly, a *slit* (B) is a tiny crack, cut, or separation in something, and can be called a small *gap*.

**34. D**

*Quixotic* means impractical, after the hero of *Don Quixote*. A *realist* is a person who is especially realistic. *Realistic* is the opposite of *quixotic,* so a realist is never quixotic. In (A), *pedantic* people show off their learning. Many scholars are pedantic, so this won't work. In (B), a *fool* is foolish—a synonym for *idiotic.* The same relationship holds true for (C)—an *idler* is a *lethargic* person. (D) looks good—a *tormentor* is vicious or cruel. The opposite sort of person would be kinder and more *sympathetic*—a tormentor is never sympathetic.

**35. C**

A *badge* is the identification worn by a *policeman*. In (A), a *placard* is a sign carried by a *demonstrator*. There's a link here but a placard isn't an official ID and a demonstrator doesn't necessarily carry a placard. (B) is incorrect because although there is a tradition for a *sailor* to have a *tattoo*, a tattoo isn't an official identification of a sailor. In (C), a *soldier* wears a *dog-tag* on his uniform to identify him, so this is plausible. In (D), the *pedigree* of a *dog* is the dog's lineage or genealogy, not something worn by the dog as identification.

**36. B**

To *scrutinize* means to *observe* intently, so the relationship is one of degree. In (A), to *pique* interest is to *excite* interest. The words mean the same thing. In (B), to *beseech* means to *request* with great fervor—this is more like it. In (C), to *search* is the process you go through to *discover* something. That's different from the stem pair. In (D) to *grin* is to *smile* broadly—this reverses the original pair.

**37. D**

If you didn't know what *epicurean* means, you might have had trouble here, but you can still eliminate some choices. There must be some relationship between *epicurean* and *indulge*. Could (A) have the same relationship? No, because there really is no relationship between *frightened* and *ugly*. Something ugly doesn't necessarily frighten

people. Same with (C)—there's no relationship between *hesitate* and *unproductive.* There are good relationships for the other choices but let's see if we can eliminate them. In (B), *revocable* means something can be taken back, so the relationship is, "Something *revocable* can be *retracted*." That leaves us with (D), and there our relationship is something like, "someone *vindictive* is likely to *revenge* himself," and that sounds better. In fact, an epicurean person is one who is likely to indulge himself, so (D) is correct here.

**38. D**

To *stare* is to look at intently or searchingly, so the relationship here is one of degree or intensity: to stare is to look more penetratingly or intently. In choice (A), *peek* might be a less intense form of *glare*, but this is the reverse of the bridge we want. The same is true of choice (B); *wanting* is a lesser, not a greater, degree of *craving*. In choice (C), *befriend* is the opposite of *alienate*, not a more intense form of it. In choice (D), to *despair*, or to abandon all hope, is a more intense form of *worry*; this is the bridge we want.

**39. A**

A *pancreas* is, by definition, a type of *organ*. Let's plug the choices into this bridge, and see which one fits. Choice (A) sounds good; a *knee* is a type of *joint*. Choice (B) doesn't work; the *stomach* is not a type of *obesity*. In choice (C), an *artery* and a *vein* are both types of blood vessels, but an *artery* is not a type of *vein*. Choice (D) uses the same bridge as the stem pair, but the words are in the wrong order. A *molar* certainly is a type of *tooth*, but a *tooth* is not a type of *molar*.

**40. D**

The first pair has a degree bridge where *enunciate*, or articulate, means to pronounce more clearly and precisely. We can eliminate choices (A) and (B), because *recite* and *impress* have no definitive relationship, and *reiterate*, meaning to repeat, has no necessary relationship with *bother*. Next, we can eliminate choice (C) because there is no degree difference between the words. In choice (C), to *inquire* means to *ask*. Choice (D) is the correct answer because to *elaborate*, which means to clarify or to discuss in depth, is, by definition, to *explain* something more clearly and precisely.

**41. A**

To *meander* is to walk aimlessly or idly: this is a "type" bridge. Choice (A) has the same bridge—to *prattle* is to *talk* aimlessly or idly. To *mutilate*, choice (B), is pointedly to disfigure, that is, to *destroy* in a specific way, not to *destroy* aimlessly. To *legislate*, choice (C), may be to *mandate* through the creation of laws, but once again, there is no sense of idleness or aimlessness. To *draw*, choice (D), is certainly not to *write* aimlessly.

**42. D**

*Diluvial* means having to do with a *flood*. You may have heard the word *antediluvian,* meaning before the flood, Noah's flood, that is—in other words, a long time ago. So our bridge has to do with that. In (A), *criminal* can mean having to do with crime but it doesn't mean having to do with *punishment*. In (B), *biological* means having to do with living things. *Bacteria* are living things but to define *biological* as having to do with bacteria would be too narrow. In (C), *judicial* means having to do with the administration of justice. A *verdict* is the decision about the guilt or innocence of a defendant, a small part of the judicial process. This leaves (D) and *cardiac* means having to do with the *heart*, so (D) is correct.

**43. D**

A *penitent* person tends to regret. Starting at the top, in (A), you can't *detect* something *imperceptible*. (B), *zealous* and *doubt*, and (C), *exuberant* and *socialize*, have weak bridges. In choice (D), a *querulous* or habitually whining person tends to *complain*, or argue over minor details.

**44. D**

One who *vegetates* is inert or not *active*. If this gave you trouble, think of vegetables, which are markedly inactive living things, or perhaps the expression "veg out" meaning to stagnate, not think or do anything. Similarly, one who *accepts* (D) takes things as they are without doubting, doesn't call things into question; he or she is therefore not *questioning*.

**45. A**

To *debilitate* means, by definition, to make weak. By definition, to *empower*, choice (A), means to make *strong*. To *countermand*, (B), by definition, does not mean to make something *illegal*; it means to cancel or reverse an order.

*Abominate*, choice (C), does not mean to make *absent*; it means to hate. To *instigate*, choice (D), does not mean to make *guilty*; it means to urge on. (D) is the only choice that works, and it's correct.

**46. D**

The correct spelling is *appalling*.

**47. B**

The correct spelling is *recognizable*.

**48. D**

The correct spelling is *height*.

**49. B**

The correct spelling is *irrational*.

**50. A**

The correct spelling is *avoidable*.

**51. D**

The correct spelling is *limited*.

**52. D**

The correct spelling is *emphasize*.

**53. C**

The correct spelling is *appearance*.

**54. B**

The correct spelling is *vacuum*.

**55. D**

The correct spelling is *campaign*.

**56. A**

The correct spelling is *a lot*.

**57. C**

The correct spelling is *advice*.

**58. B**

The correct spelling is *assured*.

**59. D**

No mistake.

**60. B**

The correct spelling is *oversight*.

**61. C**

The correct spelling is *then*.

**62. C**

The correct spelling is *correspondence*.

**63. B**

The correct spelling is *amazement*.

**64. A**

The correct spelling is *willingly*.

**65. A**

No mistake.

## Mathematics

**1. C**

To round off to the nearest 100, look at the tens digit. If it is 5 or greater, round the hundreds digit up. If the tens digit is 4 or smaller, keep the same hundreds digit. Here, the tens digit is 9, so you must round the hundreds digit up to 3 and replace the digits to the right with zeros.

**2. C**

This question has several steps. First, determine the amount of overtime dollars the worker earned. Do this by figuring how much she earned over a 40-hour work week. If she makes $16 for 40 hours, she would earn $16 \times \$40 = \$640$. However, she earned $60 more than that. ($700 − $640 = $60.) How many extra hours did she work to earn that $60 if she earns time and a half for each hour over 40? If she earned $16 per hour, then she made $\$16 \times 1.5 = \$24$ per hour in overtime. Therefore, $\frac{\$60}{\$24} = 2.5$ hours worked overtime.

**3. A**

This is a translation problem. You're told that Janice has $B$ books. Lisa has 40 less than 3 times the number of books Janice has, which you can translate as $L = 3B − 40$. The total number they have together equals $B + 3B − 40$ or $4B − 40$ which is choice (A).

**4. C**

The value of $x$ is an even integer greater than 8 but less than 17. Thus, $x$ could be 10, 12, 14, or 16. The mean of all its possible values $\frac{10 + 12 + 14 + 16}{4} = \frac{52}{4} = \frac{26}{2} = 13$. Be sure to read each question carefully. This question required two steps. If you read too quickly, you might have missed the second step that was finding the mean of all the possible values of $x$.

**5. C**

We know that $x$ is odd and $y$ is even. Let's say that $x = 3$ and $y = 4$.

(A) $2x + y$; $2(3) + 4 = 6 + 4 = 10$; 10 is even, so this isn't correct.

(B) $2(x + y)$; $2(3 + 4) = 2(7) = 14$; 14 is even.

(C) $x^2 + y^2$; $3^2 + 4^2 = 9 + 16 =$ because 25; 25 is odd, so (C) is correct.

**6. B**

Remember to count the number of negatives to determine whether the product of negative and positive integers is either negative or positive. An odd number of negatives will yield a negative number, while an even number of negatives will yield a positive number. Since choice (B) is a positive integer, it is not the product of a negative and a positive integer.

**7. D**

Let $x =$ the number of ties the Tigers had. It lost 5 times as many games as it tied, $5x$. It had no wins so the total number of games played by the Tigers $= 5x + x = 6x$. So, the number of games the Tigers played must be a multiple of 6; the only choice that is a multiple of 6 is choice (D).

## 8.  A

Remember PEMDAS. Perform the operation in parenthesis first. $2^3(3 - 1)^2 + (-4)^2 = 2^3(2)^2 + (-4)^2$. Exponents next, $8(4) + 16$. Multiplication next, and addition or subtraction last: $32 + 16 = 48$.

## 9.  C

Let $x =$ the part of the novel Ruth has finished.

$$x = \frac{3}{8} + \frac{1}{10}$$

Change these two fractions to a common denominator of 80 and add them.

$$\frac{30}{80} + \frac{8}{80} = \frac{38}{80}$$

Reduce the fraction to $\frac{19}{40}$.

## 10.  C

This is a simple arithmetic problem if $m \angle ABD = 145°$, then $x = 145 - (48 + 45)$. $x = 145 - 93 = 52°$.

## 11.  A

This problem looks harder than it really is. If $90 \div x = 9n$, then $9n \cdot x = 90$, or $9nx = 90$ and $nx = 10$.

## 12.  B

The perimeter of triangle $ABC$ is 28, so $AB + BC + AC = 28$. Plug in the algebraic expression given for the length of each side in meters:

$$(3a - 1) + (2a + 1) + (5a - 2) = 28$$
$$10a - 2 = 28$$
$$10a = 30$$
$$a = 3$$

The length of $AC$ is represented by the expression $5a - 2$, so $AC = 5(3) - 2 = 13$.

## 13.  B

The time it takes to complete the entire exam is the sum of the time spent on the first half of the exam and the time spent on the second half. We know the time spent on the first half is $\frac{2}{3}$ of the time spent on the second half. If $S$ represents the time spent on the second half, then the total time spent is $\frac{2}{3}S + S$ or $\frac{5}{3}S$. We know this total time is one hour, or 60 minutes. So we can set up a simple equation and solve for $S$.

$$\frac{5}{3}S = 60$$
$$\frac{3}{5} \times \frac{5}{3}S = \frac{3}{5} \times 60$$
$$S = 36, \text{ so } \frac{2}{3}s = 24.$$

## 14.  D

Set up a simple proportion on questions like this one:

$$\frac{150 \text{ bottles}}{20 \text{ minutes}} = \frac{60 \text{ bottles}}{x \text{ minutes}}.$$

$$150x = 1,200$$

Divide both sides by 150:

$$x = \frac{1,200}{150} = 8$$

(D)  is correct.

## 15.  B

Multiply through and solve for $y$ by isolating it on one side of the equation:

$$4(y - 5) = 2(y + 3)$$
$$4y - 20 = 2y + 6$$
$$4y - 20 - 6 = 2y$$
$$4y - 26 - 4y = 2y - 4y$$
$$\frac{-26}{-2} = \frac{-2y}{-2}$$
$$13 = y$$

## 16.  B

To learn the man's overtime rate of pay, we have to figure out his regular rate of pay. Divide the amount of money made, $200, by the time it took to make it, 40 hours. $200 \div 40 \text{ hours} = \$5$ per hour. That is the normal rate. The man is paid $1\frac{1}{2}$ times his regular rate during overtime, so when working more than 40 hours he makes $\frac{3}{2} \times \$5$ per hour $= \$7.50$ per hour. Now we can figure out how long it takes the man to make $230. It takes him 40 hours to make the first $200. The last $30 are made at the overtime rate. Since it takes the man one hour to make $7.50 at this rate, we can figure out the number of extra hours by dividing $30 by $7.50 per hour. $30 ÷ $7.50 per hour = 4 hours. The total time needed is 40 hours plus 4 hours, or 44 hours.

### 17.  D

The way to calculate this is:

Percent × Whole = Part

Percent × 25 = 16

Percent = $\frac{16}{25}$ × 100% = 64%

### 18.  B

Don't fall for the answer choice trap and assume that the average of $\frac{1}{20}$ and $\frac{1}{30}$ is $\frac{1}{25}$. Instead, use the average formula: Average = $\frac{\text{Sum of the terms}}{\text{Number of terms}}$ . So, in this case,

Average = $\dfrac{\frac{1}{20} + \frac{1}{30}}{2} = \dfrac{\frac{3}{60} + \frac{2}{60}}{2} = \dfrac{\frac{5}{60}}{2} = \dfrac{5}{120} = \dfrac{1}{24}$.

### 19.  (A)

If a full barrel can hold 75 gallons, when it is $\frac{3}{5}$ full it will hold $\frac{3}{5}$ of 75 gallons. $\frac{3}{5}$ × 75 = 45 gallons.

### 20.  C

This question is just testing your knowledge of definitions. The *supplement* of an angle is the angle that when added to the original angle equals 180°. So if an angle measures $y°$, its supplement is $180 - y$.

### 21.  A

Pick numbers to solve this one. Let's say that $n = 2$. That means the tree grew 5 feet, or 60 inches, in 2 years, which means it grew at a rate of 30 inches per year. Plug in 2 for $n$ into the answer choices, and only (A) gives the answer of 30 that you are looking for.

### 22.  A

To find the area of the entire figure, determine the area of each rectangle and add these values together. *ABFG* has an area of 8 × 4 = 32 square units. *CDEF* has a length of 2, and, since *C* bisects *BF* which = 4, *CDEF* also has a width of 2. In other words, it is a square. If you eyeballed the diagram, rather than doing the math, you probably would

not have arrived at the correct value. Remember, diagrams are not drawn to scale. The area of *CDEF* then is $2^2$ = 4 square cm. The area of the entire figure = 32 + 4 = 36 square cm.

### 23.  D

You can't find the value of either variable alone, but you don't need to. Rearranging the equation, you get:

$$13 + a = 25 + b$$
$$13 = 25 + b - a$$
$$13 - 25 = b - a$$
$$b - a = -12$$

### 24.  A

If one kilogram is approximately 2.2 pounds, then you would need to divide one pound by 2.2 pounds to determine how many pounds were in one kilogram:

$$\frac{1 \text{ pound}}{2.2 \text{ pounds}} = \frac{10}{22} = \frac{5}{11}, \text{ choice (A)}$$

### 25.  A

To find the average, add the weights and divide by the number of people.

Average $\dfrac{150 + 153 + 154 + 157 + 151}{5} = \dfrac{765}{5} = 153$.

### 26.  C

This problem needs to be done in several steps. First find out what the sale price of the radio was. The discount was 20%, so the sale price was 80% of the original price.

Percent × Whole = Part

0.80 × $118 = Sale price

$94.40 = Sale price

Now figure out how much tax Brad paid. The tax was 8% of the sale price.

Percent × Whole = Part

0.08 × $94.40 = Tax

$7.5520 = Tax

$7.55 = Tax

Now just add the tax to the sale price.

$94.40 + $7.55 = $101.95.

**KAPLAN**

**27. C**

Here you're looking for an extremely rough approximation (the answer choices all have a range of 100), so you could square the upper bounds of the ranges in the answer choices, until you find the range that encompasses 104,906. For instance, starting with the upper bound of (A), $(200)^2 = 40,000$, which is less than 104,906. Now try (B): $(300)^2 = 90,000$, which is still too low. Now check (C): $(400)^2 = 160,000$. 104,906 is between 90,000 and 160,000, so (C) is the answer.

**28. C**

If the ratio of males to females is 3:5, then there are 8 parts total in the ratio. The total number of students must be a multiple of 8. Only choice (C), 152, is a multiple of 8.

**29. C**

If 48 of 60 seats are occupied, then 12 of 60 seats are unoccupied (since $60 - 48 = 12$).What percent of the seats are unoccupied?

$$\text{Percent} = \frac{\text{part}}{\text{whole}} \times 100\% = \frac{12}{60} \times 100\% = \frac{1}{5} \times 100\% =$$

20%, choice (C).

**30. B**

You could translate the English into math to get:

$0.36 \times 18 = 0.18 \times n$, so $n = 0.36 \times \dfrac{18}{0.18} = 2 \times 18 = 36$.

Of course, you don't have to go through all that work if you realize that $x\%$ of $y = y\%$ of $x$.

**31. B**

If the charge for one pound is $25.00, then the charge for $\frac{4}{5}$ of a pound would be $\frac{4}{5} \times \$25.00 = \$20.00$ plus 8% sales tax. 8% of $20.00 $= 0.08(\$20.00) = \$1.60$. $20.00 + $1.60 = \$21.60$, choice (B).

**32. C**

If a truck takes 6 hours to complete a trip at 20 miles per hour, the total distance for the trip must be $6 \times 20 =$ 120 miles. When traveling 120 miles at a rate of 30 miles per hour, the truck would take $\dfrac{120}{30} = 4$ hours. So instead of

taking 6 hours, the truck took 4 hours. That saves 2 hours, so choice (C) is correct.

**33. A**

To solve this problem, set up an algebraic equation. Let $BC = x$. $AB$ is twice the length of $BC$, so it can be represented by $2x$. $BC = CD$, so $CD = x$. $DE$ is three times the length of $CD$, or $3x$. Since $AE = 49$, $2x + x + x + 3x = 49$, $7x = 49$ and $x = 7$. $BD$ is composed of segments $BC$ and $CD$, so its length is $7 + 7 = 14$ units.

**34. B**

Solve a question like this using algebra if it's a strong area for you. Otherwise, work backwards from the answer choices. To solve this question using algebra, we'll need to set up equations and solve for $R$ which is Robert's money. We're told that Ed has 100 more dollars than Robert.

$$E = R + 100.$$

Ed then spends 20 dollars and has 5 times as much money as Robert.

$$E - 20 = 5R$$

Substitute $R + 100$ for $E$ and solve. So:

$$R + 80 = 5R.$$
$$80 = 4R.$$
$$R = \$20, \text{ choice (B)}.$$

If you were to backsolve, choose a value like $20 or $24 for Robert's money. Then see which value would work for all the information we're given in the question. Only choice (B), $20, works.

**35. D**

If $2m > 24$, then $m > 12$. But so are all the answer choices, so check out the other inequality. If $3m < 48$, then $m < 16$. Thus, (D), 16, could not be a possible value for $m$.

**36. D**

Isolate $x$ on one side of the equation:

$$\frac{1}{2} + x = 6.5$$
$$-\frac{1}{2} + x = 6.5 - \frac{1}{2}$$
$$x = 6$$

This problem is easy when you remember the decimal equivalent of $\frac{1}{2}$ is 0.5.

**37. C**

When you multiply terms that have exponents over the same base, you add the exponents and multiply the coefficients, so in this case you get:

$3x^2 \times 5x^3 = (3 \times 5)x^{2+3} = 15x^5$.

**38. C**

The numbers 2, 37, and 67 are all prime. $51 = 3 \times 17$, so it is not prime. Knowing the *rules of divisibility* can help you when dealing with problems involving prime numbers, multiples, or factors. For instance, here one should be able to see quickly that 51 is divisible by 3, because its digits— that is, 5 and 1—add up to 6, which is a multiple of 3. (C) is correct.

**39. B**

Draw a chart or table to help organize the information. Newark is in a time zone that is 2 hours ahead of the time in Denver, so if the time in Denver when Harry arrives is 2:30 P.M., then the time in Newark when he arrives in Denver is 4:30 P.M. The flight takes 5 hours, so the time he began in Newark is 5 hours earlier than 4:30 P.M., or 11:30 A.M., choice (B).

**40. D**

Since $AE$ is a line segment, all the lengths are additive, so $AE = AD + DE$. We're told that $AD = 6$ and $AE = 8$. So $DE = AE - AD = 8 - 6 = 2$. We're also told that $BE = 6$. So $BD = BE - DE = 6 - 2 = 4$. We have the length of $BD$, but still need the length of $BC$. Since $CD = 3(BC)$, the situation looks like this:

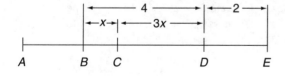

Here $x$ stands for the length of $BC$. Since $BD = 4$, we can write:

$$x + 3x = 4$$
$$4x = 4$$
$$x = 1$$

So $BC = 1$, answer choice (D).

**41. C**

If 75% of $x$ is 150, then $0.75(x) = 150$ or $\frac{3}{4}(x) = 150$. Multiply both sides by $\frac{4}{3}$ and you find that $x = 200$, choice (C). You could also work backwards from the answer choices. Only choice (C), 200, works. If $x = 200$, then $0.75(x) = 150$ since $0.75(200) = 150$.

**42. D**

If $\frac{\sqrt{n}}{3}$ is an even integer, then $\frac{\sqrt{n}}{3} = 2k$, where $k$ is an integer because any even integer is equal to 2 multiplied by an integer. Since $\frac{\sqrt{n}}{3} = 2k$, $\sqrt{n} = 6k$. Squaring both sides of $\sqrt{n} = 6k$, we have $\left(\sqrt{n}\right)^2 = (6k)^2$, and $n = 36k^2$. So $n$ must be a multiple of 36. Only choice (D), 144, is a multiple of 36. $144 = 4 \times 36$. Checking choice (D), $\frac{\sqrt{144}}{3} = \frac{12}{3} = 4$ and 4 is an even integer. Choice (D) is correct.

Another way to solve this problem is to work backward. When you plug 144 in for $n$ you get $\frac{\sqrt{144}}{3}$. When you plug 144 in $\frac{\sqrt{144}}{3} = \frac{12}{3} = 4$. 4 is an even integer.

**43. D**

Multiply through and then find $a$ in terms of $m$ by isolating $a$ on one side of the equation:

$$2(a + m) = 5m - 3 + a$$
$$2a + 2m = 5m - 3 + a$$
$$2a + 2m - a - 2m = 5m - 3 + a - 2m - a$$
$$a = 3m - 3$$

**44. D**

Be careful and translate the words into math: "the product of 3 and $x$ is equal to 2 less than $y$" becomes $3x = y - 2$. But all of the equations in the answer choices set the right side of the equation to zero, so let's do that to our equation:

$$3x = y - 2$$
$$3x - y = -2$$
$$3x - y + 2 = 0.$$

**45. B**

Miles per gallon $= \dfrac{\text{miles}}{\text{gallons}} = \dfrac{414}{18}$, so the answer is $414 \div 18$. But let's say you would rather not divide 414 by 18. In that case you could now backsolve until you find an answer choice that when multiplied by 18 will give you 414. Let's start with (B), 23: $23 \times 18 = 414$, so (B) is the answer.

**46. B**

The three interior angles of any triangle add up to 180°, and the parts of the ratio here add up to $1 + 2 + 3 = 6$. So to know what to multiply the ratio part numbers by to get numbers that add up to 180, divide 180 by 6, which gives you 30. Now you know that the three angles have degree measures of $1 \times 30 = 30$, $2 \times 30 = 60$, and $3 \times 30 = 90$. So the difference in the degree measures between the largest and the smallest angles is $90 - 30 = 60$.

**47. C**

$5 \times 5 \times 5 = 125$, and $125 \times 125 = 15,625$, which is the smallest power of 5 that's greater than 10,000. So $(5 \times 5 \times 5) \times (5 \times 5 \times 5)$, or $5^6 = 5^n$, and $n = 6$.

**48. C**

Be careful with the units again. Change 12 feet into inches. $12 \times 12 = 144$ inches. If you subtract $3 \times 17$ inch pieces from 144, that will give you the length of the remaining board. $144 - 3(17) = 144 - 51 = 93$. Choice (C) is correct.

**49. A**

If the first year begins with Town A at 9,400 and Town B at 7,600, the populations are $9,400 - 7,600 = 1,800$ apart. Each year after 2000 beginning in 2001, the gap will close by 200. So it would take 9 more years for the gap to close entirely. So by 2009, the populations will be equal, choice (A).

**50. B**

You are given values for all the variables, so just plug those values into the equation you are given. $x^2 - 4yz - z^2 = \sqrt{5^2} - 4\frac{1}{3}(3) + 3^2 = 5 - 4 + 9 = 10$.

**51. B**

Work through the clock systematically: First reading at 12 P.M., second at 4 P.M., third at 8 P.M., fourth at midnight, fifth at 4 A.M., sixth at 8 A.M., 7th at 12 P.M., eighth at 4 P.M., ninth and final reading at 8 P.M., choice (B).

**52. D**

Be careful with units of measure on this one. You're given feet as units of length and width, but then are asked for square yardage rather than square footage in your answer choices. One easy way to handle this question is to begin by converting feet into yards. 18 ft × 24 ft is the same as 6 yd × 8 yd. If the length and width are 6 × 8, then the area of the room would be $6 \times 8 = 48$ square yards, choice (D).

**53. B**

There are 360° in a circle and 60 minutes in an hour, so you could solve this question by setting up a proportion.

$\dfrac{45}{360} = \dfrac{n}{60}$, where $n$ is the number of minutes. $n = 45 \times \dfrac{60}{360} = 7.5$, so the answer is (B).

**54. C**

To determine the number of minutes in a week, begin with the number of minutes in an hour and work your way up from there. There are 60 minutes per hour. 24 hours per day, so there are $60 \times 24 = 1,440$ minutes per day. There are 7 days per week, so there are $1,440 \times 7 = 10,080$ minutes per week. (C) is correct.

## 55. A

The average formula is:

$$\text{Average} = \frac{\text{Sum of the Terms}}{\text{Number of terms}}$$

Don't just average the old average and the last test score —that would give the last score as much weight as all the other scores combined. The best way to deal with changing averages is to use the sums. Use the old average to figure out the total of the first 6 scores:

Sum of first 6 scores = (83)(6) = 498

Then add the 7th score and divide:

$$\frac{498 - 97}{7} - \frac{595}{7} = 85.$$

## 56. B

Begin by writing the division problem as a fraction:

$\frac{7.6}{0.019} = x$. Now move the decimal points on the top and the bottom of the fraction the same number of places to the right until you are dealing with whole numbers:

$\frac{7.6}{0.019} = \frac{7,600}{19}$. Now go ahead and divide:

$$\frac{7,600}{19} = 400.$$

## 57. D

You're given two inequalities here: $a < b$ and $b < c$, which we can combine into one, $a < b < c$. We need to go through the answer choices to see which *must* be true. Choice (D): $a + b < 2c$. We know that $a < c$ and $b < c$. If we add the corresponding sides of these inequalities we'll get $a + b < c + c$, or $a + b < 2c$. This statement is *always* true, so it must be the correct answer.

## 58. C

The key to this question is that while the value of the stock decreases and increases by the same *amount*, it doesn't decrease and increase by the same *percent*. When the stock first decreases, that amount of change is part of a larger whole. If the stock were to increase to its former value, that same amount of change would be a larger percent of a smaller whole. Pick a number for the original value of the stock, such as $100. (Since it's easy to take percents of 100, it's usually best to choose 100.) The

25% decrease represents $25, so the stock decreases to a value of $75. Now in order for the stock to reach the value of $100 again, there must be a $25 increase. What percent of $75 is $25? It's $\frac{\$25}{\$75} \times 100\%$, or $\frac{1}{3} \times 100\%$, or $33\frac{1}{3}\%$.

## 59. D

Circumference of a circle $= 2\pi r$, where $r$ is the radius of the circle. So, a circle with a circumference of $18\pi$ has a radius of 9 in.

## 60. D

This question is actually a remainder question in disguise. If 587 people are to be divided among a number of buses that each seat 48 people, we need to divide 587 by 48 to see how many buses we would fill completely. The remainder would be the number of people in the unfilled bus. $587 \div 48 = 12$ and the remainder is 11, so (D) is correct.

## 61. C

Approach this problem in the following way: $81 = 3 \times 3 \times 3 \times 3 = 3^4$, so $3^{n-7} = 3^4$. Since the exponents are equivalent, that means $n - 7 = 4$, so $n = 7 + 4 = 11$, choice (C).

## 62. A

The circumference of a circle $= 2\pi(\text{radius})$, so the radius of a circle with a circumference of 8 is $\frac{8}{2\pi} = \frac{4}{\pi}$. The area of a circle $= \pi(\text{radius})^2$, so the area of a circle with a radius of $\frac{4}{\pi}$ is $\pi\left(\frac{4}{\pi}\right)^2 = \pi\left(\frac{16}{\pi^2}\right) = \frac{16}{\pi}$, choice (A).

## 63. C

Distribute the numbers outside the parentheses and solve for $y$.

$$4(y - 1) = 2(y + 2)$$
$$4y - 4 = 2y + 4$$
$$2y = 8$$
$$y = 4$$

(C) is correct.

**KAPLAN**

**64. C**

Joan can shovel the whole driveway in 50 minutes, so each minute she does $\frac{1}{50}$ of the driveway. Mary can shovel the whole driveway in 20 minutes; in each minute she does $\frac{1}{20}$ of the driveway. In one minute they do:

$$\frac{1}{50} + \frac{1}{20} = \frac{2}{100} + \frac{5}{100} = \frac{7}{100}$$

If they do $\frac{7}{100}$ of the driveway in one minute, they do the entire driveway in $\frac{100}{7}$ minutes. So all that remains is to round $\frac{100}{7}$ off to the nearest integer. Since $\frac{100}{7} = 14\frac{2}{7}$, $\frac{100}{7}$ is approximately 14. It takes about 14 minutes for both of them to shovel the driveway.

**65. D**

You can pick numbers to make sense of this geometry problem. You are asked to increase the sides of a square by 10%, so you want to pick a number for the original sides of the square which is easy to take 10%. For instance, you could say that the original square is $10 \times 10$. 10% of 10 is 1, so the dimensions of the increased square are $11 \times 11$. In this case, the area of the original square is 100, and the area of the new square is 121, which represents a 21% increase, choice (D).

**66. A**

The key to answering this question is realizing that 2 is the only even prime number. Since at least two of the three numbers will be odd, the sum of those two numbers will be even (odd + odd = even), which means that the third number must be even for the sum of the three numbers to be even (even + even = even). Therefore one of the numbers must be 2, which also happens to be the smallest prime number, so the answer is (A).

**67. C**

This one's tricky since it's asking for the number of rectangular tiles, each 12 cm × 18 cm, needed to cover *four* flat rectangular surfaces, each 60 cm × 180 cm. To determine the number of smaller tiles needed, divide the total area of the four bigger rectangles by the area of one of

the smaller rectangles. $\frac{4 \times 60 \times 180}{12 \times 18} = 4 \times 5 \times 10 = 200$, and choice (C) is correct.

**68. D**

Since we are told the value of $d$, we can plug it into the equation $\frac{c}{d} = 3$ to find the value of $c$. We are told that $d = 1$, so $\frac{c}{d} = 3$ can be rewritten as $\frac{c}{1} = 3$. Since $\frac{c}{1}$ is the same as $c$, we can rewrite the equation as $c = 3$. Now we can plug in the values of $c$ and $d$ into the expression: $3(3) + 1 = 10$.

**69. C**

Work backward from your answer choices on this one. Begin with choice (C). If the smaller number is 21 (and the larger number is 35), does the math from the question make sense? If (C) is correct, then the average of 21 and 35 is equal to twice the positive difference between the two numbers. The average of 21 and 35 = $\frac{21 + 35}{2} = \frac{56}{2} = 28$. The positive difference between 21 and 35 is 14. Twice the positive difference would be 2(14) or 28. As we've already seen, this is also the average of the numbers, so (C) is correct.

**70. A**

First find how long the trip takes him at each of the two different rates, using the formula:

$$\text{Time} = \frac{\text{Distance}}{\text{Rate}}$$

He travels the first 10 km at 30 km per hour, so he takes $\frac{10}{30} = \frac{1}{3}$ hour for this portion of the journey. He travels the remaining 30 km at 15 km per hour, so he takes $\frac{30}{15} = 2$ hours for this portion of the journey. So the whole journey takes him $2 + \frac{1}{3} = 2\frac{1}{3}$ hours. Now we need to compare this to the amount of time it would take to make the same trip at a constant rate of 20 km per hour. If he traveled the whole 40 km at 20 km per hour, it would take $\frac{40}{20} = 2$ hours. Now $2\frac{1}{3}$ hours is more than 2 hours by $\frac{1}{3}$ hour, or 20 minutes.

## 71. C

First factor out an *x* from each term, and then rearrange the terms and factor what's left:

$$2x + 3x^2 + x^3 = x(2 + 3x + x^2)$$
$$= x(x^2 + 3x + 2)$$
$$= x(x + 1)(x + 2)$$

## 72. A

This question states that each seat of the Ferris wheel can hold 3 people and that all but 3 of the 12 cars are full. Therefore, the 9 full cars containing 3 people each contain a total of 27 people. In addition, one of the remaining cars is empty and 2 cars contain 2 people each, adding 4 people to the 27 in the full cars for a total of 31 people on the Ferris wheel.

## 73. C

This is a proportion question.

$$\frac{4 \text{ ft object}}{9 \text{ ft shadow}} = \frac{x \text{ ft object}}{21 \text{ ft shadow}}$$

Cross-multiply to solve.

$$4 \times 21 = 9x$$
$$\frac{84}{9} = \frac{9x}{9}$$
$$x = 9\frac{1}{3}$$

Choice (C) is correct.

## 74. B

Pay attention to your calculations on this one. Proceed carefully, one step at a time. You're told that Eileen earns $280 per week. Kelly earns $50 more than Eileen, so Kelly earns $280 + $50 = $330 per week. June's salary is $70 less than Kelly's, so June earns $330 − $70 = $260 per week, and (B) is correct.

## 75. A

Jim runs 1 mile per 5 minutes, so in 40 minutes he will run 8 miles. Rebecca runs 1 mile per 8 minutes, so in 40 minutes she will run 5 miles. Thus, if they start out at the same point and run in the same direction, after 40 minutes Jim will be 8 − 5 = 3 miles ahead of Rebecca.

## Science

### 1. C

In the $AA \times aa$ cross, the F1 generation will be 100% $Aa$, a heterozygous genotype with a dominant phenotype. In the F2 generation, there will be a 1:2:1 ratio of $AA{:}Aa{:}aa$. Therefore, the F1 generation is entirely dominant heterozygous. Answer choices I and II can be eliminated, leaving only III.

### 2. D

The bony skeleton serves as a support system within all vertebrate organisms. Muscles are attached to the bones, permitting movement. The skeleton also provides protection for vital organs. For example, the rib cage protects the heart and the lungs, while the skull and vertebral column protect the brain and the spinal cord. The hollow cavity formed within many bones is filled with bone marrow, the site of formation of blood cells.

### 3. C

The breathing center in the medulla oblongata monitors the increase in $CO_2$ through its sensory cells. It will also detect a decrease in pH in the blood, which is indicative of an increase of $CO_2$ levels in the blood. A decrease in $O_2$ is monitored peripherally by chemoreceptors, located in the carotid bodies in the carotid arteries and in the aortic bodies in the aorta. In (A), the cerebrum is involved in sensory interpretation, memory, and thought, while the cerebellum (B) is involved in fine motor coordination, balance, and equilibrium. Finally, the spinal cord (D) relays sensory and motor information to and from the brain.

### 4. D

In the nucleus, DNA is produced during cell division, while RNA is produced by transcription of DNA. MRNA travels from the nucleus into the cytoplasm, where it is translated into polypeptides on the ribosomes.

### 5. D

This is a basic cross using Drosophila melanogaster. You're told that the gene for wing type is located on an autosomal chromosome, a non–sex chromosome, which means that it is NOT inherited as a sex-linked trait. You're also told that the dominant allele codes for wild-type wings; "wild type" simply means that this is the phenotype that predominates in nature. The recessive allele codes for the vestigial wing

**KAPLAN**

type, which is a stumpy wing. The gender of the flies is of no relevance here; gender only comes into play for sex-linked traits. So, our male fly is homozygous dominant for wing type and our female fly is homozygous recessive. A cross between a homozygous dominant and a homozygous recessive yields 100% heterozygous individuals, which in this case means that 100% of the progeny will have wild-type wings.

**6. A**

Members of an order are more alike than members of a class.

**7. B**

The process by which plants convert carbon dioxide and water into sugar and oxygen is called photosynthesis. The reverse process, by which animals convert oxygen and sugars into carbon dioxide and water, is called respiration.

**8. A**

Oxytocin is released by the posterior pituitary. It increases uterine contractions during childbirth.

**9. C**

Type O blood, also known as the "universal donor" type, can be donated to anyone.

**10. B**

A typical human gamete contains half the number of chromosomes as a normal cell, or 23.

**11. D**

If color-blindness is a recessive sex-linked chromosome found on the $X$ chromosome, the incidence of color-blindness among men indicates the incidence of the color-blindness gene, which is 1 in 20. Because females have two $X$ chromosomes, for a female to be color-blind, both $X$ chromosomes would have to contain the recessive gene. Thus the probability that a female in the population would be color-blind would be $\frac{1}{20} \times \frac{1}{20} = \frac{1}{400}$.

**12. C**

Most digestion takes place in the small intestine.

**13. C**

The Primate order includes man, who also belongs to the phylum Chordata, the class Mammalia, and the family Homidae.

**14. C**

Insulin is created in the body's pancreas.

**15. D**

If two brown-eyed parents have a blue-eyed child, the probability that their next child will have blue eyes is 1 in 4. The blue-eyed gene (B) is recessive to the brown-eyed gene (B), so if both parents have brown eyes and one of the children has blue eyes, both parents carry the recessive blue-eyed gene (Bb), and thus the chances of any more of their children being blue-eyed (bb) is 1 in 4.

**16. A**

Tough elastic tissues found in the joints that connect bones to bones are called ligaments. Tendons are connective tissue that unite a muscle with some other part, such as a bone. Cartilage is a somewhat elastic tissue (unlike bone) that in adults is found in some joints, respiratory passages, and the external ear. Finally, muscles are body tissue consisting of long cells that contract when stimulated to produce motion.

**17. D**

Marsupial mammals differ from placental mammals in that marsupials bear premature embryos which complete development in their mothers' pouches.

**18. D**

Rods and cones are light sensitive cells inside the eye's retina.

**19. B**

Striated muscles, also known as skeletal muscles, are controlled by conscious thought, unlike cardiac muscles or the smooth muscles of the digestive system, which are controlled by the autonomic nervous system.

**20. B**

The study of interactions between organisms and their interrelationships with the physical environment is known as ecology. Cytology is the study of cells, physiology is the study of the organism, and embryology is the study of embryos and their development.

**21. C**

Most of the nutrients in food are absorbed in the body's small intestine.

**22. C**

Carbohydrates include both starches and sugars, which makes choice (C), both (A) and (B), correct.

**23. B**

The phylum that includes man is called Chordata, meaning vertebrate animals.

**24. C**

Protein synthesis does require mRNA. tRNA (A) brings the amino acid to the ribosome, where it interacts with the mRNA that has the appropriate sequence. As for (B), tRNA molecules do in fact have an amino acid bound to their 3' end. The mRNA is read from 5' to 3' as the ribosome moves along the message. (D) is also true.

**25. D**

During meiosis, the gamete reduces its genetic component from $2n$ to $n$, resulting in a haploid cell with half the normal chromosome number. When a haploid egg and sperm unite, they form a diploid organism known as a zygote. All ova will contain an $X$ chromosome and all sperm will contain either an $X$ or a $Y$ chromosome. These gametes are formed during the two reductional divisions called meiosis. During metaphase I of meiosis I, tetrads form, and sister chromatids undergo the homologous recombination known as crossing over.

**26. A**

Red blood cells are produced in the bone marrow. They lose their nuclei to make room for more hemoglobin, which means that they cannot reproduce, repair themselves, or make proteins. Red blood cells actually greatly outnumber leukocytes (white blood cells) (C); as for (D), the spleen stores a reservoir of red blood cells and acts as a biological and physical filter for the blood, but it does not make red blood cells.

**27. C**

tRNA carries its specific amino acid to the ribosome, where it attaches to the growing polypeptide chain coded for by mRNA.

**28. D**

Oogenesis produces only one viable egg and two or three polar bodies. This is a result of unequal distribution of the cytoplasm during meiosis. Interstitial cells (A) are stimulated by LH to produce testosterone. FSH and testosterone then initiate the development of sperm in the seminiferous tubules. As for (B), eggs develop in follicles in the ovaries under the control of FSH. It is obvious in (C) that FSH plays a role in gamete production in both sexes.

**29. D**

Insulin is the hormone secreted by the beta cells of the pancreas in response to high blood glucose levels. Insulin decreases blood glucose by stimulating cells to uptake glucose, and by stimulating the conversion of glucose into its storage form, glycogen, in the liver and muscle cells. An overdose of insulin can, and often does, lead to a sharp decrease in blood glucose concentration.

**30. A**

Saliva in the mouth often begins the process of breaking down starch. Fats and proteins begin breaking down later in the digestive process.

**31. D**

Spermatogenesis and oogenesis are both examples of gametogenesis in that both produce haploid gametes through reductional division (meiosis) of diploid cells. These processes occur in the gonads. They differ in that in spermatogenesis, the cytoplasm is equally divided during meiosis and four viable sperm are produced from one diploid cell. In oogenesis, on the other hand, the cytoplasm is divided unequally, and only one ovum, with the bulk of the cytoplasm, is produced in addition to two or three inert polar bodies. Spermatogenesis is also continuous, meaning that it occurs throughout life and not only during puberty. Meanwhile, oogenesis freezes at the end of meiosis I and does not complete meiosis II until fertilization.

**32. C**

A Turner's female has the genotype *XO*; she carries only one *X* chromosome, has underdeveloped ovaries, and is sterile, but is female in appearance. These individuals are often shorter than normal and may have varying degrees of mental development problems.

**33. C**

According to the heterotroph hypothesis, the first forms of life lacked the ability to synthesize their own nutrients, requiring preformed molecules. Gradually, the molecules spontaneously formed by the environment began to prove inadequate to meet their energy needs, and autotrophs developed in response.

**34. D**

AB is known as the universal acceptor. It does not have antibodies to either the A or B antigens. Therefore, AB patients can receive blood from A, B, AB, or O people.

**35. D**

Progesterone is secreted by the corpus luteum. Its function is to thicken the uterine lining, preparing it for implantation of the fertilized egg.

**36. D**

A female has two *X* chromosomes, one inherited from her mother and one inherited from her father, while a given male has one *X* chromosome inherited from his mother and one *Y* chromosome inherited from his father. If a male expresses an *X*-linked trait, he must have inherited it from his mother. If normal parents have a color-blind son, he *must* have inherited the color blind gene, which is *X*-linked, from his mother. His mother *must* be a carrier of the color blind allele. The probability that a color blind son inherited the gene for color blindness from his mother is 100%.

**37. B**

Iron forms rust when water (or an even better electrolyte) turns iron and oxygen into iron oxide ($Fe_2O_3$), a chemical process. Helium and neon are both inert, so they do not react chemically. Water causing soil erosion may or may not incur a chemical change, and ice melting does not alter the chemistry of $H_2O$.

**38. A**

The major portion of an atom's mass consists of neutrons and protons. Electrons, positrons, neutrinos, and other subatomic particles have practically negligible masses.

**39. B**

Orbiting around the nucleus of an atom are electrons.

**40. D**

In degrees Kelvin, the freezing pointing of water is 273°. In the Kelvin temperature scale absolute zero, which is −273° Celsius, is set at 0°, and any temperature in degrees Celsius is 273° less than the same temperature as read in degrees Kelvin. Since the freezing point of water in degrees Celsius is 0°, in degrees Kelvin it is 273°.

**41. B**

The atom of an element with an atomic number of 17 must have 17 protons.

**42. C**

An atom that is not electrically neutral is called an ion. An isotope is any of two or more species of atoms of an element that have the same atomic number and nearly identical chemical behavior but differ in atomic mass or mass number and other physical properties. A positron is a positively charged particle having the same mass and magnitude of charge as the electron and constituting the antiparticle of the electron. An allotrope is an element that has two or more different forms (as of crystals) usually in the same phase; an example of allotropy is carbon, which can exist in such different forms as graphite and diamonds.

**43. A**

Electrons are in fact required for the fusion reactions, which makes sense because the hydrogen is being converted into helium. In fact, the core of the sun is so hot, that any electrons around atoms are stripped away. The remaining three answers are all properties of the standard fusion reaction.

## 44. C

Electronegativity is a measure of the attraction an atom has for electrons in a chemical bond. The greater the electronegativity of an atom, the greater its attraction for bonding electrons.

## 45. D

The noble gases, also called the inert gases possess low boiling points and are all gases at room temperature.

## 46. D

A pH below 7 indicates a relative excess of $H^+$ ions, and therefore an acidic solution.

## 47. C

Hydrocarbons can be classified into one of four classes: alkanes, alkenes, alkynes, and aromatics.

## 48. C

Electron affinity is the energy that is released when an electron is added to a gaseous atom, and it represents the ease with which the atom can accept an electron.

## 49. B

Malleability is the ability of a metal to be hammered into shapes.

## 50. D

The average speed of a gas is defined as the mathematical average of all the speeds of the gas particles in a sample. To answer this question, you must understand the Maxwell-Boltzmann distribution curve, which shows the distribution of speeds of all the gas particles in a sample at a given temperature. The distribution curve is a bell-shaped curve that flattens and shifts to the right as the temperature increases. The flattening of the curve means that gas particles within the sample are traveling at a greater range of speeds. As a result, a smaller proportion of the molecules will move at exactly the new average speed.

## 51. B

At high altitudes, the boiling point of water is lower than at sea level, because air pressure decreases as altitude increases.

## 52. A

If an element is very highly electronegative, its electron affinity won't be near zero. Electron affinity is a measure of the ease with which an atom can accept an electron in terms of the amount of energy released when a neutral atom accepts an additional electron. An atom that is highly electronegative can, of course, accept an electron very easily, so it will release a larger amount of energy. There are two ways of measuring electron affinity. According to one convention, increasing electron affinity is indicated by increasingly high positive numbers; according to the other convention, an increase in electron affinity is indicated by more negative numbers. The reason for the second convention is that increased electron affinity means more energy is released, and energy leaving a system means that the $\Delta H$ is negative. What both these conventions have in common is that the electron affinity is closer to zero for those elements that accept an electron less readily. A highly electronegative element, therefore, will have an electron affinity that is not close to zero, so choice (A) is our answer.

## 53 C

The atomic weight is the mass in grams of one mole (mol) of atoms. A mole corresponds to about $6.022 \times 10^{23}$. The atomic weight of an element, expressed in terms of g/mol, therefore, is the mass in grams of $6.022 \times 10^{23}$ atoms of that element. This number, roughly $6.022 \times 10^{23}$, to which a mole corresponds, is known as *Avogadro's number*.

## 54. B

In electricity, a unit of resistance is called an ohm. An ampere is a unit of electric current, a volt is a unit of electromotive force, and a watt is a unit of power equal to 1 joule per second.

## 55. C

As an ambulance passes, its pitch seems to change. This perception is best explained by the Doppler effect. As the ambulance approaches, the sound waves from its siren are compressed towards the observer. The intervals between waves diminish, which translates into an increase in frequency or pitch. As the ambulance recedes, the sound waves are stretched relative to the observer, causing the siren's pitch to decrease. By the change in pitch of the siren, one can determine if the ambulance is coming nearer or speeding away.

**56. A**

Of the states of electromagnetic radiation listed, radio waves have the longest wavelength and lowest frequency.

**57. B**

Weight is dependent on mass and acceleration due to gravity ($W = mg$).

**58. D**

Resistance is measured in ohms, and the symbol for an ohm is $\Omega$.

**59. A**

Using the formula $W = F \times d$, it can be seen that 1 pound of force applied through a distance of 1 foot will result in 1 foot-pound of work being done.

**60. C**

An insulator is a material that does not conduct electricity.

**61. B**

The principle of conservation of energy tells us that the amount of energy in the universe is constant.

**62. B**

A boulder that begins to roll down a hill is an example of an energy conversion from potential energy to kinetic energy.

**63. A**

Newton's Third Law of Motion tells us that when the bullet is fired, the bullet exerts that same amount of force on the gun as the gun exerts on the bullet.

**64. B**

Meters per second is a quantity that is related to speed. Acceleration and acceleration due to gravity are both measured in meters-per-second$^2$.

**65. D**

The energy of movement is known as kinetic energy.

# Learning Resources

# Math In a Nutshell

We've highlighted the 100 most important concepts that you'll need for almost any math test, including your nursing school entrance exam, and listed them in this learning resource. Use this list to remind yourself of the key areas you'll need to know. Do four concepts a day, and you'll be ready within a month. If a concept continually causes you trouble, circle it and refer back to it when correcting your practice tests.

## Number Properties

### 1. Number Categories

**Integers** are **whole numbers;** they include negative whole numbers and zero.

A **rational number** is a number that can be expressed as a **ratio of two integers. Irrational numbers** are real numbers—they have locations on the number line—but they **can't be expressed precisely as a fraction or decimal.** For the purposes of the SAT, the most important **irrational numbers** are $\sqrt{2}$, $\sqrt{3}$, and $\pi$.

### 2. Adding/Subtracting Signed Numbers

To **add a positive and a negative,** first ignore the signs and find the positive difference between the number parts. Then attach the sign of the original number with the larger number part. For example, to add 23 and −34, first ignore the minus sign and find the positive difference between 23 and 34—that's 11. Then attach the sign of the number with the larger number part—in this case it's the minus sign from the −34. So, 23 + (−34) = −11.

Make **subtraction** situations simpler by turning them into addition. For example, you can think of −17 − (−21) as −17 + (+21).

To **add or subtract a string of positives and negatives,** first turn everything into addition. Then combine the positives and negatives so that the string is reduced to the sum of a single positive number and a single negative number.

### 3. Multiplying/Dividing Signed Numbers

To multiply and/or divide positives and negatives, treat the number parts as usual and **attach a minus sign if there were originally an odd number of negatives.** For example, to multiply −2, −3, and −5, first multiply the number parts: $2 \times 3 \times 5 = 30$. Then go back and note that there were *three*—an *odd* number—negatives, so the product is negative: $(-2) \times (-3) \times (-5) = -30$.

### 4. PEMDAS

When performing multiple operations, remember to perform them in the right order: **PEMDAS,** which means **Parentheses** first, then **Exponents,** then **Multiplication** and **Division** (left to right), and lastly **Addition** and **Subtraction** (left to right). In the expression $9 - 2 \times (5 - 3)^2 + 6 \div 3$, begin with the parentheses: $(5 - 3) = 2$. Then do the exponent: $2^2 = 4$. Now the expression is: $9 - 2 \times 4 + 6 \div 3$. Next do the multiplication and division to get: $9 - 8 + 2$, which equals 3. If you have difficulty remembering PEMDAS, use this sentence to recall it: **P**lease **E**xcuse **M**y **D**ear **A**unt **S**ally.

**KAPLAN**

### 5. Counting Consecutive Integers

To count consecutive integers, **subtract the smallest from the largest and add 1.** To count the integers from 13 through 31, subtract: $31 - 13 = 18$. Then add 1: $18 + 1 = 19$.

## Number operations and concepts

### 6. Exponential Growth

If $r$ is the ratio between consecutive terms, $a_1$ is the first term, $a_n$ is the $n$th term, and $S_n$ is the sum of the first $n$ terms, then $a_n = a_1 r^{n-1}$ and $S_n = \dfrac{a_1 - a_1 r^n}{1 - r}$.

### 7. Union and Intersection of Sets

The things in a set are called elements or members. The union of Set $A$ and Set $B$, sometimes expressed as $A \cup B$, is the set of elements that are in either or both of Set $A$ and Set $B$. If Set $A = \{1, 2\}$ and Set $B = \{3, 4\}$, then $A \cup B = \{1, 2, 3, 4\}$. The intersection of Set $A$ and Set $B$, sometimes expressed as $A \cap B$, is the set of elements common to both Set $A$ and Set $B$. If Set $A = \{1, 2, 3\}$ and Set $B = \{3, 4, 5\}$, then $A \cap B = \{3\}$.

## Divisibility

### 8. Factor/Multiple

The **factors** of integer $n$ are the positive integers that divide into $n$ with no remainder. The **multiples** of $n$ are the integers that $n$ divides into with no remainder. For example, 6 is a factor of 12, and 24 is a multiple of 12. 12 is both a factor and a multiple of itself, since $12 \times 1 = 12$ and $12 \div 1 = 12$.

### 9. Prime Factorization

To find the prime factorization of an integer, just keep breaking it up into factors until **all the factors are prime.** To find the prime factorization of 36, for example, you could begin by breaking it into $4 \times 9$: $36 = 4 \times 9 = 2 \times 2 \times 3 \times 3$.

### 10. Relative Primes

Relative primes are integers that have no common factor other than 1. To determine whether two integers are relative primes, break them both down to their prime factorizations. For example: $35 = 5 \times 7$, and $54 = 2 \times 3 \times 3 \times 3$. They have **no prime factors in common,** so 35 and 54 are relative primes.

### 11. Common Multiple

A common multiple is a number that is a multiple of two or more integers. You can always get a common multiple of two integers by **multiplying** them, but, unless the two numbers are relative primes, the product will not be the *least* common multiple. For example, to find a common multiple for 12 and 15, you could just multiply: $12 \times 15 = 180$.

To find the **least common multiple,** check out the **multiples of the larger integer** until you find one that's **also a multiple of the smaller.** To find the LCM of 12 and 15, begin by taking the multiples of 15: 15 is not divisible by 12; 30 is not; nor is 45. But the next multiple of 15, 60, *is* divisible by 12, so it's the LCM.

### 12. Greatest Common Factor (GCF)

To find the greatest common factor, break down both integers into their prime factorizations and multiply **all the prime factors they have in common.** $36 = 2 \times 2 \times 3 \times 3$, and $48 = 2 \times 2 \times 2 \times 2 \times 3$. What they have in common is two 2s and one 3, so the GCF is $2 \times 2 \times 3 = 12$.

### 13. Even/Odd

To predict whether a sum, difference, or product will be even or odd, just **take simple numbers like 1 and 2 and see what happens.** There are rules—"odd times even is even," for example—but there's no need to memorize them. What happens with one set of numbers generally happens with all similar sets.

### 14. Multiples of 2 and 4

An integer is divisible by 2 (even) if the **last digit is even.** An integer is divisible by 4 if the **last two digits form a multiple of 4.** The last digit of 562 is 2, which is even, so 562 is a multiple of 2. The last two digits form 62, which is *not* divisible by 4, so 562 is not a multiple of 4. The integer 512, however is divisible by four because the last two digits form 12, which is a multiple of 4.

### 15. Multiples of 3 and 9

An integer is divisible by 3 if the **sum of its digits is divisible by 3.** An integer is divisible by 9 if the **sum of its digits is divisible by 9.** The sum of the digits in 957 is 21, which is divisible by 3 but not by 9, so 957 is divisible by 3 but not by 9.

### 16. Multiples of 5 and 10

An integer is divisible by 5 if the **last digit is 5 or zero.** An integer is divisible by 10 if the **last digit is zero.** The last digit of 665 is 5, so 665 is a multiple of 5 but *not* a multiple of 10.

### 17. Remainders

The remainder is the **whole number left over after division.** 487 is 2 more than 485, which is a multiple of 5, so when 487 is divided by 5, the remainder will be 2.

## Fractions and Decimals

### 18. Reducing Fractions

To reduce a fraction to lowest terms, **factor out and cancel** all factors the numerator and denominator have in common.

$$\frac{28}{36} = \frac{4 \times 7}{4 \times 9} = \frac{7}{9}$$

### 19. Adding/Subtracting Fractions

To add or subtract fractions, first find a **common denominator,** then add or subtract the numerators.

$$\frac{2}{15} + \frac{3}{10} = \frac{4}{30} + \frac{9}{30} = \frac{4+9}{30} = \frac{13}{30}$$

### 20. Multiplying Fractions

To multiply fractions, **multiply** the numerators and **multiply** the denominators.

$$\frac{5}{7} \times \frac{3}{4} = \frac{5 \times 3}{7 \times 4} = \frac{15}{28}$$

### 21. Dividing Fractions

To divide fractions, **invert** the second one and **multiply.**

$$\frac{1}{2} \div \frac{3}{5} = \frac{1}{2} \times \frac{5}{3} = \frac{1 \times 5}{2 \times 3} = \frac{5}{6}$$

### 22. Mixed Numbers and Improper Fractions

To convert a mixed number to an improper fraction, **multiply** the whole number part by the denominator, then **add** the numerator. The result is the new numerator (over the same denominator). To convert $7\frac{1}{3}$, first multiply 7 by 3, then add 1, to get the new numerator of 22. Put that over the same denominator, 3, to get $\frac{22}{3}$.

To convert an improper fraction to a mixed number, divide the denominator into the numerator to get a **whole number quotient with a remainder.** The quotient becomes the whole number part of the mixed number, and the remainder becomes the new numerator—with the same denominator. For example, to convert $\frac{108}{5}$, first divide 5 into 108, which yields 21 with a remainder of 3. Therefore, $\frac{108}{5} = 21\frac{3}{5}$.

### 23. Reciprocal

To find the reciprocal of a fraction, **switch the numerator and the denominator.** The reciprocal of $\frac{3}{7}$ is $\frac{7}{3}$. The reciprocal of 5 is $\frac{1}{5}$. The product of reciprocals is 1.

### 24. Comparing Fractions

One way to compare fractions is to **re-express them with a common denominator.** $\frac{3}{4} = \frac{21}{28}$ and $\frac{5}{7} = \frac{20}{28}$. $\frac{21}{28}$ is greater than $\frac{20}{28}$, so $\frac{3}{4}$ is greater than $\frac{5}{7}$. Another method is to **convert them both to decimals.** $\frac{3}{4}$ converts to 0.75, and $\frac{5}{7}$ converts to approximately 0.714.

### 25. Converting Fractions and Decimals

To convert a fraction to a decimal, **divide the bottom into the top.** To convert $\frac{5}{8}$, divide 8 into 5, yielding 0.625.

To convert a decimal to a fraction, set the decimal over 1 and **multiply the numerator and denominator by 10** raised to the number of digits to the right of the decimal point.

To convert 0.625 to a fraction, you would multiply $\frac{0.625}{1}$ by $\frac{10^3}{10^3}$ or $\frac{1000}{1000}$. Then simplify: $\frac{625}{1000} = \frac{5 \times 125}{8 \times 125} = \frac{5}{8}$.

### 26. Repeating Decimal

To find a particular digit in a repeating decimal, note the **number of digits in the cluster that repeats.** If there are 2 digits in that cluster, then every second digit is the same. If there are 3 digits in that cluster, then every third digit is the same. And so on. For example, the decimal equivalent of $\frac{1}{27}$ is 0.037…, which is best written $0.\overline{037}$. There are 3 digits in the repeating cluster, so every third digit is the same: 7. To find the 50th digit, look for the multiple of 3 just less than 50—that's 48. The 48th digit is 7, and with the 49th digit the pattern repeats with zero. The 50th digit is 3.

### 27. Identifying the Parts and the Whole

The key to solving most fractions and percents story problems is to identify the part and the whole. Usually you'll find the **part** associated with the verb *is/are* and the **whole** associated with the word *of.* In the sentence, "Half of the boys are blonds," the whole is the boys ("*of the boys*"), and the part is the blonds ("*are* blonds").

## Percents

### 28. Percent Formula

Whether you need to find the part, the whole, or the percent, use the same formula:

**Part = Percent × Whole**

**Example:** What is 12% of 25?
**Setup:** Part = 0.12 × 25

**Example:** 15 is 3% of what number?
**Setup:** 15 = 0.03 × Whole

**Example:** 45 is what percent of 9?
**Setup:** 45 = Percent × 9

### 29. Percent Increase and Decrease

To increase a number by a percent, **add the percent to 100%,** convert to a decimal, and multiply. To increase 40 by 25%, add 25% to 100%, convert 125% to 1.25, and multiply by 40. 1.25 × 40 = 50.

### 30. Finding the Original Whole

To find the **original whole before a percent increase or decrease,** set up an equation. Think of the result of a 15% increase over *x* as 1.15*x*.

**Example:** After a 5% increase, the population was 59,346. What was the population before the increase?
**Setup:** 1.05*x* = 59,346

### 31. Combined Percent Increase and Decrease

To determine the combined effect of multiple percent increases and/or decreases, **start with 100 and see what happens.**

**Example:** A price went up 10% one year, and the new price went up 20% the next year. What was the combined percent increase?

**Setup:** First year: 100 + (10% of 100) = 110. Second year: 110 + (20% of 110) = 132. That's a combined 32% increase.

## Ratios, Proportions, and Rates

### 32. Setting up a Ratio

To find a ratio, put the number associated with the word *of* **on top** and the quantity associated with the word *to* **on the bottom** and reduce. The ratio of 20 oranges to 12 apples is $\frac{20}{12}$, which reduces to $\frac{5}{3}$.

### 33. Part-to-Part Ratios and Part-to-Whole Ratios

If the parts add up to the whole, a part-to-part ratio can be turned into two part-to-whole ratios by putting **each number in the original ratio over the sum of the numbers.**

If the ratio of males to females is 1 to 2, then the males-to-people ratio is $\frac{1}{1+2} = \frac{1}{3}$ and the females-to-people ratio is $\frac{2}{1+2} = \frac{2}{3}$. In other words, $\frac{2}{3}$ of all the people are female.

### 34. Solving a Proportion

To solve a proportion, **cross multiply:**

$$\frac{x}{5} = \frac{3}{4}$$

$$4x = 3 \times 5$$

$$x = \frac{15}{4} = 3.75$$

### 35. Rate

To solve a rates problem, **use the units** to keep things straight.

**Example:** If snow is falling at the rate of 1 foot every 4 hours, how many inches of snow will fall in 7 hours?

**Setup:**

$$\frac{1 \text{ foot}}{4 \text{ hours}} = \frac{x \text{ inches}}{7 \text{ hours}}$$

$$\frac{12 \text{ inches}}{4 \text{ hours}} = \frac{x \text{ inches}}{7 \text{ hours}}$$

$$4x = 12 \times 7$$

$$x = 21$$

### 36. Average Rate

Average rate is *not* simply the average of the rates.

$$\text{Average } A \text{ per } B = \frac{\text{Total } A}{\text{Total } B}$$

$$\text{Average Speed} = \frac{\text{Total distance}}{\text{Total time}}$$

To find the average speed for 120 miles at 40 mph and 120 miles at 60 mph, **don't just average the two speeds.** First, figure out the total distance and the total time. The total distance is 120 + 120 = 240 miles. The times are 2 hours for the first leg and 3 hours for the second leg, or 5 hours total. The average speed, then, is $\frac{240}{5} = 48$ miles per hour.

## Averages

### 37. Average Formula

To find the average of a set of numbers, **add them up and divide by the number of numbers.**

$$\text{Average} = \frac{\text{Sum of the Terms}}{\text{Number of Terms}}$$

To find the average of the 5 numbers 12, 15, 23, 40, and 40, first add them: $12 + 15 + 23 + 40 + 40 = 130$. Then, divide the sum by 5: $130 \div 5 = 26$.

### 38. Average of Evenly Spaced Numbers

To find the average of evenly spaced numbers, just **average the smallest and the largest.** The average of all the integers from 13 through 77 is the same as the average of 13 and 77:

$$\frac{13 + 77}{2} = \frac{90}{2} = 45$$

### 39. Using the Average to Find the Sum

**Sum = (Average) × (Number of terms)**

If the average of 10 numbers is 50, then they add up to $10 \times 50$, or 500.

### 40. Finding the Missing Number

To find a missing number when you're given the average, **use the sum.** If the average of 4 numbers is 7, then the sum of those 4 numbers is $4 \times 7$, or 28. Suppose that 3 of the numbers are 3, 5, and 8. These 3 numbers add up to 16 of that 28, which leaves 12 for the fourth number.

### 41. Median and Mode

The median of a set of numbers is the **value that falls in the middle of the set.** If you have 5 test scores, and they are 88, 86, 57, 94, and 73, you must first list the scores in increasing or decreasing order: 57, 73, 86, 88, 94.

The median is the middle number, or 86. If there is an even number of values in a set (6 test scores, for instance), simply take the average of the 2 middle numbers.

The mode of a set of numbers is the **value that appears most often.** If your test scores were 88, 57, 68, 85, 99, 93, 93, 84, and 81, the mode of the scores would be 93 because it appears more often than any other score. If there is a tie for the most common value in a set, the set has more than one mode.

## Possibilities and Probability

### 42. Counting the Possibilities

The fundamental counting principle: If there are *m* **ways** one event can happen and *n* **ways** a second event can happen, then there are *m* × *n* **ways** for the 2 events to happen. For example, with 5 shirts and 7 pairs of pants to choose from, you can have $5 \times 7 = 35$ different outfits.

### 43. Probability

$$\text{Probability} = \frac{\text{Favorable Outcomes}}{\text{Total Possible Outcomes}}$$

For example, if you have 12 shirts in a drawer and 9 of them are white, the probability of picking a white shirt at random is $\frac{9}{12} = \frac{3}{4}$. This probability can also be expressed as 0.75 or 75%.

## Powers and Roots

### 44. Multiplying and Dividing Powers

To multiply powers with the same base, **add the exponents and keep the same base:**

$$x^3 \times x^4 = x^{3+4} = x^7$$

To divide powers with the same base, **subtract the exponents and keep the same base:**

$$y^{13} \div y^8 = y^{13-8} = y^5$$

### 45. Raising Powers to Powers

To raise a power to a power, **multiply the exponents:**

$$(x^3)^4 = x^{3 \times 4} = x^{12}$$

### 46. Simplifying Square Roots

To simplify a square root, **factor out the perfect squares** under the radical, unsquare them, and put the result in front.

$$\sqrt{12} = \sqrt{4 \times 3} = \sqrt{4} \times \sqrt{3} = 2\sqrt{3}$$

### 47. Adding and Subtracting Roots

You can add or subtract radical expressions **when the part under the radicals is the same:**

$$2\sqrt{3} + 3\sqrt{3} = 5\sqrt{3}$$

Don't try to add or subtract when the radical parts are different. There's not much you can do with an expression like:

$$3\sqrt{5} + 3\sqrt{7}$$

### 48. Multiplying and Dividing Roots

The product of square roots is equal to the **square root of the product:**

$$\sqrt{3} \times \sqrt{5} = \sqrt{3 \times 5} = \sqrt{15}$$

The quotient of square roots is equal to the **square root of the quotient:**

$$\frac{\sqrt{6}}{\sqrt{3}} = \sqrt{\frac{6}{3}} = \sqrt{2}$$

### 49. Negative Exponent and Rational Exponent

To find the value of a number raised to a negative exponent, simply rewrite the number, without the negative sign, as the bottom of a fraction with 1 as the numerator of the fraction: $3^{-2} = \frac{1}{3^2} = \frac{1}{9}$. If $x$ is a positive number and $a$ is a

nonzero number, then $x^{\frac{1}{a}} = \sqrt[a]{x}$. So $4^{\frac{1}{2}} = \sqrt[2]{4} = 2$. If $p$ and $q$ are integers, then $x^{\frac{p}{q}} = \sqrt[q]{x^p}$. So $4^{\frac{3}{2}} = \sqrt[2]{4^3} = \sqrt{64} = 8$.

## Absolute Value

### 50. Determining Absolute Value

The absolute value of a number is the distance of the number from zero on the number line. Because absolute value is a distance, it is always positive. The absolute value of 7 is 7; this is expressed $|7| = 7$. Similarly, the absolute value of $-7$ is 7: $|-7| = 7$. Every positive number is the absolute value of 2 numbers: itself and its negative.

## Algebraic Expressions

### 51. Evaluating an Expression

To evaluate an algebraic expression, **plug in** the given values for the unknowns and calculate according to **PEMDAS.** To find the value of $x^2 + 5x - 6$ when $x = -2$, plug in $-2$ for $x$: $(-2)^2 + 5(-2) - 6 = -12$.

### 52. Adding and Subtracting Monomials

To combine like terms, **keep the variable part unchanged while adding or subtracting the coefficients:**

$$2a + 3a = (2 + 3)a = 5a$$

### 53. Adding and Subtracting Polynomials

To add or subtract polynomials, **combine like terms.**

$$(3x^2 + 5x - 7) - (x^2 + 12) =$$
$$(3x^2 - x^2) + 5x + (-7 - 12) =$$
$$2x^2 + 5x - 19$$

### 54. Multiplying Monomials

To multiply monomials, **multiply the coefficients and the variables separately:**

$$2a \times 3a = (2 \times 3)(a \times a) = 6a^2$$

### 55. Multiplying Binomials: FOIL

To multiply binomials, use **FOIL.** To multiply $(x + 3)$ by $(x + 4)$, first multiply the **F**irst terms: $x \times x = x^2$. Next the **O**uter terms: $x \times 4 = 4x$. Then the **I**nner terms: $3 \times x = 3x$. And finally the **L**ast terms: $3 \times 4 = 12$. Then add and combine like terms:

$$x^2 + 4x + 3x + 12 = x^2 + 7x + 12$$

### 56. Multiplying Other Polynomials

FOIL works only when you want to multiply two binomials. If you want to multiply polynomials with more than two terms, make sure you **multiply each term in the first polynomial by each term in the second.**

$$(x^2 + 3x + 4)(x + 5) =$$
$$x^2(x + 5) + 3x(x + 5) + 4(x + 5) =$$
$$x^3 + 5x^2 + 3x^2 + 15x + 4x + 20 =$$
$$x^3 + 8x^2 + 19x + 20$$

After multiplying two polynomials together, the number of terms in your expression before simplifying should equal the number of terms in one polynomial multiplied by the number of terms in the second. In the example, you should have $3 \times 2 = 6$ terms in the product before you simplify like terms.

## Factoring Algebraic Expressions

### 57. Factoring out a Common Divisor

A factor common to all terms of a polynomial can be **factored out.** All three terms in the polynomial $3x^3 + 12x^2 - 6x$ contain a factor of $3x$. Pulling out the common factor yields $3x(x^2 + 4x - 2)$.

### 58. Factoring the Difference of Squares

One of the test maker's favorite factorables is the **difference of squares.**

$$a^2 - b^2 = (a - b)(a + b)$$

$x^2 - 9$, for example, factors to $(x - 3)(x + 3)$.

### 59. Factoring the Square of a Binomial

Recognize polynomials that are squares of binomials:

$$a^2 + 2ab + b^2 = (a + b)^2$$
$$a^2 - 2ab + b^2 = (a - b)^2$$

For example, $4x^2 + 12x + 9$ factors to $(2x + 3)^2$, and $n^2 - 10n + 25$ factors to $(n - 5)^2$.

### 60. Factoring Other Polynomials: FOIL in Reverse

To factor a quadratic expression, **think about what binomials you could use FOIL on to get that quadratic expression.** To factor $x^2 - 5x + 6$, think about what **F**irst terms will produce $x^2$, what **L**ast terms will produce $+6$, and what **O**uter and **I**nner terms will produce $-5x$. Some common sense—and a little trial and error—lead you to $(x - 2)(x - 3)$.

### 61. Simplifying an Algebraic Fraction

Simplifying an algebraic fraction is a lot like simplifying a numerical fraction. The general idea is to **find factors common to the numerator and denominator and cancel them.** Thus, simplifying an algebraic fraction begins with factoring.

For example, to simplify $\dfrac{x^2 - x - 12}{x^2 - 9}$, first factor the numerator and denominator:

$$\frac{x^2 - x - 12}{x^2 - 9} = \frac{(x - 4)(x + 3)}{(x - 3)(x + 3)}$$

Canceling $x + 3$ from the numerator and denominator leaves you with $\dfrac{x - 4}{x - 3}$.

## Solving Equations

### 62. Solving a Linear Equation

To solve an equation, do whatever is necessary to both sides to **isolate the variable.** To solve the equation $5x - 12 = -2x + 9$, first get all the $x$'s on one side by adding $2x$ to both sides: $7x - 12 = 9$. Then add 12 to both sides: $7x = 21$. Then divide both sides by 7: $x = 3$.

### 63. Solving "In Terms Of"

To solve an equation for one variable **in terms of** another means to **isolate the one variable on one side of the equation,** leaving an expression containing the other variable on the other side of the equation. To solve the equation $3x - 10y = -5x + 6y$ for $x$ in terms of $y$, isolate $x$:

$$3x - 10y = -5x + 6y$$

$$3x + 5x = 6y + 10y$$

$$8x = 16y$$

$$x = 2y$$

### 64. Translating from English into Algebra

To translate from English into algebra, look for the key words and systematically turn phrases into algebraic expressions and sentences into equations. Be careful about order, especially when subtraction is called for.

**Example:**    The charge for a phone call is $r$ cents for the first 3 minutes and $s$ cents for each minute thereafter. What is the cost, in cents, of a phone call lasting exactly $t$ minutes? $(t > 3)$

**Setup:**    The charge begins with $r$, and then something more is added, depending on the length of the call. The amount added is $s$ times the number of minutes past 3 minutes. If the total number of minutes is $t$, then the number of minutes past 3 is $t - 3$. So the charge is $r + s(t - 3)$.

### 65. Solving a Quadratic Equation

To solve a quadratic equation, put it in the "$ax^2 + bx + c = 0$" form, **factor** the left side (if you can), and set each factor equal to 0 separately to get the two solutions. To solve $x^2 + 12 = 7x$, first rewrite it as $x^2 - 7x + 12 = 0$. Then factor the left side:

$$(x - 3)(x - 4) = 0$$

$$x - 3 = 0 \text{ or } x - 4 = 0$$

$$x = 3 \text{ or } 4$$

### 66. Solving a System of Equations

You can solve for 2 variables only if you have 2 distinct equations. 2 forms of the same equation will not be adequate. **Combine the equations** in such a way that **one of the variables cancels out.** To solve the 2 equations $4x + 3y = 8$ and $x + y = 3$, multiply both sides of the second equation by $-3$ to get: $-3x - 3y = -9$. Now add the 2 equations; the $3y$ and the $-3y$ cancel out, leaving: $x = -1$. Plug that back into either one of the original equations and you'll find that $y = 4$.

### 67. Solving an Inequality

To solve an inequality, do whatever is necessary to both sides to **isolate the variable.** Just remember that when you **multiply or divide both sides by a negative number, you must reverse the sign.** To solve $-5x + 7 < -3$, subtract 7 from both sides to get: $-5x < -10$. Now divide both sides by $-5$, remembering to reverse the sign: $x > 2$.

### 68. Radical Equations

A radical equation contains at least one radical expression. Solve radical equations by using standard rules of algebra. If $5\sqrt{x} - 2 = 13$, then $5\sqrt{x} = 15$ and $\sqrt{x} = 3$, so $x = 9$.

## Functions

### 69. Function Notation and Evaluation

Standard function notation is written $f(x)$ and read "$f$ of 4." To evaluate the function $f(x) = 2x + 3$ for $f(4)$, replace $x$ with 4 and simplify: $f(4) = 2(4) + 3 = 11$.

### 70. Direct and Inverse Variation

In direct variation, $y = kx$, where $k$ is a nonzero constant. In direct variation, the variable $y$ changes directly as $x$ does. If a unit of Currency $A$ is worth 2 units of Currency $B$, then $A = 2B$. If the number of units of $B$ were to double, the number of units of $A$ would double, and so on for halving, tripling, etc. In inverse variation, $xy = k$, where $x$ and $y$ are variables and $k$ is a constant. A famous inverse relationship is $rate \times time = distance$, where distance is constant. Imagine having to cover a distance of 24 miles. If you were to travel at 12 miles per hour, you'd need 2 hours. But if you were to halve your rate, you would have to double your time. This is just another way of saying that rate and time vary inversely.

### 71. Domain and Range of a Function

The domain of a function is the set of values for which the function is defined. For example, the domain of $f(x) = \dfrac{1}{1 - x^2}$ is all values of $x$ except 1 and $-1$, because for those values the denominator has a value of 0 and is therefore undefined. The range of a function is the set of outputs or results of the function. For example, the range of $f(x) = x^2$ is all numbers greater than all or equal to zero, because $x^2$ cannot be negative.

## Coordinate Geometry

### 72. Finding the Distance Between Two Points

To find the distance between points, **use the Pythagorean theorem** or **special right triangles.** The difference between the $x$'s is one leg and the difference between the $y$'s is the other.

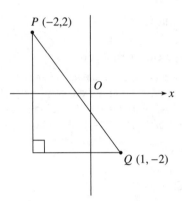

In the figure above, $PQ$ is the hypotenuse of a 3-4-5 triangle, so $PQ = 5$.

You can also use the **distance formula:**

$$d = \sqrt{(x_1 - x_2)^2 + (y_1 - y_2)^2}$$

To find the distance between $R(3, 6)$ and $S(5, -2)$:

$$d = \sqrt{(3 - 5)^2 + [6 - (-2)^2]}$$

$$= \sqrt{(-2)^2 + (8)^2}$$

$$= \sqrt{68} = 2\sqrt{17}$$

### 73. Using Two Points to Find the Slope

$$\text{Slope} = \frac{\text{Change in } y}{\text{Change in } x} = \frac{\text{Rise}}{\text{Run}}$$

The slope of the line that contains the points $A(2, 3)$ and $B(0, -1)$ is:

$$\frac{y_A - y_B}{x_A - x_B} = \frac{3 - (-1)}{2 - 0} = \frac{4}{2} = 2$$

### 74. Using an Equation to Find the Slope

To find the slope of a line from an equation, put the equation into the **slope-intercept** form:

$$y = mx + b$$

The **slope is** *m*. To find the slope of the equation $3x + 2y = 4$, rearrange it:

$$3x + 2y = 4$$

$$2y = -3x + 4$$

$$y = -\frac{3}{2}x + 2$$

The slope is $-\frac{3}{2}$.

### 75. Using an Equation to Find an Intercept

To find the *y*-intercept, you can either put the equation into **y = mx + b** (**slope-intercept**) form—in which case **b is the y-intercept**—or you can just **plug x = 0** into the equation and **solve for y**. To find the *x*-intercept, **plug y = 0** into the equation and **solve for x**.

### 76. Finding the Midpoint

The midpoint of two points on a line segment is the average of the *x*-coordinates of the endpoints and the average of the *y*-coordinates of the endpoints. If the endpoints are $(x_1, y_1)$ and $(x_2, y_2)$, the midpoint is $\left(\frac{x_1 + x_2}{2}, \frac{y_1 + y_2}{2}\right)$. The midpoint of (3, 5) and (9, 1) is $\left(\frac{3 + 9}{2}, \frac{5 + 1}{2}\right)$.

## Lines and Angles

### 77. Intersecting Lines

When two lines intersect, **adjacent angles are supplementary and vertical angles are equal.**

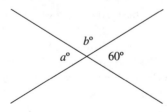

In the previous image, the angles marked *a°* and *b°* are adjacent and supplementary, so $a + b = 180$.
Furthermore, the angles marked *a°* and 60° are vertical and equal, so $a = 60$.

### 78. Parallel Lines and Transversals

A transversal across parallel lines forms **four equal acute angles and four equal obtuse angles.**

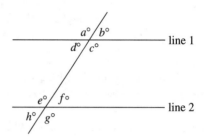

In the figure above, line 1 is parallel to line 2. Angles *a, c, e,* and *g* are obtuse, so they are all equal. Angles *b, d, f,* and *h* are acute, so they are all equal.

Furthermore, **any of the acute angles is supplementary to any of the obtuse angles.** Angles *a* and *h* are supplementary, as are *b* and *e, c* and *f,* and so on.

## Triangles: General

### 79. Interior and Exterior Angles of a Triangle

The 3 angles of any triangle **add up to 180°.**

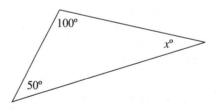

In the figure above, $x + 50 + 100 = 180$, so $x = 30$.

An exterior angle of a triangle is equal to the **sum of the remote interior angles.**

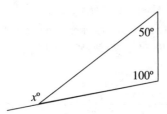

In the figure above, the exterior angle labeled $x°$ is equal to the sum of the remote angles: $x = 50 + 100 = 150$.

The 3 exterior angles of a triangle add up to 360°.

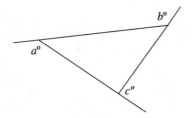

In the figure above, $a + b + c = 360$.

## 80. Similar Triangles

Similar triangles have the same shape: **corresponding angles are equal and corresponding sides are proportional.**

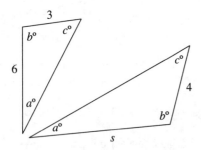

The triangles above are similar because they have the same angles. The 3 corresponds to the 4 and the 6 corresponds to the $s$.

$$\frac{3}{4} = \frac{6}{s}$$
$$3s = 24$$
$$s = 8$$

## 81. Area of a Triangle

$$\text{Area of Triangle} = \frac{1}{2}(\text{base})(\text{height})$$

The height is the perpendicular distance between the side that's chosen as the base and the opposite vertex.

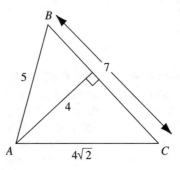

In the triangle above, 4 is the height when the 7 is chosen as the base.

$$\text{Area} = \frac{1}{2}bh = \frac{1}{2}(7)(4) = 14$$

## 82. Triangle Inequality Theorem

The length of one side of a triangle must be **greater than the difference and less than the sum** of the lengths of the other two sides. For example, if it is given that the length of one side is 3 and the length of another side is 7, then you know that the length of the third side must be greater than $7 - 3 = 4$ and less than $7 + 3 = 10$.

## 83. Isosceles and Equilateral Triangles

An isosceles triangle is a triangle that has **2 equal sides.** Not only are 2 sides equal, but the angles opposite the equal sides, called **base angles**, are also equal.

Equilateral triangles are triangles in which **all 3 sides are equal.** Since all the sides are equal, all the angles are also equal. All 3 angles in an equilateral triangle measure 60°, regardless of the lengths of sides.

# RIGHT TRIANGLES

### 84. Pythagorean Theorem

For all right triangles:

$$(leg_1)^2 + (leg_2)^2 = (hypotenuse)^2$$

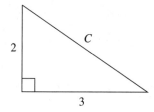

If one leg is 2 and the other leg is 3, then:

$$2^2 + 3^2 = c^2$$
$$c^2 = 4 + 9$$
$$c = \sqrt{13}$$

### 85. The 3-4-5 Triangle

If a right triangle's leg-to-leg ratio is 3:4, or if the leg-to-hypotenuse ratio is 3:5 or 4:5, it's a 3-4-5 triangle and you don't need to use the Pythagorean theorem to find the third side. Just figure out what multiple of 3-4-5 it is.

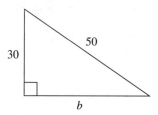

In the right triangle shown, one leg is 30 and the hypotenuse is 50. This is 10 times 3-4-5. The other leg is 40.

### 86. The 5-12-13 Triangle

If a right triangle's leg-to-leg ratio is 5:12, or if the leg-to-hypotenuse ratio is 5:13 or 12:13, then it's a 5-12-13 triangle and you don't need to use the Pythagorean theorem to find the third side. Just figure out what multiple of 5-12-13 it is.

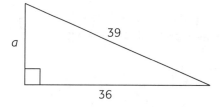

Here one leg is 36 and the hypotenuse is 39. This is 3 times 5-12-13. The other leg is 15.

### 87. The 30-60-90 Triangle

The sides of a 30-60-90 triangle are in a ratio of $x : x\sqrt{3} : 2x$. You don't need the Pythagorean theorem.

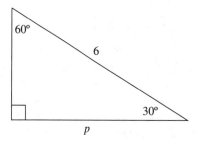

If the hypotenuse is 6, then the shorter leg is half that, or 3; and then the longer leg is equal to the short leg times $\sqrt{3}$, or $3\sqrt{3}$.

### 88. The 45-45-90 Triangle

The sides of a 45-45-90 triangle are in a ratio of $x : x : x\sqrt{2}$.

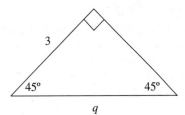

If one leg is 3, then the other leg is also 3, and the hypotenuse is equal to a leg times $\sqrt{2}$, or $3\sqrt{2}$.

## Other Polygons

### 89. Characteristics of a Rectangle

A rectangle is a **four-sided figure with four right angles.** Opposite sides are equal. Diagonals are equal.

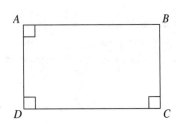

Quadrilateral *ABCD* above is shown to have three right angles. The fourth angle therefore also measures 90°, and *ABCD* is a rectangle. The perimeter of a rectangle is equal to the sum of the lengths of the four sides, which is equivalent to 2(length + width).

### Area of Rectangle = Length × width

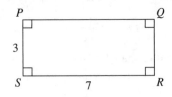

The area of a 7-by-3 rectangle is $7 \times 3 = 21$.

### 90. Characteristics of a Parallelogram

A parallelogram has **two pairs of parallel sides.** Opposite sides are equal. Opposite angles are equal. Consecutive angles add up to 180°.

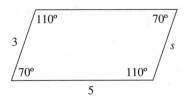

In the figure above, *s* is the length of the side opposite the 3, so $s = 3$.

### Area of Parallelogram = Base × height

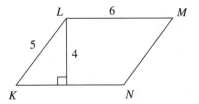

In parallelogram *KLMN* above, 4 is the height when *LM* or *KN* is used as the base. Base × height = $6 \times 4 = 24$.

### 91. Characteristics of a Square

A square is a **rectangle with four equal sides.**

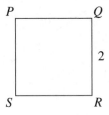

If *PQRS* is a square, all sides are the same length as *QR*. The perimeter of a square is equal to four times the length of one side.

### Area of Square = (Side)²

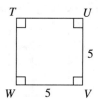

The square above, with sides of length 5, has an area of $5^2 = 25$.

### 92. Interior Angles of a Polygon

The **sum of the measures of the interior angles of a polygon = $(n - 2) \times 180$**, where $n$ is the number of sides.

$$\text{Sum of the Angles} = (n - 2) \times 180$$

The eight angles of an octagon, for example, add up to $(8 - 2) \times 180 = 1,080$.

## Circles

### 93. Circumference of a Circle

$$\text{Circumference} = 2\pi r$$

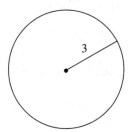

In the circle above, the radius is 3, and so the circumference is $2\pi(3) = 6\pi$.

### 94. Length of an Arc

An **arc** is a piece of the circumference. If $n$ is the degree measure of the arc's central angle, then the formula is:

$$\text{Length of an Arc} = \left(\frac{n}{360}\right)(2\pi r)$$

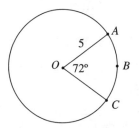

In the figure above, the radius is 5 and the measure of the central angle is 72°. The arc length is $\frac{72}{360}$ or $\frac{1}{5}$ of the circumference:

$$\left(\frac{72}{360}\right)(2\pi)(5) = \left(\frac{1}{5}\right)(10\pi) = 2\pi$$

### 95. Area of a Circle

$$\text{Area of a Circle} = \pi r^2$$

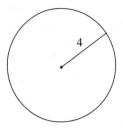

The area of the circle is $\pi(4)^2 = 16\pi$.

### 96. Area of a Sector

A **sector** is a piece of the area of a circle. If $n$ is the degree measure of the sector's central angle, then the formula is:

$$\text{Area of a Sector} = \left(\frac{n}{360}\right)(\pi r^2)$$

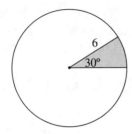

In the figure above, the radius is 6 and the measure of the sector's central angle is 30°. The sector has $\frac{30}{360}$ or $\frac{1}{12}$ of the area of the circle:

$$\left(\frac{30}{360}\right)(\pi)(6^2) = \left(\frac{1}{12}\right)(36\pi) = 3\pi$$

### 97. Tangency
When a line is tangent to a circle, the radius of the circle is perpendicular to the line at the point of contact.

## Solids

### 98. Surface Area of a Rectangular Solid
The surface of a rectangular solid consists of three pairs of identical faces. To find the surface area, find the area of each face and add them up. If the length is $l$, the width is $w$, and the height is $h$, the formula is:

$$\text{Surface Area} = 2lw + 2wh + 2lh$$

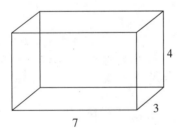

The surface area of the box above is:
$2 \times 7 \times 3 + 2 \times 3 \times 4 + 2 \times 7 \times 4 = 42 + 24 + 56 = 122$

### 99. Volume of a Rectangular Solid

$$\text{Volume of a Rectangular Solid} = lwh$$

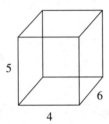

The volume of a $4 = 5 = 6$ box is

$4 \times 5 \times 6 = 120$.

A cube is a rectangular solid with length, width, and height all equal. If $e$ is the length of an edge of a cube, the volume formula is:

$$\text{Volume of a Cube} = e^3$$

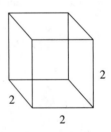

The volume of this cube is $2^3 = 8$.

### 100. Volume of a Cylinder

$$\text{Volume of a Cylinder} = \pi r^2 h$$

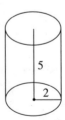

In the cylinder above, $r = 2$, $h = 5$, so:

$\text{Volume} = \pi(2^2)(5) = 20\pi$.

# State Boards of Nursing

In this section, you will find the contact information for each of the State Boards of Nursing. These boards will have the most up-to-date and relevant information pertaining to education and licensing in your field, so you should contact them as needed. Please note that mailing addresses, phone numbers, website addresses, and other contact information are all subject to change.

## Alabama Board of Nursing

P.O. Box 303900
Montgomery, AL 36130-3900
(334) 242-4060
(334) 242-4360 (fax)
http://www.abn.state.al.us/

## Alaska Board of Nursing

Robert B. Atwood Building
550 West 7th Avenue
Suite 1500
Anchorage, AK 99501-3567
(907) 269-8161
(907) 269-8196 (fax)
http://www.dced.state.ak.us/occ/pnur.htm

## Arizona Board of Nursing

4747 N. 7th St., Suite 200
Phoenix, AZ 85014
(602) 889-5150
(602) 889-5155 (fax)
http://www.azbn.gov

## Arkansas State Board of Nursing

University Tower Bldg.
1123 South University, Suite 800
Little Rock, AR 72204-1619
(501) 686-2700
(501) 686-2714 (fax)
http://www.arsbn.org

## State of California Board of Registered Nursing

P.O. Box 944210
Sacramento, CA 94244-2100
(916) 322-3350
(916) 574-7697 (fax)
http://www.rn.ca.gov/

## Colorado Board of Nursing

1560 Broadway, Suite 1350
Denver, CO 80202
(303) 894-2430
(303) 894-2821 (fax)
http://www.dora.state.co.us/nursing/

## Connecticut Board of Nursing

410 Capitol Avenue, P.O. Box 340308
Hartford, CT 06134-0308
(860) 509-7624
(860) 509-7553 (fax)
http://www.ct.gov/dph/site/default.asp

## Delaware Board of Nursing

Cannon Building, Suite 203
861 Silver Lake Blvd.
Dover, DE 19904-2467
(302) 744-4516
(302) 739-2711 (fax)
http://www.dpr.delaware.gov/boards/nursing

## District of Columbia Board of Nursing

Department of Health
Health Professional Licensing Administration
717 14th Street, NW, Suite 600
Washington, DC 20005
(202) 244-1689
(202) 727-8471 (fax)
http://hpla.doh.dc.gov/hpla/site/default.asp

## Florida Board of Nursing

4052 Bald Cypress Way, BIN C02
Tallahassee, FL 32399
(850) 245-4125
(850) 245-4172 (fax)
http://www.doh.state.fl.us/mqa/nursing

## Georgia Board of Nursing (RN)

237 Coliseum Drive
Macon, GA 31217-3858
(478) 207-2440
(478) 207-1354 (fax)
http://www.sos.georgia.gov/plb/rn

## Georgia Board of Licensed Practical Nurses

237 Coliseum Drive
Macon, GA 31217-3858
(478) 207-1300
(478) 207-1363 (fax)
http://www.sos.georgia.gov/plb/rn

## Guam Board of Nurse Examiners

P.O. Box 2816
Agana, Guam 96932
(671) 475-0251
(671) 477-4733 (fax)

## Hawaii Board of Nursing

Professional & Vocational Licensing Division
P.O. Box 3469
Honolulu, HI 96801
(808) 586-3000
(808) 586-2689 (fax)
http://hawaii.gov/dcca/areas/pvl/boards/nursing

## State of Idaho Board of Nursing

280 North 8th Street, Suite 210
Boise, ID 83720-0061
(208) 334-3110
(208) 334-3262 (fax)
http://www2.idaho.gov/ibn/about.htm

## Illinois Department of Professional Regulation

320 West Washington

Springfield, IL 62786

(217) 785-0800

(217) 782-7645 (fax)

http://www.idfpr.com/

## Indiana State Board of Nursing

402 West Washington Street, Room W072

Indianapolis, IN 46204

(317) 234-2043

(317) 233-4236 (fax)

http://www.in.gov/pla/2373.htm

## Iowa Board of Nursing

400 S.W. 8th Street, Suite B

Des Moines, IA 50309-4685

(515) 281-3255

(515) 281-4825 (fax)

http://www.iowa.gov/nursing

## Kansas State Board of Nursing

900 SW Jackson St., Suite 1051

Topeka, KS 66612-1230

(785) 296-4929

(785) 296-3929 (fax)

http://www.ksbn.org/

## Kentucky State Board of Nursing

312 Whittington Parkway, Suite 300

Louisville, KY 40222-5172

(502) 429-3300

(502) 429-3311 (fax)

http://www.kbn.ky.gov

## Louisiana State Board of Nursing

17373 Perkins Road

Baton Rouge, LA 70809

(225) 755-7500

(225) 755-7585 (fax)

http://www.lsbn.state.la.us/

## Maine Board of Nursing

158 State House Station

Augusta, ME 04333

(207) 287-1133

(207) 287-1149 (fax)

http://www.maine.gov/boardofnursing

## Maryland Board of Nursing

4140 Patterson Avenue

Baltimore, MD 21215-2254

(410) 585-1900

(410) 358-3530 (fax)

http://www.mbon.org/

## Massachusetts Board of Nursing

239 Causeway Street, 2nd Floor

Boston, MA 02114

(617) 973-0800

(617) 973-0984 (fax)

http://www.mass.gov/dpl/boards/rn

## Michigan CIS/Bureau of Health Services

Ottawa Towers North

611 W. Ottawa, 1st Floor

Lansing, MI 48933

(517) 335-0918

(517) 373-2179 (fax)

http://www.michigan.gov/healthlicense

## State of Minnesota Board of Nursing

2829 University Avenue SE, #200
Minneapolis, MN 55414-3253
(612) 617-2270
(612) 617-2190 (fax)
http://www.nursingboard.state.mn.us/

## Mississippi Board of Nursing

1935 Lakeland Drive, Suite B
Jackson, MS 39216-5014
(601) 987-4188
(601) 364-2352 (fax)
http://www.msbn.state.ms.us/

## Missouri State Board of Nursing

3605 Missouri Boulevard
P. O. Box 656
Jefferson City, MO 65102-0656
(573) 751-0681
(573) 751-0075 (fax)
http://www.pr.mo.gov/nursing.asp

## Montana Board of Nursing

301 South Park, Suite 401
Helena, MT 59620-0513
(406) 841-2300
(406) 841-2305 (fax)
http://www.nurse.mt.gov

## Nebraska Board of Nursing

Dept. of Regulation & Licensure, Nursing Section
301 Centennial Mall South, 3rd Floor
Lincoln, NE 68509-4986
(402) 471-4376
(402) 471-1066 (fax)
http://www.hhs.state.ne.us/crl/nursing/nursingindex.htm

## Nevada State Board of Nursing

5011 Meadowood Mall Way, suite 300
Reno, NV 89502
(775) 688-2620
(775) 688-2628 (fax)
http://www.nursingboard.state.nv.us/

## New Hampshire Board of Nursing

21 South Fruit Street, Suite 16
Concord, NH 03301-2431
(603) 271-2323
(603) 271-6605 (fax)
http://www.state.nh.us/nursing/

## New Jersey Board of Nursing

P.O. Box 45010
124 Halsey Street, 6th Floor
Newark, NJ 07101
(973) 504-6430
(973) 648-3481 (fax)
http://www.state.nj.us/lps/ca/medical/nursing.htm

## New Mexico Board of Nursing

6301 Indian School NE, Suite 710
Albuquerque, NM 87110
(505) 841-8340
(505) 841-8347 (fax)
http://www.bon.state.nm.us

## New York State Board of Nursing

Education Bldg.
89 Washington Avenue
2nd Floor West Wing
Albany, NY 12234-1000
(518) 474-3817 ext. 280
(518) 474-3398 (fax)
http://www.nysed.gov/nurse.htm

## North Carolina Board of Nursing

3724 National Drive, Suite 201

Raleigh, NC 27602-2129

(919) 782-3211

(919) 781-9461 (fax)

http://www.ncbon.com/

## North Dakota Board of Nursing

919 South 7th Street, Suite 504

Bismarck, ND 58504-5881

701-328-9777

701-328-9785 (fax)

http://www.ndbon.org/

## Ohio Board of Nursing

17 South High Street, Suite 400

Columbus, OH 43215-7410

(614) 466-3947

(614) 466-0388 (fax)

http://nursing.ohio.gov/

## Oklahoma Board of Nursing

2915 N. Classen Boulevard, Suite 524

Oklahoma City, OK 73106

(405) 962-1800

(405) 962-1821 (fax)

http://www.youroklahoma.com/nursing/

## Oregon Board of Nursing

17938 SW Upper Boones Ferry Rd.

Portland, OR 97224

(971) 673-0685

(971) 673-0684 (fax)

http://www.osbn.state.or.us/

## Pennsylvania Board of nursing

P.O. Box 2649

Harrisburg, PA 17105-2649

(717) 783-7142

(717) 783-0822 (fax)

http://www.dos.state.pa.us/bpoa/cwp/view.asp?a=1104&q=432869

## Puerto Rico Board of Nurse Examiners

800 Roberto H. Todd Avenue, Room 202, Stop 18

Santurce, PR 00908

(787) 725-7506

(787) 725-7903 (fax)

## Rhode Island Board of Nurse Registration and Nursing Education

105 Cannon Building

Three Capitol Hill, Room 205

Providence, RI 02908

(401) 222-5700

(401) 222-3352 (fax)

http://www.health.ri.gov

## South Carolina Board of Nursing

P. O. Box 12367

Columbia, SC 29211

(803) 896-4550

(803) 896-4525 (fax)

http://www.llr.state.sc.us/pol/nursing/

## South Dakota Board of Nursing

4305 S. Louise Ave., Suite 201

Sioux Falls, SD 57106-3115

(605) 362-2760

(605) 362-3666 (fax)

http://www.state.sd.us/doh/nursing/

## Tennessee State Board of Nursing

227 French Landing, Suite 300

Heritage Place Metro Center

Nashville, TN 37243

(615) 532-5166

http://health.state.tn.us/Boards/Nursing/

## Texas State Board of Nurse Examiners

333 Guadalupe, Ste. 3-460

Austin, TX 78701

(512) 305-7400

(512) 305-7401 (fax)

http://www.bne.state.tx.us/

## Utah Division of Occupational and Professional Licensing

Herbert M. Wells Bldg., 4th Floor

160 East 300 South

Salt Lake City, UT 84111-6741

(801) 530-6628

(801) 530-6511 (fax)

http://www.dopl.utah.gov/licensing/nursing.html

## Vermont Board of Nursing

Office of Professional Regulation

National Life Building North, Fl. 2

Montpelier, VT 05620

(802) 828-2396

(802) 828-2484 (fax)

http://vtprofessionals.org/opr1/nurses/

## Virgin Islands Board of Nurse Licensure

P.O. Box 304247

Veterans Drive Station

St. Thomas, VI 00803

(340) 776-7397

(340) 777-4003 (fax)

## Virginia Board of Nursing

Department of Health Professions

Perimeter Center

9960 Maryland Drive, Suite 300

Richmond, VA 23233

(804) 367-4515

(804) 527-4455 (fax)

http://www.dhp.virginia.gov/nursing/

## Washington State Nursing Care Quality Assurance Commission

Department of Health

HPQA#6

310 Israel Rd. SE

Tumwater, WA 98501-7864

(360) 236-4738 (fax)

https://fortress.wa.gov/doh/hpqa1/hps6/Nursing/default.htm

## West Virginia Board of Examiners for Registered Professional Nurses

101 Dee Drive, Suite 102

Charleston, WV 25311-1620

(304) 558-3596

(304) 558-3666 (fax)

http://www.wvrnboard.com

### West Virginia State Board of Examiners for Licensed Practical Nurses

101 Dee Drive, Suite 102

Charleston, WV 25311-1620

(304) 558-3572

(304) 558-3666 (fax)

http://www.lpnboard.state.wv.us

### Wisconsin Department of Regulation and Licensing

1400 E. Washington Avenue, Rm. 173

Madison, WI 53708–8935

(608) 266-2112

(608) 261-7083 (fax)

http://www.drl.state.wi.us

### Wyoming State Board of Nursing

1810 Pioneer Avenue

Cheyenne, WY 82001

(307) 777-7601

(307) 777-3519 (fax)

http://nursing.state.wy.us/